LIFE UNIVERSITY
1269 BARCLAY CIRCLE
MARIETTA, GA 30060
(770) 426-2688

LIFE UNIVERSITY
1269 BARCLAY CIRCLE
MARIETTA, GA 30060
(770) 426-2688

DRUG THERAPY 1999

Notice

Medicine is an ever-changing science. As new research and clinical experience broaden our knowledge, changes in treatment and drug therapy are required. The editors and the publisher of this work have checked with sources believed to be reliable in their efforts to provide information that is complete and generally in accord with the standards accepted at the time of publication. However, in view of the possibility of human error or changes in medical sciences, neither the editors nor the publisher nor any other party who has been involved in the preparation or publication of this work warrants that the information contained herein is in every respect accurate or complete, and they are not responsible for any errors or omissions or for the results obtained from use of such information. Readers are encouraged to confirm the information contained herein with other sources. For example and in particular, readers are advised to check the product information sheet included in the package of each drug they plan to administer to be certain that the information contained in this book is accurate and that changes have not been made in the recommended dose or in the contraindications for administration. This recommendation is of particular importance in connection with new or infrequently used drugs.

DRUG THERAPY 1999

A CRITICAL REVIEW OF THERAPEUTICS

MILO GIBALDI, PH.D.

SCHOOL OF PHARMACY
DEPARTMENT OF PHARMACEUTICS
UNIVERSITY OF WASHINGTON
SEATTLE, WASHINGTON

WITH THE EDITORIAL ADVICE OF
BRIAN RASMUSSEN

McGraw-Hill
Health Professions Division

New York   St. Louis   San Francisco   Auckland   Bogotá   Caracas
Lisbon   London   Madrid   Mexico City   Milan   Montreal
New Delhi   San Juan   Singapore   Sydney   Tokyo   Toronto

McGraw-Hill

A Division of The McGraw·Hill Companies 

1234567890 DOCDOC 99

ISBN 0-07-134990-1

This book was set in Galliard by The PRD Group, Inc.
The editors were Steve Zollo and Peter McCurdy.
The production supervisor was Heather Barry;
project management was performed by the PRD Group, Inc.
The cover and text designer was Tom Scheuerman.
The index was prepared by Virginia Dais.
R. R. Donnelley & Sons, Inc. was the printer and binder.

This book is printed on acid-free paper.
Cataloging-in-Publication data is on file for this title at the Library of Congress.

To Florence, Ann, and Frodo Baggins

CONTENTS

Contents

RESPIRATORY DISEASE

WOMEN'S HEALTH

MEN'S HEALTH

OTHER INDICATIONS

LATE BREAKING REPORTS

CHAPTER 2
DRUG EVALUATION: CONTROLLED CLINICAL STUDIES

CARDIOVASCULAR DISEASE

DIABETES

NEUROLOGICAL DISEASE

OBESITY

ONCOLOGY

PAIN MANAGEMENT

RESPIRATORY DISEASE

OTHER INDICATIONS

LATE BREAKING REPORTS

CHAPTER 3
DRUG EVALUATION: OTHER STUDIES AND REPORTS

CARDIOVASCULAR DISEASE

DIABETES

GASTROINTESTINAL DISEASE

INFECTIOUS DISEASE

INFLAMMATORY DISEASE

MENTAL HEALTH

OBESITY

ONCOLOGY

CHILDREN'S HEALTH

HEALTH IN THE ELDERLY

OTHER STUDIES AND REPORTS

ADVERSE DRUG EFFECTS

PHARMACOECONOMICS

LATE BREAKING REPORTS

CHAPTER 4
IN THE PIPELINE

CARDIOVASCULAR DISEASE

GASTROINTESTINAL DISEASE

INFECTIOUS DISEASE

MENTAL HEALTH

NEUROLOGICAL DISEASE

OBESITY

ONCOLOGY

PAIN MANAGEMENT

RESPIRATORY DISEASE

SUBSTANCE ABUSE

TRANSPLANTATION

WOMEN'S HEALTH

OTHER INDICATIONS

LATE BREAKING REPORTS

CHAPTER 5
VACCINES

INTRODUCTION

NEW PRODUCTS

IN THE PIPELINE

THERAPEUTIC STRATEGIES

APOPTOSIS

ANGIOGENESIS

REGULATORY ISSUES

OTHER REPORTS

LATE BREAKING REPORTS

CHAPTER 8
REGULATORY ACTIONS AND ISSUES

DRUG RECALLS AND WARNINGS

Regulatory Issues

Late Breaking Reports

OTHER ISSUES

LATE BREAKING REPORTS

INDEX   463

Sources Cited

The information contained in *Drug Therapy 1999* was drawn from a wide array of sources. The leading medical journals—the *New England Journal of Medicine, Lancet, JAMA,* and *Annals of Internal Medicine*—were routinely reviewed for pertinent material. The same is true for two important biomedical journals—*Nature Medicine* and *Nature Biotechnology. Current Contents* offered a window to reviews and reports in other medical and biomedical periodicals. The journals *Science* and *Chemical & Engineering News* also provided timely information. A wealth of material was gleaned from two trade papers—*The Pink Sheet* and *Scrip*—as well as from two medical newsletters—*The Medical Letter* and the *Prescriber's Letter.* The national newspapers, *The Wall Street Journal* and *The New York Times,* were a critical source of information, often offering a societal or business point of view. Most of the monographs were informed by more than one source and present multiple perspectives.

Throughout *Drug Therapy 1999,* both trade and nonproprietary drug names have been used. Because pharmaceutical advertising is so pervasive, physicians, pharmacists, patients, and the general public are more accustomed to trade names, especially for relatively new drugs still available only from the originating manufacturer. However, all indexing services and most publications use nonproprietary names. Whenever appropriate, both nonproprietary (roman type) and trade (italic type) names have been used for readers' benefit.

PREFACE

Drug therapy is now the cornerstone of medicine, vital to every medical subspecialty. Even transplant procedures, the pinnacle of surgery today, would not be possible without drugs to prevent graft rejection. Keeping up with new developments in drug therapy is increasingly daunting. Health care professionals—doctors, pharmacists, and nurses—seek information that is easily assimilated and applicable. Professional caregivers often turn to information provided by the *Physicians Desk Reference* (PDR), by drug companies and their sales representatives, and by ads in trade journals. While these sources are useful, information is usually decontextualized; all too often, professionals are left with the challenge of piecing together several sound bites.

The general public is increasingly aware of health-related issues and demands more information on medical technology and treatment. The media meets much of this demand. It is indeed uncommon when an issue of *The Wall Street Journal* or *The New York Times* does not contain an article on a pharmaceutical product. Even local papers have a reporter doing double duty in science and health. The media, however, frequently presents isolated, uncritical information, often providing no more than an edited version of a press release.

As pharmaceutical products loom large in the overall scheme of health care, pharmaceutical companies are now a darling of Wall Street. Business-oriented dailies and periodicals are diligent in reporting news of pharmaceutical developments, especially about novel products and potential blockbusters that await regulatory approval. The reports tell of successes and failures, but many times do not present the entire picture.

In light of the increasing importance of pharmaceutical products in our society, there is a need to have an ongoing chronicle of drug therapy—an annual review of important new products; or new ways to safely use marketed products; of new ways to use drugs for the elderly, young children, and women; of breakthroughs in biotechnology; of new regulations that affect the development and marketing of pharmaceuticals; of the impact of drug therapy on health care costs; of ethical issues that influence the conduct of clinical trials; of important matters in the marketing and promotion of pharmaceuticals; and of new information on vitamins, other dietary supplements, and herbal medications. There has been no compilation of such information, no chronicle of progress. Now there is one—*Drug Therapy 1999.*

MILO GIBALDI

DRUG THERAPY
1999

1 New Drugs

CARDIOVASCULAR DISEASE

Clopidogrel (*Plavix*): A Rich Man's Aspirin
Glycoprotein IIb/IIIa Receptor Blockers: Superaspirins for
    Acute Coronary Syndromes
Lepirudin (*Refludan*) for Heparin-Induced Thrombocytopenia
Angiotensin II Receptor Antagonists for Hypertension
Fenoldopam (*Corloplam*) for Severe Hypertension
Fenofibrate (*Tricor*) for Elevated Triglyceride Levels
Cilostazol (*Pletal*): A New Drug for Intermittent Claudication

Clopidogrel (Plavix): A Rich Man's Aspirin. Clopidogrel (*Plavix*) is a new oral anti-platelet agent recently approved by the FDA for secondary prevention of atherosclerotic events [*Med Letter* 1998;40:59–60]. The clinical evidence for the effectiveness of *Plavix* is based on data from the CAPRIE trial, a controlled study in more than 19,000 patients with a previous stroke or myocardial infarction (MI) or with peripheral vascular disease. The trial compared *Plavix* with aspirin and found that patients receiving *Plavix* had a 5.32% risk of having a heart attack, a stroke, or dying from vascular death, compared with a 5.83% risk for people treated with aspirin. The difference between treatments (less than 10%) is statistically significant but clinically trivial. Critics have criticized the CAPRIE trial for its failure to include a comparison of aspirin with a combination of aspirin and *Plavix*.

Plavix is similar to ticlopidine (*Ticlid*) and, like ticlopidine, inhibits platelet aggregation by blocking the adenosine diphosphate (ADP) pathway for platelet activation. Aspirin, on the other hand, works by blocking the cyclooxygenase pathway. The three drugs are about equally effective. *Ticlid* may be somewhat more effective than aspirin in preventing re-occlusion after coronary angioplasty and stenting. *Plavix* may be marginally better than aspirin for patients with peripheral arterial disease. However, it is no more effective than aspirin in preventing recurrent heart attacks.

There are important differences in the safety profiles of the three agents. *Ticlid* is the most problematic as it may cause a precipitous decline in neutrophils and platelets, aplastic anemia, and thrombotic thrombocytopenic purpura (TTP) in some patients [*Ann Intern Med* 1998;128:541–44]. Because severe neutropenia or TTP has not been reported with *Plavix*, some experts recommend that it replace *Ticlid* as an aspirin alternative. The wholesale cost of a one-month supply of *Plavix* is 28 times the cost of an equal supply of *Bayer Aspirin.*

As expected, cardiologists in the US are switching from ticlopidine to clopidogrel to prevent restenosis in patients undergoing coronary artery revascularization and stenting [*Scrip,* October 21, 1998, p 26]. About 70% of the more than one million angioplasties performed worldwide include the use of stents. Interventional cardiologists report that ticlopidine and clopidogrel have equivalent efficacy in this setting.

Glycoprotein IIb/IIIa Receptor Blockers: Superaspirins for Acute Coronary Syndromes. Platelet activation and aggregation, which leads to an arterial thrombus, are pivotal in the pathophysiology of acute coronary syndromes— unstable angina and non-Q wave MI. Aspirin is an effective anti-platelet agent but there is a great deal of room for improvement. Pharmaceutical researchers, seeking a more effective aspirin, have focused on agents that inhibit the platelet glycoprotein IIb/IIIa receptor. Binding of fibrinogen to the IIb/IIIa receptor on the surface of platelets is the final step in platelet aggregation.

The effectiveness of IIb/IIIa inhibitors to prevent acute ischemic complications related to abrupt vessel closure after angioplasty is well documented. Studies have also shown that blockade of the receptor may be useful to treat patients with unstable angina. These patients are now managed with drug therapy—aspirin and sometimes warfarin. Many, however, eventually require angioplasty. A recent review describes the impact of platelet glycoprotein IIb/IIIa receptor blockade in cardiovascular medicine [*Japanese Circulation Journal* 1998;62:233–43]. Abciximab (*ReoPro)* is a FAB fragment of a monoclonal antibody and was the first drug in the class to reach the US market. Two more intravenous agents, eptifibatide (*Integrilin*), a cyclic heptapeptide, and tirofiban (*Aggrastat*), a non-peptide, now joint it. Both agents are given with aspirin, if not contraindicated.

On April 3, 1998, the FDA announced its intention to approve Cor Therapeutics' *Integrilin* for patients undergoing coronary angioplasty and for patients with unstable angina. Several weeks later, the agency also approved Merck's *Aggrastat* for the same indications. *The Wall Street Journal* [April 3, 1998, B5] reported that the approvals open a large and almost untapped market of people who have severe chest pain. Market analysts estimate that about 1.3 million episodes of unstable angina occur each year in the US, compared with about 500,000 angioplasties. The unstable angina indication will give *Integrilin* and *Aggrastat* a significant advantage in the anti-platelet market. While Centocor/Lilly's *ReoPro* is well established as a successful medication to prevent acute closure after coronary angioplasty, it is approved only for angioplasty, although label indications do include patients with unstable angina undergoing revascularization. About half of all patients with unstable angina undergo angioplasty. The new IIb/IIIa receptor inhibitors may reduce the need for angioplasty for such patients. Although there are no head-to-head trials, the available data suggest that *ReoPro* may be more effective than either *Integrilin* or *Aggrastat* for preventing restenosis after revascularization.

Aggrastat is approved for use in combination with heparin to prevent cardiac ischemic events in patients with acute coronary syndromes. This includes patients undergoing angioplasty or atherectomy. Unlike *ReoPro, Aggrastat* is not approved for those patients undergoing elective angioplasty who do not have unstable angina. Supporting the unstable angina indication is the PRISM study [*N Engl J Med* 1998;338:1498–505], which involved more than 3000 patients with unstable angina or non-Q wave MI. They randomly received a 48-hour intravenous infusion of either *Aggrastat* or heparin. All patients also received aspirin. The primary end point—a composite of death, MI, or refractory ischemia at 48 hours—occurred in 5.6% of the patients treated with heparin and 3.8% of patients treated with *Aggrastat,* a 32% reduction in risk. Although the benefits of *Aggrastat* waned at 30 days, mortality was still lower among the group receiving *Aggrastat* than among those receiving only heparin and aspirin.

Also supporting approval is the PRISM-PLUS study with a similar patient population and the same end point as the PRISM study [*N Engl J Med* 1998;338:1488–97]. This trial compared 72-hour infusions of *Aggrastat,* heparin, and *Aggrastat* with heparin administered to more than 1900 patients who also received aspirin. *Aggrastat* combined with heparin and aspirin decreased the incidence of ischemic events by 28% at 7 days and by 18% at 30 days, compared with heparin and aspirin alone.

Integrilin has broader indications than either *ReoPro* or *Aggrastat,* having received approval for unstable angina and both emergency and elective angioplasty. Supporting the indications for *Integrilin* are the results of the PURSUIT trial [*N Engl J Med* 1998;339:436–43] in nearly 11,000 patients with acute coronary syndromes, many of whom also underwent angioplasty, and the findings of the IMPACT II study, which included about 4000 coronary angioplasty patients [*Lancet* 1997;349:1422–28].

Aggrastat and *Integrilin* cost about $350 per day, and are expected to be infused for two to three days for a patient suffering an episode of unstable angina and for 24 hours after angioplasty. Although not considered as effective as *ReoPro, Aggrastat* and *Integrilin* could capture some of the emergency angioplasty market, as they may be given to patients presenting with unstable angina, who then undergo angioplasty. Some institutions may select *Integrilin* as an all-purpose glycoprotein IIb/IIIa receptor blocker because the new agent costs less than *ReoPro* [*Scrip,* June 3, 1998, p 31]. And although *ReoPro* is not cleared for the treatment of unstable angina, it may be effective for this indication.

A critical review of the new agents in the *Medical Letter* [1998;40:89–90], concludes: "Tirofiban, eptifibatide, and abciximab can all decrease the incidence of cardiac events associated with acute coronary syndromes; direct comparisons are needed to establish which, if any, is superior. For angioplasty, until more data become available, abciximab appears to be the drug of choice."

Both *Aggrastat* and *Integrilin* signify an important advance in the treatment of patients with acute coronary syndromes. Their cost and mode of administration, however, are not practical for long-term treatment of unstable angina. This advance awaits the development of agents that can be given orally or by subcutaneous injection. Several drug companies are now investigating orally effective glycoprotein IIb/IIIa receptor inhibitors.

Lepirudin (Refludan) for Heparin-Induced Thrombocytopenia. Lepirudin (*Refludan*), is a direct inhibitor of thrombin and the first hirudin-derived anticoagulant to receive marketing approval [*Med Letter* 1998;40:94–95]. The drug is indicated for treatment of the 1% to 2% of patients who develop thrombocytopenia and thromboembolic complications during treatment with heparin. The problem occurs when antibodies, formed against a heparin-platelet protein complex, activate platelets and rapidly cause severe thrombocytopenia and damage vascular endothelium. Untreated, heparin-induced thrombocytopenia (HIT) can lead to thrombosis, pulmonary embolism, acute MI, peripheral arterial occlusion, and stroke, with a mortality rate of 20% to 30%. Low molecular weight heparins can also cause serious thrombocytopenia.

The package insert describes two studies in a total of 198 patients with HIT, in whom heparin was stopped and replaced with intravenous lepirudin. Effective anticoagulation was achieved in about 80% of patients. The cumulative risk of death 35 days after starting treatment was 9% in the lepirudin-treated patients, compared with 18% in historical controls. The cumulative risk of new thromboembolic complications was 6% with lepirudin and 22% in historical controls.

Angiotensin II Receptor Antagonists for Hypertension. Angiotensin-converting-enzyme (ACE) inhibitors are a major advance in the treatment of patients with heart failure and left ventricular dysfunction. These agents are also widely used for the treatment of hypertension. They are broadly effective, either alone or combined with a low-dose diuretic and, except for a nagging cough experienced by some patients, are very well tolerated. However, patent protection is running out on ACE inhibitors and drug companies are looking to a new class of drugs—angiotensin II receptor antagonists—to offset the anticipated rapid decline in sales when relatively inexpensive generic versions of ACE inhibitors become available.

ACE inhibitors work by blocking the conversion of angiotensin I to angiotensin II, a potent vasoconstrictor, but other enzymes that are not blocked by ACE inhibitors may also form II. Angiotensin II receptor antagonists, by binding to angiotensin II receptors, completely block the effects of II. Two angiotensin II receptor antagonists—losartan (*Cozaar*) and valsartan (*Diovan*)—have been available in the US for the treatment of hypertension. SmithKline Beecham's eprosartan (*Teveten*) is also approved in the US, but not yet marketed. *Cozaar* is the market leader.

Irbesartan (*Avapro*) and candesartan (*Atacand*) have received approval and join the others in the marketplace. *Avapro* and *Atacand,* like the earlier agents, are effective in reducing systolic and diastolic blood pressure, are less effective in black patients, and are more effective when combined with a thiazide diuretic. Two studies show that *Avapro* is more effective than *Cozaar* in reducing elevated systolic and diastolic blood pressures. *Atacand,* like *Avapro,* may be one of the more effective members of the drug class.

Toward the end of the year, FDA also approved the fifth angiotensin II receptor blocker telmisartan (*Micardis*) for once-daily treatment of hypertension [*Scrip,* November 18, 1998, p 22]. Telmisartan has a longer half-life than do other agents in the class. Boerhinger Ingelheim says that because of the greater persistence of telmisartan it is a, ". . . true once-a-day antihypertensive agent."

ACE inhibitors also block the breakdown of bradykinin and substance P, which accumulate and contribute to the cough reported by some patients. Angiotensin II receptor antagonists are not burdened with this problem. On the other hand, bradykinin and substance P may contribute to the protective effects of ACE inhibitors on the heart and kidneys. Whether angiotensin II receptor antagonists also have long-term protective effects on vital organ function remains to be established [*Med Letter* 1998:40:18–19].

Fenoldopam (Corloplam) for Severe Hypertension. Severe hypertension (hypertensive crises), defined as diastolic blood pressure of 120 mm Hg or higher, demands prompt intravenous treatment with potent antihypertensive agents. Patients with severe hypertension receive treatment with drugs having an array of pharmacological mechanisms, including angiotensin converting enzyme inhibitors, adrenergic blockers, calcium channel blockers, and vasodilators. Vasodilators used for treatment include diazoxide, nitroglycerin, and sodium nitroprusside.

Fenoldopam (*Corloplam*) is the latest agent approved for parenteral use to lower blood pressure [*Med Letter* 1998;40:57–58]. *Corloplam* induces arteriolar vasodilation mainly through stimulation of dopamine-1 receptors. Neurex, the manufacturer, claims that unlike other parenteral antihypertensive agents, *Corloplam* also maintains or improves renal function. Vasodilation of the renal vasculature leads to an increase in renal blood flow in spite of the decrease in arterial pressure.

With intravenous infusion of *Corloplam*, effects are seen in about five minutes. Clinical trials show that *Corloplam* is as effective as nitroprusside. Other studies report that patients with renal impairment have improved function when treated with fenoldopam. Adverse effects of *Corloplam* are related to vasodilation (e.g., hypotension, headache, and an increase in heart rate). Whether physicians will view fenoldopam as having significant advantages over nitroprusside and other agents remains to be seen.

Fenofibrate (Tricor) for Elevated Triglyceride Levels. Clinical data provide evidence that elevated plasma triglyceride levels and reduced high-density lipoprotein (HDL) cholesterol may be associated with an increase in the risk of coronary artery disease (CAD). The independent contribution of plasma triglycerides to ameliorate CAD, however, remains controversial [*Circulation* 1998;97:1027–28]. The FDA has recently approved micronized fenofibrate (*Tricor*), a new agent for once-a-day treatment of hypertriglyceridemia. Micronization significantly improves the absorption of fenofibrate after oral administration. The new drug is structurally similar to gemfibrozil (*Lopid*). Fibrates increase lipoprotein lipase activity and the clearance of triglycerides. They also increase serum HDL-cholesterol levels by decreasing the transfer of cholesterol from high-density lipoprotein to very-low-density lipoprotein. Reduction of triglycerides also leads to a less atherogenic form of LDL-cholesterol.

A clinical trial in patients with elevated levels of both cholesterol and triglycerides shows that fenofibrate decreases LDL-cholesterol almost as well as simvastatin (*Zocor*) and pravastatin (*Pravachol*) but has a much greater effect on triglyceride levels. *Tricor* is also more effective than atorvastatin (*Lipitor*) in reducing triglycerides and increasing HDL-cholesterol levels but not as effective as *Lipitor* in reducing LDL-cholesterol levels. *Tricor* seems to have a greater effect on elevated LDL-cholesterol levels than does *Lopid* [*Med Letter* 1998;40:68–69].

There is no information concerning the effects of fenofibrate on morbidity and mortality from coronary heart disease. Clinical trials with other fibrates suggest that these agents slow the progression of coronary atherosclerosis and decrease the incidence of coronary events, but do not affect mortality [*Lancet* 1996;347:849–53; *Circulation* 1997;96:2137–43].

Cilostazol (Pletal): A New Drug for Intermittent Claudication. In July, an FDA advisory panel considered the endorsement of cilostazol (*Pletal*), a phosphodiesterase (PDE) inhibitor, for the treatment of intermittent claudication [*Scrip*, July 15, 1998, p 24]. This painful vascular condition severely limits walking. The panel was impressed with the effectiveness of cilostazol, as measured by walking distance on a treadmill, but on the first vote a majority of the members voted against it.

In the pivotal trial assessing the effectiveness and safety of cilostazol in about 2500 patients, investigators found that the mortality rate among patients assigned cilostazol was slightly higher than among those assigned to placebo—an absolute difference of 0.15%. Ordinarily, such a small difference would not raise eyebrows. However, cilostazol is a PDE3 inhibitor, and long-term treatment of heart-failure patients with other PDE3 inhibitors—amrinone, milrinone, and vesnarinone—has been associated with increased mortality. A majority of the panel members were persuaded to vote approval of the drug only when FDA representatives suggested to the panel that patients should not be denied the opportunity to decide whether they would risk death in exchange for being able to walk an extra city block or two.

Members of the advisory committee urged the FDA to require more information on drug interactions before approving cilostazol [*The Pink Sheet* 1998;60(No 29):5]. The drug is metabolized by cytochrome P450 3A4 and potent 3A4 inhibitors will increase blood levels. There is concern that cilostazol may also inhibit 3A4 and increase blood levels and toxicity of other drugs taken at the same time. The panel was particularly concerned about interactions of cilostazol and the cholesterol-lowering agents simvastatin (*Zocor*) and lovastatin (*Mevacor*). This problem was encountered with the calcium antagonist mebfradil (*Posicor*) and led to its withdrawal from the market.

Pentoxifylline (*Trental*) is the only drug currently approved to treat the estimated four million people in the US with intermittent claudication. In a comparative study, pentoxifylline was no more effective than placebo, whereas cilostazol increased walking distance about two-thirds compared with the other two groups.

DIABETES

Repaglinide (*Prandin*) for Type 2 Diabetes
Recombinant Glucagon for Hypoglycemia

Repaglinide (Prandin) for Type 2 Diabetes. When patients with type 2 diabetes fail to control blood glucose with diet and exercise, most physicians turn to an oral agent, typically a sufonylurea such as glipizide, glyburide, or glimepiride. These agents stimulate secretion of insulin by the pancreas. They can also precipitate dangerously low blood glucose levels. Metformin (*Glucophage*), which decreases production and increases uptake of glucose, is as effective as sulfonylureas, without the danger of hypoglycemia. Rarely, metformin can cause lactic acidosis and care must be taken when prescribing the drug for patients with renal impairment. Troglitazone (*Rezulin*), which decreases insulin resistance, is very effective in some patients, particularly in combination with another oral agent or with insulin. Type 2 diabetics who require insulin may find that the addition of troglitazone permits them to reduce their dose of insulin. In some patients, troglitazone has eliminated the need for insulin. Although troglitazone carries no risk of hypoglycemia, complicating its use is the need to closely monitor liver enzyme levels to avoid hepatotoxicity.

Repaglinide (*Prandin, NovoNorm*) is the newest oral agent approved to treat patients with type 2 diabetes [*Med Letter* 1998;40:55–56], and the first of a new class of drugs called prandial glucose regulators. Novartis is developing another prandial glucose inhibitor called nateglinide.

Repaglinide may be used alone or in combination with metformin. Although structurally and mechanistically different from sulfonylureas, repaglinide also increases secretion of insulin by the pancreas. *Prandin's* advantages are rapid absorption from the gastrointestinal tract and a short duration of action. Taken with meals, *Prandin* decreases peak glucose concentrations after a meal more effectively than sulfonylureas and is less likely to cause symptomatic hypoglycemia, as its effects wear off soon after the peak. Clinical trials comparing *Prandin* with a sulfonylurea report that the incidence of severe hypoglycemia is lower when patients are treated with *Prandin* (1.4% vs. 2.8%).

The safety profile of *Prandin* seems favorable. Because repaglinide is to be taken only with a meal and skipped if a meal is missed, some patients may find it convenient. On the other hand, other patients may find the need to take *Prandin* two to four times daily to be disadvantageous compared with the once-a-day dosing schedule for products such as *Rezulin, Glucotrol XL* (glipizide), and *Amaryl* (glimepiride).

Studies presented at an international meeting on diabetes in September suggest that repaglinide is more effective than glipizide and at least as effective as glibenclamide in maintaining glycemic control in type 2 diabetic patients. In the comparative trial, patients who took repaglinide at each meal had a smaller mean increase in glycosylated hemoglobin compared with those on glipizide. Also reported is that repaglinide combined with metformin improves glycemic control to a greater extent than the sum of the changes with each drug taken alone. Overall, 59% of patients on combination therapy achieved a glycosylated hemoglobin level less that 7.1% compared with 20% and 22% for the metformin alone and repaglinide alone groups, respectively [*Scrip,* September 18, p 22].

Recombinant Glucagon for Hypoglycemia. Novo Nordisk is looking for a marketing partner to launch its recombinant DNA glucagon product called *GlucaGen.* The new product is for patients with diabetes who develop severe hypoglycemia following an injection of insulin. Eli Lilly's version of recombinant glucagon has also been approved by the FDA and may be the first to reach the US market. Recombinant glucagon eliminates the risk of acquiring bovine spongiform encephalitis from animal-derived product.

Glucagon induces the breakdown of glycogen, thereby releasing glucose from the liver. Glucose levels increase within 10 minutes and peak at about 30 minutes after injection of glucagon. Once a patient is awake and able to swallow, he or she should be given carbohydrates to restore depleted glycogen stores [*The Pink Sheet* 1998;60 (No 26):7–8].

Infectious Disease

Ribavirin Increases Effectiveness of Interferon in Hepatitis C. About 100 million patients worldwide, including about 4 million Americans, are infected with hepatitis C virus (HCV). Up to half may develop cirrhosis. Destruction of the liver by HCV is the most common reason for liver transplants [*Lancet* 1998;351:351–55].

On May 4,1998, a FDA advisory panel unanimously recommended that the agency approve a combination of ribavirin (*Rebetol*) and α-interferon (*Intron A*) for patients with chronic HCV infection who relapse while receiving α-interferon therapy alone [*Scrip,* May 6/8, 1998, p 20]. Four weeks later, the FDA agreed [*Scrip,* June 10,1998, p 22]. Effective therapy requires a six-month course of interferon injections and ribavirin capsules. The product consists of a kit called *Rebetron Combination Therapy.* Physicians will probably prescribe the combination more widely than its approved indication, but care is needed because both drugs have significant side effects. Schering-Plough is preparing to file a supplemental New Drug Application for the use of *Rebetron* in patients who have not previously received antiviral therapy.

Clinical trials uniformly favor the combination over *Intron A* monotherapy [*Lancet* 1998;351:78–79]. Adding ribavirin to α-interferon increases the number of patients who show eradication of virus during treatment from about 5% to 50%. Although not as dramatic, histologic improvement in liver biopsy also significantly favors ribavirin/α-interferon over interferon alone. One study shows that twice as many patients with chronic hepatitis C have a sustained virological response with the combination than with interferon alone [*Lancet* 1998;351:83–87]. Frequently reported adverse events, which are greater in severity with combination therapy compared with interferon-only therapy, include headache, myalgia, fatigue, and nausea. Fifteen to twenty percent of patients on either therapy complain of insomnia, depression, and irritability.

In October 1998, *The Lancet* [1998;352:1426–32] carried the results of a 48-week trial comparing interferon α-2b plus ribavirin with interferon α-2b plus placebo in 832 adult patients with untreated chronic hepatitis C viral infection. The investigators found that only 19% of patients treated for 48 weeks with interferon α-2b plus placebo showed a sustained virological response. In contrast, 43% of the patients receiving combination therapy for 48 weeks and 35% of patients receiving interferon α-2b for 48 weeks and ribavirin for 24 weeks demonstrated a sustained response.

In November 1998, *The New England Journal of Medicine* published two more reports on combination therapy, one that compared interferon α-2b alone or in combination with ribavirin for treatment of chronic hepatitis C after relapse and the other that compared them as initial treatment for chronic hepatitis C. The first report concludes that in patients with chronic hepatitis C who relapse after treatment with interferon, combination therapy with interferon and oral ribavirin is more effective than the re-administration of interferon [*N Engl J Med* 1998;339:1493–99]. After treatment for six months, serum levels of HCV RNA were undetectable in 141 of the 173 patients who were treated with interferon and ribavirin and in 80 of 172 patients who were treated with interferon alone. Serum HCV RNA levels remained undetectable 24 weeks after treatment in 49% of patients in the combination therapy group, but in only 5% of patients in the interferon group.

The second report demonstrates that initial therapy with interferon and ribavirin is more effective for patients with chronic hepatitis C than is initial therapy with interferon alone [*N Engl J Med* 1998;339:1485–92]. Serum HCV RNA levels were undetectable in 6% of patients treated with interferon alone for 24 weeks and in 13% of those treated for 48 weeks. By comparison, HCV RNA was undetectable in 31% of patients treated with interferon and ribavirin for 24 weeks and in 38% treated for 48 weeks. In December, the FDA approved the expanded use of Rebetron for initial treatment of patients with hepatitis C. Expanded use was approved over the objections of patient advocates who accuse Schering of bundling ribavirin with interferon, thereby keeping physicians from prescribing oral ribavirin alone [*The New York Times,* December 12, 1998, p C2].

An editorial on the reports says that the findings of both studies represent an important advance in the treatment of hepatitis C. The author observes: "Many other antiviral compounds in addition to interferon may soon be available for the treatment of hepatitis C. . . . As has been true in the search for the best therapy for HIV infection, it will be a daunting challenge to develop the most effective and least costly combination therapies for HCV infections" [*N Engl J Med* 1998;339:1549-50].

Ribavirin is also sold in the US in aerosolized form as *Virazole* for the treatment of respiratory syncytial virus. An alternative treatment for hepatitis C is interferon alfacon-1 (*Infergen*) approved in 1997 as monotherapy not only for patients who have relapsed, but also as first-line therapy for newly diagnosed patients. A high dose of *Infergen* seems as effective as *Rebetron* for relapsed patients. However, truly effective therapy for HCV infection awaits the development of new agents with more specific antiviral activity against HCV.

Anti-HIV Drug for Chronic Hepatitis B. An advisory panel has unanimously recommended that the FDA approve lamivudine (*Epivir-HBV*) as the first oral agent indicated for the treatment of chronic hepatitis B infection [*The Wall Street Journal*, October 7, 1998, p B7]. The virus affects about 300 million people worldwide. About 75% of all cases occur in Asia.

Current treatment for hepatitis B is based on injections of α-interferon given several times a week for four to six months. *Epivir-HBV* is taken once a day. For the treatment of hepatitis B, patients would receive only one-third the dose of lamivudine used to treat HIV infection. Clinical trials with low-dose lamivudine demonstrate a loss of hepatitis B virus (HBV DNA), loss of hepatitis antigen (HbeAg), and a gain of hepatitis B antibody (HBeAb). A Glaxo official said that clinical studies show that *Epivir-HBV* is more effective than α-interferon.

FDA's Antiviral Drugs Advisory Committee recommended that therapy with *Epivir-HBV* should continue until surrogate markers indicate the loss of effect. The lack of a fixed duration of treatment differentiates lamivudine from α-interferon. Some members of the committee urged studies comparing interferon plus lamivudine with interferon alone [*The Pink Sheet* 1998;60(No41):7–8]. Committee members expressed some reservations about the durability of lamivudine's effect and said Glaxo should conduct post-marketing studies to follow the long-term course of the disease. In December, Glaxo Wellcome reported that the FDA had approved lamivudine for the treatment of hepatitis B. The drug will have a wholesale price of $1250 a year in the US.

Trovafloxacin (Trovan): A New Fluoroquinolone for a Wide Variety of Infections. Fluoroquinolones are active *in vitro* against gram-negative and gram-positive bacteria. Trovafloxacin (*Trovan*) is the sixth fluoroquinolone to reach the US market, but has great potential. Pfizer was able to wrest 14 indications from the FDA—a record. *Trovan* has the best *in vitro* activity of any fluoroquinolone. Its indications include treatment of hospital- and community-acquired pneumonia. *Trovan* has good activity against pneumococci and other respiratory pathogens such as *Chlamydia pneumoniae, Legionella,* and *Mycoplasma.* It is about as active as ciprofloxacin (*Cipro*) against *Pseudomonas aeruginosa.*

Trovafloxacin is available for once-a-day oral or intravenous administration. The injectable contains a prodrug of trovafloxacin called altrofloxacin (*Trovan IV*). After intravenous injection, altrofloxacin is converted rapidly to trovafloxacin. Trovafloxacin offers the possibility of single-agent coverage for a wide range of infections. Because of concerns about superinfection and emergence of resistant organisms, infectious disease experts recommend limiting use of the drug to mixed infections in which anaerobes may be involved [*Med Letter* 1998;40:30–31]. Some observers think that the big market for *Trovan* will be in respiratory infections. They believe that the nursing home market could be important, with its need for drugs that cover broad ranges of potential respiratory pathogens, including nosocomials.

Synercid : A Drug Combination for Resistant Organisms. In the last decade the occurrence of antibiotic-resistant infections has surged. Certain species, such as *Enterococcus faecium* and glycopeptide-intermediate *Staphylococcus aureus* (GISA), have become resistant to so many antibiotics they have been described as "untreatable" pathogens. More than 30% of bacterial isolates of *Streptococcus pneumoniae* obtained from hospitalized patients in the US are partially or completely resistant to penicillins. The rate of methicillin-resistant *Staphylococcus aureus* has also steadily increased to nearly 30% nationwide. Now we are confronted with organisms resistant to vancomycin, the drug many consider the last line of defense.

The first product to address the problem of resistance is *Synercid,* a combination of quinupristin and dalfopristin. These agents belong to a family of natural compounds, streptogramins, derived from *Streptomyces pristi-*

naespiralis. They are given by injection and synergistically inhibit bacterial protein synthesis. The synergy displayed by the combination results in bactericidal activity, whereas the individual components are only bacteriostatic. The hope is that if the synergism of the combination is conserved despite resistance to one of the components, evolution towards resistance to the other and therefore to the combination should not occur or should at least be delayed [*Lancet* 1998;352:591–92].

Synercid is active against most gram-positive bacteria and most respiratory pathogens. Recent trials suggest that the combination is active against more than 90% of vancomycin-resistant *Enterococci faecium*. In comparison, ampicillin, oxacillin, and erythromycin are virtually inactive against resistant strains of *E. faecium* [*The Scientist,* 1998;12(No 8): pp 1,6,7]. On the basis of its activity *in vitro* and clinically, the drug combination was submitted to the FDA for approval for treatment of severe infections including complicated skin infections, nosocomial pneumonia, and infections caused by glycopeptide-resistant *E. faecium* (GREF).

In February 1998, FDA's advisory panel on anti-infective drugs recommended *Synercid* to treat complicated skin infections, vancomycin-resistant *E. faecium* infection, and hospital-acquired pneumonia. The panel did not recommend *Synercid* for community-acquired pneumonia, the largest potential market for the drug. The panel unanimously expressed concern that in the community setting, resistance to *Synercid* might develop rapidly [*Scrip,* February 25, 1998, No 2312, p 19]. If used wisely, *Synercid* could be a needed understudy to vancomycin. Used indiscriminately, it will surely result in more unwanted strains of drug-resistant bacteria.

Rifapentine (Priftin): New Treatment for Tuberculosis. After consistently declining for 40 years, the incidence of tuberculosis in the US increased 20% from 1985 to 1992. Public health officials attribute the increase to the AIDS epidemic, increased immigration, and cuts in funding for prevention and treatment programs. Those with HIV infection have a 100-times greater risk for developing active tuberculosis after exposure to the bacilli than HIV-free individuals.

Of still greater concern, the number of cases of drug-resistant tuberculosis increased even more sharply during the same period. Patients who do not complete an extended course of treatment are major contributors to the development of drug-resistant tuberculosis. In response, public health officials instituted directly observed therapy, wherein health care workers give patients the prescribed drugs directly and watch them swallow the medication. This has proved to be a very effective strategy

The FDA recently approved Hoechst Marion Roussel's rifapentine (*Priftin*), the first new drug for the treatment of pulmonary tuberculosis in twenty-five years [*The Pink Sheet* 1998;60(No 26): 6–7]. Rifapentine is taken twice weekly during the first two months of treatment and then only once a week during the last four months of therapy. By making it easier for patients to complete treatment, rifapentine may reduce the development of drug-resistant strains. The simplified dosing regimen also facilitates and reduces the cost of directly observed therapy.

A comparative trial with rifapentine and a standard rifampin regimen of two to three doses weekly, shows that both treatments cured 82% to 88% of infected patients. Patients in both groups also received three other antitubercular drugs for the first two months—isoniazid, pyrazinamide, and ethambutol. Polytherapy is standard in the treatment of tuberculosis. Rifapentine must always be used with at least one other antitubercular drug to which the isolate is susceptible. Rifapentine is not effective in patients who have developed drug resistance to rifampin.

Patients with HIV infection seem to need more frequent dosing of rifapentine to avoid relapse. Those receiving protease inhibitors should probably avoid rifapentine because, like rifampin, rifapentine accelerates the metabolism of these life-prolonging drugs. For the same reason, rifapentine may decrease the reliability of hormone contraceptives. Rifapentine, like several other antitubercular agents, is associated with adverse hepatic effects.

Sustiva: Another NNRTI for the Treatment of HIV Infection. DuPont's *Sustiva* (efavirenz), cleared by the FDA in September, was the first anti-HIV drug to receive approval in 1998 and the third non-nucleoside reverse transcriptase inhibitor (NNRTI) to reach the market. The others are nevirapine (*Viramune*) and delavirdine (*Rescriptor*). *Sustiva* is approved for use in combination with other antiretroviral agents in the treatment of HIV-infected adults and children.

FDA approval of *Sustiva* is based on viral load data. One study compared the combination of zidovudine and lamivudine plus *Sustiva* or indinavir (*Crixivan*). The *Sustiva* combination suppressed HIV RNA to undetectable levels in a greater proportion of patients than the indinavir combination. The difference appeared to be related to a greater frequency of dropouts due to adverse events in the indinavir group than in the *Sustiva* group [*The Pink Sheet* 1998;60(No38):3–4].

The use of *Sustiva* will decrease the number of pills patients must take to keep the virus under control. Unlike other components of combination therapy, *Sustiva* is taken only once a day. According to *The Wall Street Journal* [September 21, 1998, p B5], DuPont plans to promote the drug to be as effective as protease inhibitors when combined with nucleoside RTIs (NRTIs). Merck, anticipating competition from *Sustiva,* studied the effectiveness of its protease inhibitor indinavir given only twice a day, but has now abandoned those efforts. An interim analysis showed that the three times a day regimen was more effective than the simpler dosing scheme.

The *Prescriber's Letter* [October 1998, p 58] notes that *Sustiva* penetrates and reduces HIV levels in the central nervous system (CNS). Penetration, however, also produces CNS side effects including dizziness, drowsiness, and impaired concentration. Patients are well advised to take *Sustiva* at bedtime for the first few weeks or longer if symptoms persist.

Also in October, *The Pink Sheet* [1998;60(No40):15] reported that DuPont is enrolling patients in a trial to study the effects of *Sustiva* in patients who are responding to protease inhibitors and who have HIV RNA levels less than 50 copies per ml. Patients participating in the trial will have their protease inhibitor replaced by *Sustiv*a. If successful, physicians could consider the switch for patients experiencing the adverse metabolic effects linked to the use of protease inhibitors, including lipodystrophy, hypertriglyceridemia, elevated cholesterol, and/or hyperglycemia.

About the same time, *Scrip* [October 14, 1998, p 26] took note of interim data from a clinical study of *Sustiva* in children, presented at an infectious disease meeting. The children were 16 years old or younger and had been treated previously with NRTIs but not NNRTIs or protease inhibitors. *Sustiva* plus an NRTI and the protease inhibitor nelfinavir (*Viracept*) replaced their current therapy. At the start of the study, less than 4% of the children had plasma HIV RNA lower than 400 copies per ml. At two weeks, this proportion increased to 52%, peaked at 78% at week 12, then fell back to 67% at week 20. At that time, the median CD4 cell count was 15% higher than baseline.

Abacavir (Ziagen): An NRTI Alternative to HIV Protease Inhibitors. An FDA advisory panel in November 1998 recommended accelerated approval of Glaxo's abacavir (*Ziagen*), an unusually effective NRTI, in combination with other agents for the treatment of HIV infection in children and adults. The advisory committee, on examining the evidence, concluded that abacavir would be useful as a second-line therapy in HIV patients for whom protease inhibitors are contraindicated [*The Wall Street Journal,* November 3, 1998, p B4].

The panel's vote, however, was not unanimous. One dissenter did not think that a regimen containing three nucleoside analogs alone provides appropriate therapy. Another was concerned by evidence of serious, and potentially fatal, allergic reactions to abacavir in about 3% of patients. The reactions are characterized by fever, rash, gastrointestinal symptoms, and malaise. If the syndrome is not recognized, continued treatment can lead to organ failure and death. Patients presenting with symptoms of hypersensitivity should be told to stop abacavir therapy immediately.

Glaxo Wellcome plans to distribute a wallet-card describing hypersensitivity reactions to abacavir as part of its marketing of the drug. The card contains both patient and physician information. The company also plans to make a targeted education effort for physicians who are not specialists in the management of patients with HIV infection that emphasizes the potential risks posed by the drug. Labeling for *Ziagen* will include a boxed warning citing the potential for hypersensitivity reactions [*The Pink Sheet* 1998;60(No45):27–28].

Four clinical studies support the approval of *Ziagen*. They show that triple therapy that includes abacavir is more effective in reducing virus levels and elevating CD4 cell counts than the combination of zidovudine and lamivudine alone and at least as effective as the standard cocktail containing indinavir, zidovudine, and lamivudine.

INFLAMMATORY DISEASE

Hyaluronic Acid Derivatives for Osteoarthritis
Leflunomide (*Arava*) for Rheumatoid Arthritis

Hyaluronic Acid Derivatives for Osteoarthritis. The *Medical Letter* [1998;40:69–70] reports the approval of two hyaluronic acid derivatives for intra-articular injection in patients with knee pain stemming from osteoarthritis. *Hyalgan* is simply sodium hyaluronate and *Synvisc,* hylan G-F, is a cross-linked derivative of hyaluronic acid. Synovial fluid in an osteoarthritic joint has an inadequate concentration of hyaluronic acid and low viscoelasticity, which leads to loss of lubrication and reduced protection from mechanical stress. Injections of hyaluronic acid reduce inflammation and may stimulate hyaluronic acid synthesis in the joint. Recommended treatment with *Synvisc* is three injections into the knee, one week apart. *Hyalgan* is given once weekly for five weeks.

Two studies suggest *Hyalgan* is more effective than placebo, one of which also shows that the drug is marginally more effective than nonsteroidal anti-inflammatory agents (NSAIDs). No study has compared the new agents with acetaminophen, the most commonly used drug for osteoarthritis. In a telephone survey, patients treated with *Synvisc,* with or without an NSAID, reported lower pain scores than those treated with placebo and NSAID. Patients who were treated with *Synvisc* and an NSAID had the lowest pain scores.

Medical Letter editors conclude that the new agents might decrease pain in some patients, but they are expensive; the cost to pharmacists is more than $600 for a single course of treatment. They also find that results from published studies are unimpressive and warn that these agents may produce inflammatory reactions and carry the threat of anaphylaxis.

Leflunomide (Arava) for Rheumatoid Arthritis. Hoechst Marion Roussel (HMR) has launched a new agent for relief of the signs and symptoms of rheumatoid arthritis. The product offers an alternative to methotrexate [*The Pink Sheet* 1998;60(No 32):29]. Like methotrexate, leflunomide is classified as a disease-modifying anti-rheumatic drug (DMARD). It is an immune modulator, inhibiting pyrimidine synthesis and blocking the expansion of T lymphocytes [*Scrip,* August 12, 1998, p 19].

HMR told FDA's arthritis advisory panel that in a 12-month US trial in 482 patients, leflunomide produced a clinical response in 41% of patients, compared with a 16% response rate in patients assigned to placebo. A 6-month, 358-patient multinational trial produced similar results. The US trial showed equivalence of leflunomide to methotrexate and the international study showed equivalence to sulfasalazine. Adverse events were said to be mild to moderate. Diarrhea was the most frequent complaint and occurred in one of four patients taking leflunomide.

The panel strongly supported approval, including an indication for retardation of structural damage due to the disease. The claim is based on X-ray studies of hands and feet before and after treatment. Patients on *Arava* show slowing of joint erosion and joint space narrowing compared to those receiving placebo. Panel members also agreed that leflunomide improves physical function for at least one year. They cautioned, however, that women should not become pregnant while on *Arava,* and that the drug should not be used in patients with significant liver disease. The panel further urged that a pregnancy registry be established to monitor possible teratogenic effects of *Arava* [*The Pink Sheet* 1998;60(No33):21].

Arava labeling includes a black box warning stating that pregnancy must be excluded before the start of treatment. Women who do become pregnant while on *Arava* should take the resin cholestyramine to sequester the drug in the gastrointestinal tract and hasten its elimination from the body. *Arava* is also not recommended for use in women who are nursing [*The Pink Sheet* 1998;60(No37):3–4]. The *Prescriber's Letter* recommends that patients be told that *Arava* may cause diarrhea, hair loss, and rash and that patients be monitored for elevated liver enzymes every month for the first few months of therapy.

HMR will also seek an indication for prevention of disease-related disability, but it is likely that the FDA will ask for continued or additional studies of longer drug exposure before granting approval. A planned combination trial may justify expanding the use of *Arava* to patients not adequately controlled with methotrexate. Patients would receive methotrexate alone, methotrexate plus a low dose of leflunomide, or placebo. A preliminary study shows that *Arava* provided benefit to 28 of 30 patients when given in combination with methotrexate [*The Pink Sheet* 1998;60(No33):20–21].

Mental Health

Citalopram (Celexa): A New SSRI for the Treatment of Depression. Forest Laboratories has received an approvable letter from the Food and Drug Administration and is getting ready to launch its selective serotonin receptor inhibitor (SSRI) antidepressant citalopram (*Celexa*) [*Scrip,* June 10, 1998, p 24]. Warner-Lambert will co-promote the drug. Forest licenses the drug from Lundbeck, a European drug company. Despite the competitive field of marketed agents, observers say *Celexa* may be a major product because it has benefits not seen with other SSRIs.

Celexa may work more quickly than other antidepressants and may have fewer side effects than other SSRIs, but there is little documentation for these claims. Another potential advantage is that citalopram—only a weak inhibitor of drug-metabolizing enzymes—has few drug interactions compared with competing agents. Labeling for fluoxetine (*Prozac*), sertraline (*Zoloft*), and fluvoxamine (*Luvox*), and to a lesser extent paroxetine (*Paxil*), suggests caution when prescribing them with drugs metabolized by cytochrome P450 2D6. The only significant interaction associated with *Celexa* is with monoamine oxidase inhibitors. *Celexa's* low potential for interactions with cardiovascular drugs makes it particularly useful for the elderly. Forest and Warner-Lambert will heavily promote the drug for that audience. On the other hand, the metabolism of citalopram itself may be slowed if given with potent inhibitors of cytochrome P450 3A4 (e.g., ketoconazole and erythromycin) and potent inhibitors of cytochrome P450 2C19 (e.g., omeprazole) [*The Pink Sheet* 1998;60(No30): 3–4]. Citalopram is the leading SSRI in several countries in Europe, where it is sold under the name *Cipramil*. In the US, *Celexa* will also compete on the basis of price.

The safety profile of citalopram is very good. Among SSRIs, citalopram has the lowest number of what the FDA defines as "commonly observed side-effects"—those that occur in 5% of patients and at a rate at least double that of placebo. The only commonly observed side-effect associated with *Celexa* use in clinical studies is ejaculation disorder, which occurred in 6% of patients assigned to the drug, compared with an occurrence of 1% in those given placebo. There is some concern that overdoses with citalopram may result in more morbidity and mortality than is seen with other SSRIs but this concern has been dismissed by Forest, which takes the position that there is no difference among SSRIs in terms of overdose.

Limiting the commercial potential of *Celexa* is only five years of market exclusivity because of patent expirations. Citalopram is a racemic mixture and observers say that Lundbeck and Forest will try to extend *Celexa's* protected life by marketing a single isomer, which has patent protection until 2009. Forest suggests that the S-enantiomer of the drug could potentially have better antidepressant activity.

NEUROLOGICAL DISEASE

Tolcapone (*Tasmar*): First COMT Inhibitor for
   Parkinson's Disease
New Triptans for Migraine
Tiagabine (*Gabitril*) for Partial Seizures

Tolcapone (Tasmar): First COMT Inhibitor for Parkinson's Disease. Therapy with levodopa and carbidopa, a peripheral aromatic amino acid decarboxylase inhibitor, is the cornerstone of treatment of Parkinson's disease. Carbidopa inhibits the metabolism of levodopa and sustains its effects. Almost inevitably, however, within a few years of starting levodopa therapy with the usual two to four doses per day, patients report that clinical benefit wanes at the end of each dosing interval. This phenomenon is related in part to levodopa's short half-life and short duration of action. Increasing the daily dose of levodopa at this stage of the disease reduces the wearing-off time, but also increases the frequency and severity of dyskinesia.

In addition to decarboxylation, methylation, catalyzed by catechol-O-methyltransferase (COMT), is another important pathway for the elimination of levodopa. Hoffmann-La Roche's tolcapone (*Tasmar*) is the first COMT inhibitor approved in the US [*Med Letter* 1998;40:60–61]. It is marketed as an adjunct to levodopa/carbidopa for treatment of Parkinson's disease in both stable patients and those with end-of-dose wearing off of levodopa effects. *Tasmar* has no intrinsic antiparkinson activity.

By inhibiting the COMT pathway, *Tasmar* results in a more favorable pharmacokinetic profile—an increase in plasma half-life and area under the curve (AUC) of levodopa, and a reduction in peak to trough fluctuations. These changes lead to improved motor function and activity scores in patients with stable Parkinson's disease and permit a decrease in levodopa dosage. In patients treated with levodopa/carbidopa but experiencing the wearing-off effect, *Tasmar* decreases off time by up to 50%. The more off time the patient experiences, the more benefit that may accrue from COMT inhibition. The new agent should outperform controlled-release levodopa preparations, which slow absorption, increase the time to peak concentration after a dose, and reduce oral bioavailability [*Lancet* 1998;351:1221–22].

In October, *Tasmar* suffered a setback when the European Medicines Evaluation Agency announced a revision in prescribing and patient information recommending more frequent monitoring following reports of severe liver dysfunction and death [*The Pink Sheet* 1998;60(No42):17]. The new labeling says that liver function should be monitored before starting therapy with *Tasmar*, then every three weeks for the first three months and every four weeks for the next three months. It also reduces the alanine aminotransferase threshold for discontinuing treatment from five to three times normal. Elevations in liver enzymes are dose-dependent and the revised labeling emphasizes that an increase to higher doses of *Tasmar* should be attempted only in exceptional circumstances. Labeling in the US had initially recommended liver enzyme monitoring once a month for the first three months, and every six weeks for the next three months. On November 17, 1998, after further consideration, the European Medicines Evaluation Agency announced the decision to suspend *Tasmar's* license.

Also in November, on analyzing reports from Europe and data in its own files, the FDA determined that *Tasmar* should carry a strict safety warning [*The Wall Street Journal*, November 17, 1998, p B6]. The new label states that the drug should be used only in patients with severe movement abnormalities who do not respond to other treatments. The label also warns that physicians should halt treatment if patients do not show substantial benefit within the first three weeks. The FDA also advises biweekly monitoring and suggests that physicians ask patients to sign a consent form alerting them to the drug's potential risks and benefits. Patients should also be asked to watch for signs of liver toxicity—jaundice, fatigue, and loss of appetite. Hoffmann-La Roche said it considered withdrawing the drug from the market but decided not to because of its considerable benefit to some patients. The FDA and the company agreed on the new labeling.

A second COMT inhibitor, entacapone (*Comtan*), is under review at the FDA. It received its first approval in the European Community. Entacapone is easier to administer than tolcapone. Labeling approved by the European Commission states that entacapone is contraindicated in patients with liver impairment but does not call for monitoring liver enzyme levels. Entacapone is taken with each dose of levodopa—the number of levodopa doses per day varies according to patient. Tolcapone is taken three times daily, independent of levodopa [*Scrip*, September 25, 1998, p 16].

New Triptans for Migraine. Glaxo's introduction several years ago of sumatriptan (*Imitrex*), a selective serotonin-receptor agonist, gave a new and needed tool to physicians to combat migraine headache. Originally marketed as an injectable, *Imitrex* is now available in oral and nasal spray formulations.

Sumatriptan works by stimulating serotonin receptors on intracranial blood vessels and the peripheral sensory nerve endings of the trigeminal vascular system. This action leads to intracranial vasoconstriction and decreased release of inflammatory neuropeptides.

Early in 1998, a second selective serotonin-receptor agonist, zolmitriptan (*Zomig*) received FDA approval [*Med Letter* 1998;40:27–28]. Zeneca acquired marketing rights to zolmitriptan when the government required divestiture of some products as a condition for the merger of Glaxo and Wellcome. Zolmitriptan is chemically and pharmacologically similar to sumatriptan. It is given orally. A large clinical trial of patients with a moderate or severe migraine headache demonstrated that headache response rates (improvement from severe or moderate to mild or no headache) after the administration of zolmitriptan were 44% at one hour, 65% at two hours, and 75% at four hours. The response rate for placebo was 30%. In some patients treated with a triptan, headache recurs but the second attack is usually milder and responds to a second dose.

A few months later, Glaxo introduced *Amerge* (naratriptan), which is similar to *Imitrex* and *Zomig* but longer acting so recurrent headaches requiring a second dose are less likely. The downside is that *Amerge* has a slower onset, taking almost three hours to work. The drug should probably be reserved for patients who get recurrent headaches.

More recently, Merck received FDA approval to market yet another triptan, *Maxalt* (rizatriptan). Merck's promotion of oral *Maxalt* will emphasize effectiveness. Merck hopes to expand the migraine drug market by getting the attention of millions of migraine sufferers who do not currently seek treatment. The company plans to launch an aggressive consumer advertising campaign [*The Wall Street Journal*, July 1, 1998, p B19]. Another version of the product, *Maxalt-MLT*, is the first migraine preparation available as a rapidly dissolving tablet. *Maxalt-MLT* disintegrates within seconds on the tongue and does not require water for ingestion. This, however, does not mean faster absorption and more rapid onset of effect because almost the entire dose is swallowed with saliva and absorbed in the gastrointestinal tract [*Prescriber's Letter* 1998;5:47]. Nevertheless, it is likely that patients perception will be that Maxalt–MLT works faster and is more convenient. A rapidly dissolving tablet of *Zomig* is also under development [*Scrip*, July 3, 1998, p 18].

All three of the new triptans claim superiority over the original product in the class—sumatriptan. The marketing battles will soon intensify, as three more products could be launched in 1999. The most interesting of these is frovatriptan because of its superior ability to reduce headache recurrence rate. Headache recurrence rate after the usual dose of frovatriptan is 13%, compared with rates of 17% to 28% reported for naratriptan and 30% to 40% for the other triptans. Frovatriptan has the longest half-life—about 25 hours—of all triptans studied to date [*Scrip*, September 11, 1998, p 20].

Triptans are not recommended for patients with ischemic heart disease or uncontrolled hypertension. Caution is needed when treating men over the age of 40, postmenopausal women, and patients with other cardiac risk factors. All triptans can constrict coronary arteries and cause chest pain.

Tiagabine (Gabitril) for Partial Seizures. Most adults with resistant epilepsy have partial seizures. Carbamazepine, phenytoin, and valproic acid, used alone or in combination, are the first-line drugs for the treatment of partial seizures. A new sustained-release form of carbamazepine decreases fluctuation in plasma levels, which results in fewer adverse effects, improved seizure control, and improved compliance.

During the past five years, three new drugs—gabapentin (*Neurontin*), lamotrigine (*Lamictal*), and topiramate (*Topamax*)—have received FDA approval for the treatment of partial seizures, but only as adjunctive therapy for refractory partial seizures in adults. A fourth new drug, felbamate (*Felbatrol*), is approved for monotherapy. One survey suggests no significant differences in efficacy or tolerability among these agents.

Felbamate can precipitate aplastic anemia and hepatic failure and should be restricted to patients with severe epilepsy who are refractory to other therapies. Gabapentin seems to work by enhancing the release of gamma-aminobutyric acid (GABA), an important inhibitory neurotransmitter. Among the drug's advantages are the absence of protein binding, no active or toxic metabolites, renal excretion, and no clinically important drug interactions. Lamotrigine has a broad spectrum of activity and a favorable safety profile. Serious toxicity, however, such as Stevens-Johnson syndrome has been reported in a small number of children receiving the drug. Topiramate also enhances GABA effects and modulates other neurological pathways. The drug is well tolerated if started at low doses. Fatigue, sleepiness, and dizziness have been reported and the drug may cause confusion in as many as 15% of patients [*JAMA* 1998;280:693–94].

Tiagabine (*Gabitril*), a GABA uptake inhibitor, is the fifth anticonvulsant approved in the past five years [*Med Letter* 1998;40:45–46]. It probably works by prolonging the effects of GABA on the central nervous system.

Well-controlled trials show that 20% to 30% of patients with complex partial seizures have a 50% or greater reduction in seizures when *Gabitril* is added to previous therapy, compared with a 5% to 10% response with placebo [*Lancet* 1998;351:203–07]. Cognitive problems—confusion and difficulty in concentrating—which have occurred with topiramate, have also been observed with *Gabitril*. Severe rash, which can occur with *Lamictal*, has not been reported for *Gabitril*. Unlike most anticonvulsant agents, *Gabitril* seems to have little penchant for inhibiting or accelerating the metabolism of co-administered drugs. Not yet answered is how *Gabitril* compares with *Neurontin*, *Lamictal*, or *Topamax* in safety and effectiveness. Preliminary evidence suggests no important differences in effectiveness among them.

Yet another anticonvulsant—vigabatrin (*Sabril*) is under review at the FDA. An advisory panel has recommended that the FDA approve the drug as add-on therapy, but final action is pending. Also of interest is a new nonpharmacologic alternative to conventional drug therapy called the vagus nerve stimulator. The device is implanted in the chest and a stimulating lead is attached to the left vagus nerve in the carotid sheath. A stimulus is given in regular on-off cycles throughout the day. A small external magnet can be used to activate the device at the beginning of an aura or seizure to abort the seizure or limit its spread [*Epilepsia* 1998;39:677–86]. The FDA approved a vagal nerve stimulator called the *NeuroCybernetic Prosthesis System* for the treatment of refractory partial epilepsy in adults in July 1997.

OBESITY

Sibutramine (Meridia) for Weight Reduction. Sibutramine (*Meridia*), which is structurally related to amphetamine, was approved by the FDA in late 1997, but not launched until February 1998 [*Med Letter* 1998;40:32]. It inhibits reuptake of norepinephrine, serotonin, and, to a lesser extent, dopamine, increasing concentrations of these neurotransmitters in the brain. *Meridia* has attracted attention because it is the first diet drug to reach the market after the embarrassing and costly withdrawal of fenfluramine (*Pondamin*) and dexfenfluramine (*Redux*) because of heart valve damage.

The FDA recommends *Meridia* for obese patients with an initial body mass index of at least 30 kg/m^2 or 27 kg/m^2 in the presence of other risk factors such as diabetes, high blood pressure, or elevated cholesterol levels. A 24-week multicenter trial in more than 1,000 obese patients on a restricted calorie diet found that patients taking a placebo lost 0.9 kg, those taking sibutramine 10 mg per day lost 5.8 kg, and those taking 15 mg per day lost 6.5 kg. One-year studies show that weight reduction reaches a maximum by six months and is maintained for another six months with some backsliding toward the end of the year.

Knoll, the drug's sponsor, emphasizes that in trials involving about 6,000 patients there were no reported cases of pulmonary hypertension, a rare but lethal side effect linked to fenfluramines, and no evidence to suggest that sibutramine causes valvular heart damage. However, *Meridia* can increase blood pressure and heart rate in normotensive people and those with controlled hypertension. This issue is addressed in the product's labeling. Physicians should not prescribe *Meridia* for patients with a history of cardiovascular disease, including uncontrolled hypertension. *Meridia* is a schedule IV substance with a low abuse potential but some patients may experience limited dependence.

Knoll recognizes that its marketing efforts must overcome the negative publicity surrounding the withdrawal of *Pondamin* and *Redux* and that it must strive to prevent overuse and misuse of *Meridia*. Physicians who had little or no compunction in prescribing fenfluramines to all comers, seem to be more cautious this time around. The market for obesity drugs is enormous. Nearly half the adult population in the US is overweight and weight-related diseases—hypertension, dyslipidemia, type 2 diabetes, and cardiovascular disease—are estimated to cost billions of dollars each year. The average price of *Meridia* to consumers is $3 to $4 per day, depending on dose [*Scrip*, February 18, 1998, p 21].

In October 1998, Knoll introduced a direct-to-consumer advertising campaign aimed at readers or viewers 25 to 45 pounds overweight. Both the print and television ads focus on *Meridia*'s contraindications and the potential for elevated blood pressure. Patient education materials include a prominent warning that advises of the need for regular blood pressure monitoring when taking *Meridia*. The materials also make clear that *Meridia* does not damage heart valves.

Oncology

Implanted Wafers for Treatment of Brain Tumors
Irinotecan (*Camptosar*) for Colorectal Cancer
Valrubicin (*Valstar*): A New Drug for Bladder Cancer
Alitretinoin Gel (*Panretin*) for Kaposi's Sarcoma
Cytarabine Liposome Injection (*DepoCyt*) for Lymphomatous
  Meningitis

Implanted Wafers for Treatment of Brain Tumors. *The Medical Letter* [1998:40:92] reports the marketing of a biodegradable polymer wafer called *Gliadel*. The dime-sized wafer is impregnated with the alkylating agent carmustine (BCNU, *Bicnu*) and used for local treatment of recurrent glioblastoma that requires surgery. The wafers are implanted into the surgical cavity left behind after resection, and release carmustine over a period of about two to three weeks. Animal data suggest that concentrations of alkylating agent in the brain tissue around the implant are hundreds of times higher than those after intravenous administration of carmustine. Only trace amounts appear in the systemic circulation [*Cancer Res* 1998;58:672–84]. One study shows that patients who received carmustine polymer implants had a median survival of 28 weeks, compared with 20 weeks for those who received placebo polymer. Six-month mortality was 36% with the *Gliadel* wafer and 56% with placebo wafer [*Neurosurgery* 1997;41:44–48]. *Gliadel* thereby provides a modest improvement in survival.

Irinotecan (Camptosar) for Colorectal Cancer. FDA's advisory committee on oncologic drugs has unanimously recommended full approval of the topoisomerase I inhibitor irinotecan (*Camptosar*) for the treatment of metastatic colorectal cancer that recurred or progressed following therapy with 5-fluorouracil (5-FU). Colorectal cancer is the second most prevalent cancer in the developed world. Experts are endorsing irinotecan as the new standard of care for metastatic colorectal cancer that has not responded to 5-FU or has relapsed within six months [*Scrip*, May 27, 1998, p 26].

In 1996, the FDA granted accelerated (conditional) approval to *Camptosar* for this indication based on studies showing that it reduces tumor size, a surrogate endpoint. To support its bid for unconditional approval, Pharmacia and Upjohn presented to the advisory panel results from two European phase III trials that focused on mortality and quality of life.

In one study, 267 eligible patients were randomly allocated irinotecan infused once every three weeks or fluorouracil by continuous infusion. Survival at one year was increased from 32% in the 5-FU group to 45% in the irinotecan group [*Lancet* 1998;352:1407–12]. In the second study, patients were allocated irinotecan or supportive care. After analyzing the results, the investigators concluded that, ". . . patients who have metastatic colorectal cancer, and for whom fluorouracil has failed, have a longer survival, fewer tumor-related symptoms, and a better quality of life when treated with irinotecan than with supportive care alone" [*Ibid*, pp 1413–18].

A commentary on the two reports warns against enthusiasm, noting that median survival was improved by only 2.3 months in one study and 2.7 months in the other. Nevertheless, the author concludes: "The prolongation of survival with irinotecan provides strong proof of principle that second-line chemotherapy can be beneficial in this disease. . ." [*Ibid*, p 1402].

Valrubicin (Valstar): A New Drug for Bladder Cancer. FDA has approved new therapy for patients with treatment-refractory localized bladder cancer. Patients who fail to respond to standard immunotherapy with Bacillus Calmette-Guerin (BCG) have a poor prognosis and usually undergo radical cystectomy, a long, complex, and high-risk procedure. Valrubicin was approved for BCG-refractory patients with chronic end-organ illness for whom cystectomy is not an immediate option. This is a sizable population because the average age at diagnosis of bladder cancer is 68 years. The new therapy is hardly a panacea. Valrubicin produced complete treatment responses in only 18% of patients who received it during clinical trials. The drug is administered locally via intravesical instillation directly into the bladder.

Alitretinoin Gel (Panretin) for Kaposi's Sarcoma. In November 1998, eight of nine members of FDA's oncologic drugs advisory committee endorsed *Panretin* gel (alitretinoin 0.1%) as topical therapy for cutaneous Kaposi's sarcoma [*Scrip*, November 20, 1998, p 19]. Among its adherents, however, there was debate as to whether the retinoid preparation should be first-line therapy for treating the disfiguring Kaposi's lesions. Some among them held that radiotherapy and other strategies seem more effective. The major element that convinced most of the panelists that *Panretin* gel has at least cosmetic value was the patient satisfaction scores that clearly favored active drug over placebo.

Cytarabine Liposome Injection (DepoCyt) for Lymphomatous Meningitis. At its November 1998 meeting, FDA's experts on oncologic drugs also recommended accelerated (conditional) approval of cytarabine liposome injection (*DepoCyt*) for the intrathecal treatment of lymphomatous meningitis [*Scrip,* November 18, 1998, p 21]. A single, 33-patient trial supported the request for approval. Response rates ranged from 20% to 70%, depending on the analysis, but were consistently better than response rates with non-liposomal cytarabine. The liposomal product requires intrathecal injection once every two weeks, compared with twice-weekly injections for cytarabine.

PAIN MANAGEMENT

Fentanyl: An Old Drug in a New Form for Serious Pain
FDA Panel Recommends Approval for COX-2
Inhibitor Celecoxib (*Celebrex*)

Fentanyl: An Old Drug in a New Form for Serious Pain. A potent analgesic, fentanyl, in the form of a self-administered lollipop (*Actiq*), has received FDA approval [*The Wall Street Journal,* November 6, 1998, p B6]. It is the first medication intended to treat sudden flare-ups of moderate to severe cancer pain. *Actiq* works within five minutes because fentanyl is rapidly absorbed from the oral cavity. Only an intravenous injection works faster. Anesta, the manufacturer, estimates that breakthrough pain affects more than 800,000 cancer patients in the US, occurring three or four times a day in between doses of regular pain medication. Regulators at the FDA worry that children might think the lozenge on a stick is candy. Consequently, Abbott Laboratories will distribute *Actiq* in child-resistant foil pouches. The product is expected to be available in March 1999.

Abbott's risk management program will target cancer pain and oncology specialists and emphasize the potential risk of ingestion by children, and the need for careful selection of patients to receive the product [*The Pink Sheet* 1998;60(No45):6]. *Actiq* should not be prescribed for the management of acute or postoperative pain. The new product is similar to *Fentanyl Oralet,* also marketed by Abbott. *Oralet*'s package, however, is not designed to prevent accidental pediatric consumption because it is used only in hospitals.

FDA Panel Recommends Approval for COX-2 Inhibitor Celecoxib (*Celebrex*). The first of a new class of NSAIDs called selective cyclooxygenase-2 (COX-2) inhibitors nears the market [*The Wall Street Journal,* December 2, 1998, p B7]. It promises effective pain relief for osteoarthritis and rheumatoid arthritis with fewer adverse gastrointestinal (GI) effects than NSAIDs now available. COX-2 inhibitors are described in more detail in Chapter 4.

While recommending the approval of celecoxib (*Celebrex*), an FDA advisory panel said that the product should still carry a warning that it could cause GI problems. The qualification was a setback for Searle who wished to promote *Celebrex* as a virtually risk-free NSAID. While Searle argued that

Celebrex had a GI safety profile similar to placebo, the FDA advisers said it was not clear whether the reduction in the number of overall ulcers, compared with conventional NSAIDs, means that there would be fewer serious ulcers that could lead to hospitalizations or fatalities. FDA staffers told the panel that *Celebrex,* like other NSAIDs, can cause hypertension and adversely affect renal function.

RESPIRATORY DISEASE

Tobramycin for Inhalation as Treatment for Cystic Fibrosis
Montelukast (*Singulair*) for Adults and Children with Asthma

Tobramycin for Inhalation as Treatment for Cystic Fibrosis. Cystic fibrosis is an incurable genetic disease that afflicts about 30,000 Americans. Most patients die of respiratory failure as thick mucus clogs airways and traps infectious bacteria. Of particular concern is *Pseudomonas aeruginosa* infection, which affects 80% of patients by adulthood and increases their risk of death eightfold. Traditionally, to combat *P. aeruginosa*, patients have received systemic antibiotic therapy with tobramycin. Treatment usually requires hospitalization because of its serious toxicity (e.g., renal failure and deafness) at the high doses needed to eradicate resistant strains.

To enhance effectiveness and safety, the FDA has approved an inhaled version of tobramycin, called *Tobi*, which is added to a nebulizer and delivered directly to the lungs with a minimum of systemic exposure and toxicity [*Scrip*, December 2, 1998, p 21]. The product has been granted orphan drug status. Clinical trials show that *Tobi* safely increases lung function and reduces hospitalization. It is used at home, thus eliminating the need for hospital-based treatment. *Tobi* is inhaled twice a day for 28 days, with a 28-day break before the next cycle. The cyclic treatment regimen may reduce the evolution of resistant strains. It may be used in adults and in children who are at least six years old. Further testing is needed in younger children.

Tobi therapy is expensive. The average wholesale price is $11,000 for a one-year supply. Before *Tobi*, many patients received inhaled tobramycin solutions mixed by physicians, using the injectable form of the drug. These solutions, however, contained preservatives that could damage lung tissue.

Montelukast (Singulair) for Adults and Children with Asthma. Montelukast (*Singulair*), the third drug to reach the US market that works by inhibiting inflammation-producing leukotrienes, may be a winner for Merck. Montelukast joins zafirlukast (*Accolate*) and zileuton (*Zyflo*). *Singulair* and *Accolate* are leukotriene receptor antagonists, whereas *Zyflo* is a 5-lipoxygenase inhibitor and thereby blocks leukotriene formation. Anti-leukotriene drugs are for long-term control of asthma and not for acute asthma attacks. They may delay and reduce the need for inhaled steroid, an especially important benefit for children. In one study, montelukast combined with as-needed bronchodilator therapy, compared with placebo and bronchodilator, decreased asthma attacks by 37% in patients 15 years of age and older [*Arch Intern Med* 1998;158:1213-20]. Studies in children ranging in age from 6 to 14 years demonstrate the safety and effectiveness of montelukast compared with placebo [*JAMA* 1998;279:1181–86].

Despite its late entry, *Singulair* has marketing advantages over its competitors. It is taken once daily as opposed to twice daily for *Accolate* and four times a day for *Zyflo*. *Singulair* may be used for children as young as six years old. The use of *Accolate* and *Zyflo* is limited to children who are at least 12 years of age. *Singulair* does not appear to inhibit the metabolism of other drugs, unlike *Accolate* and *Zyflo*. While *Accolate* should be taken at least one or two hours after a meal, *Singulair* may be taken with or without food. The labeling of *Singulair* includes data demonstrating efficacy in exercise-challenged asthma. The labeling for neither *Zyflo* nor *Accolate* mentions exercise-induced asthma.

Merck will also be able to promote *Singulair's* efficacy in combination with inhaled corticosteroids and its potential steroid-sparing effects, a benefit not yet demonstrated for *Zyflo* or *Accolate*. *Singulair's* labeling is not burdened with warnings of liver toxicity. In contrast, potential hepatotoxicity is highlighted in *Zyflo* labeling. *Accolate* was introduced with clean labeling regarding adverse effects on the liver, but the label has been updated to include a precaution about the risk of elevated liver enzymes. If this class of drugs establishes a beachhead in the treatment of asthma, *Singulair* seems to be the drug of choice.

Women's Health

Raloxifene (*Evista*): A Designer Estrogen for the
  Prevention of Osteoporosis
Estrogen/Progestin Transdermal Patch
Toremifene and Letrozole: Anti-Estrogen Therapy
  for Breast Cancer
Capecitabine (*Xeloda*): Oral Treatment for Metastatic
  Breast Cancer

Raloxifene (Evista): A Designer Estrogen for the Prevention of Osteoporosis.
Some believe that FDA's approval of Lilly's raloxifene (*Evista*) late in 1997
for the prevention of postmenopausal osteoporosis, ushers in a new era for
women's health. *Evista* is the first of a new class of drugs called selective
estrogen receptor modulators (SERMs). Until the development of tamoxifen
for the treatment of breast cancer, few people thought that one could separate
the beneficial effects of estrogen from its undesirable effects—the stimulation
of breast and endometrial tissue.

Like tamoxifen, raloxifene has estrogenic effects on bone and serum
lipids and probably protects against breast cancer. Offsetting these benefits
for tamoxifen, however, are estrogenic effects on the uterus and increased
risk of endometrial cancer. *Evista* exerts little estrogenic effect on the uterus.
Scientists at Lilly have discovered that structural differences between tamoxifen and raloxifene are responsible for differences in the effects of these compounds on the uterus. They suggest that raloxifene's molecular conformation
selectively affects the way it interacts with the two domains of the estrogen
receptor, resulting in its unique biological profile.

Compared with placebo, raloxifene increases bone density in postmenopausal women [*N Engl J Med* 1997;337:1641–47] but not as effectively as
alendronate *(Fosamax)* or conjugated estrogens (*Premarin*). Effects of *Evista*
on the risk of fracture are under investigation but not yet known. *Fosamax*
and *Premarin* hold a competitive advantage in this regard. Because of the
lack of data on fractures, *Evista* did not receive an indication for the treatment
of osteoporosis, only for prevention. Lilly hopes to file for the treatment
indication soon.

Lilly is positioning *Evista* as an alternative to hormone replacement
therapy (HRT) for women concerned about the risk of cancer. Unopposed

estrogen increases the risk of endometrial hyperplasia and endometrial cancer and also increases the risk of breast cancer, albeit to a small extent. The addition of a progestin to estrogen reduces the risk of endometrial cancer but not of breast cancer. A recent compilation of data suggests that estrogen use for five years or more may be associated with a 35% increase in the risk of breast cancer.

A two-year study in 601 postmenopausal women found that endometrial thickness was similar in the *Evista* and placebo groups at all times during the study [*N Engl J Med* 1997;337:1641–47]. An unpublished study comparing *Evista* with *Premarin* demonstrated the endometrial stimulating effect of unopposed estrogen and the lack of this effect in women receiving *Evista*. On examining their database, Lilly estimates that the incidence of breast cancer is 1.0 per 1,000 for *Evista*, 3.7 per 1,000 for placebo, and 12 per 1,000 for estrogen replacement therapy. The data suggest that *Evista* protects women from breast cancer, but FDA wants more evidence before allowing a claim.

Additional evidence of this protective effect was presented at the 1998 meeting of the American Society of Clinical Oncology. One report concerned an analysis that combined data from randomized trails of *Evista* involving more than 12,000 postmenopausal women. The investigators found a 58% reduction in breast cancer risk among women assigned to *Evista* compared with those receiving placebo. Other investigators described an osteoporosis study in 7,700 women and reported a 75% reduction in breast cancer risk in those receiving *Evista*. The incidence of breast cancer was 0.82% in the placebo group and 0.21% in the *Evista* group. The data available, however, reflect less than two years of study and include relatively few events.

A direct comparison of tamoxifen and *Evista* is about to begin under the direction of the National Cancer Institute. Under consideration is a 22,000-patient study in postmenopausal women at elevated risk for breast cancer, with five years of follow-up. Patients would be randomized to 20 mg of tamoxifen or 60 mg of *Evista* daily. Researchers postulate that both *Evista* and tamoxifen could protect against breast cancer but that *Evista* might be associated with fewer adverse events.

In its competition with *Fosamax*, Lilly will stress *Evista's* beneficial effects on cardiovascular risk factors. *Evista* decreases LDL-cholesterol and fibrinogen. Unlike conjugated estrogens, however, raloxifene does not in-crease HDL-cholesterol. The level of HDL-cholesterol is a strong inverse predictor of coronary heart disease in women. Some experts estimate that up to half of the cardiovascular benefit of estrogen therapy could be mediated by the resulting higher levels of HDL-cholesterol. A combination of *Premarin* and medroxyprogesterone decreases LDL-cholesterol to about same extent as *Evista* but has no effect on fibrinogen [*JAMA* 1998;279:1445–51].

The most serious adverse event observed during the development of *Evista* was venous thromboembolism. Compared with placebo, the relative risk for patients receiving *Evista* was 2.5 overall, with a risk of 6.7 during the first six months of use. About one in four women treated with *Evista* reported hot flashes. In light of this, women should probably avoid *Evista* in the perimenopausal period. Unlike *Premarin, Evista* does not cause resumption of menses. Unlike *Fosamax, Evista* is free of gastrointestinal side effects, and comparatively easy to administer.

Lilly is promoting *Evista* with a direct-to-consumer advertising campaign. One theme for the campaign is: "If estrogen is the answer, why are there so many questions?" Lilly stresses the "troubling side effects of HRT," such as irregular bleeding, spotting, breast tenderness, and migraines. The company also highlights recent studies showing that up to 70% of women discontinue HRT within the first year of therapy, adding that for many women the most serious question is about the possible risk of developing cancer—a concern that may keep them from ever starting therapy. Only about one-fifth of postmenopausal American women ever receive HRT, despite its established benefits. During the first few months of marketing, about two-thirds of the prescriptions written for *Evista* have been for postmenopausal women not previously on therapy.

A recent commentary observed: "The favorable effect of raloxifene on bone mineral density and serum lipid concentrations and the absence of any effect on endometrial histology are quite encouraging. The decrease in estrogen-related adverse effects with the SERMs in general and raloxifene in particular should improve compliance and decrease the incidence of cardiovascular events and fracture while not increasing breast cancer. The challenge is to realize this promise" [*N Engl J Med* 1997;337:1686–87].

The New York Times [June 21, 1998, p WH 4] reports that, ". . . nearly every major drug company is working on a version of a designer estrogen." These include droloxifene and idoxifene. Toremifene (*Fareston*), now marketed as treatment for advanced breast cancer, is also under investigation for prevention.

Estrogen/Progestin Transdermal Patch. Rhone-Poulenc Rorer (RPR) has received approval to market the first estrogen/progestin skin patch (*Combi-*

Patch), for treatment of moderate to severe postmenopausal vasomotor symptoms. The patch contains estradiol and norethindrone. RPR plans to mount a direct-to-consumer campaign to promote the product. Two regimens were evaluated against placebo in clinical trials—the continuous combined regimen and the continuous sequential regimen. The continuous combined group of perimenopausal women applied *CombiPatch* throughout three 28-day cycles, with replacement of the system twice weekly. The continuous sequential group applied an estradiol-only transdermal patch twice weekly during the first 14 days of the 28-day cycle and a *CombiPatch* twice weekly for the remaining 14 days of the cycle. Both regimens reduced the number and intensity of daily hot flushes by about the same extent. Following an estradiol-only patch with a *CombiPatch* significantly decreased the degree of endometrosis seen in women using the estradiol-only patch exclusively [*The Pink Sheet* 1998;60(No33):19].

Toremifene and Letrozole: Anti-Estrogen Therapy for Breast Cancer. Efforts to counter the unwanted effects of estrogen are a major strategy in the treatment of breast cancer. Drugs include anti-estrogens (e.g., tamoxifen), progestins (e.g., megestrol), aromatase inhibitors (e.g., anastrozole or aminoglutethimide), and luteinizing-hormone-releasing hormone agonists (e.g., leuprolide or goserelin).

Anti-estrogens compete with natural estrogen for estrogen receptors in breast tissue, thereby inhibiting the growth-stimulating effects of the hormone. The most recently approved anti-estrogen, toremifene (*Fareston*), is structurally similar to tamoxifen and, like tamoxifen, it has both anti-estrogenic and weak estrogenic activity. Large clinical trials in postmenopausal women with newly diagnosed estrogen-receptor-positive or receptor-status-unknown advanced breast cancer demonstrate the efficacy of toremifene but offer no evidence of an advantage over tamoxifen.

In postmenopausal women, natural estrogen comes mainly from conversion of androgens to estrone and estradiol, catalyzed by the enzyme aromatase (estrogen synthetase). Selective aromatase inhibitors such as newly-approved letrozole (*Femara*), decrease estrogen synthesis and receptor stimulation. Clinical trials in postmenopausal women with advanced breast cancer who failed anti-estrogen therapy show that *Femara* is more effective than megestrol and possibly more effective than aminoglutethimide. *Femara* has not been compared with anastrozole [*Med Letter* 1998;40:43–45].

Capecitabine (Xeloda): Oral Treatment for Metastatic Breast Cancer. Following accelerated approval by the FDA, Roche has launched capecitabine

(*Xeloda*) for secondary treatment of metastatic breast cancer [*Pharmacy To-day* 1998;4(No 6):3–4]. Capecitabane is metabolized to 5-fluorouracil, an anti-cancer agent that must otherwise be given intravenously. Thymidine phosphorylase, the enzyme involved in the formation of 5-FU, is found in higher concentrations in some neoplastic tissues than in surrounding tissues, which theoretically limits systemic exposure to active drug [*Med Letter* 1998;40:108]. With *Xeloda,* patients can obtain the benefits of 5-FU in an oral dosage form. Patients who are resistant to both paclitaxel (*Taxol*) and a chemotherapy regimen that includes an anthracycline (e.g., *Adriamycin*) may derive benefit from additional treatment with *Xeloda.*

Approval was based in part on response rates observed in a phase II study among 43 patients refractory to first-line drug therapy. *Xeloda* reduced tumor size by at least 50% in 11 patients. The median duration of response was 22 weeks. Side effects—lymphopenia, anemia, diarrhea, pain and swelling of the extremities, and nausea—occur frequently. The product label has guidelines for dosage adjustment in the event of serious toxicity. Accelerated approval is always conditional. In this case, to keep *Xeloda* on the market, Roche must sponsor postmarketing studies to confirm and extend effective-ness. Roche will also compare capecitabine plus docetaxel (*Taxotere*) with docetaxel alone.

MEN'S HEALTH

Viagra for Male Erectile Dysfunction
Propecia for the Prevention and Restoration of
Hair Loss in Men

Viagra for Male Erectile Dysfunction. Thanks to streamlined procedures and additional funds generated through user fees, the FDA approved a record number of new drugs and biologicals in 1998. While many new agents were more important from a therapeutic point of view, not one came close to having the impact of Pfizer's *Viagra,* the first oral agent for the treatment of impotence.

Erectile dysfunction or impotence affects up to 30 million men in the US. Prevalence rates are 39% among 40-year olds and 67% among 70-year olds. High prevalence rates are also found in men with diabetes and heart disease. Antihypertensive and antidepressant drugs are often implicated in the disorder. Before the marketing of *Viagra* (sildenafil), treatment was limited to penile prostheses or medical therapy with alprostadil, a prostaglandin, in the form of an injection directly into the male organ (*Caverject*) or a suppository for insertion into the urethra (*MUSE*). Both sildenafil and alprostadil promote the inflow and retention of blood within the body of the penis.

A normal erection depends on the relaxation of smooth muscle in the penis. Nitric oxide produced in the body of the penis on sexual arousal causes the formation of cyclic guanosine monophosphate (cGMP), which relaxes smooth muscle and leads to engorgement. The process is reversed by the conversion of cGMP to GMP, catalyzed in the body of the penis by phospho-diesterase (PDE) type 5. Impotent men seem to have an excess of this type of PDE. *Viagra,* by specifically inhibiting PDE type 5, restores the natural erectile response to sexual stimulation. The drug has little effect on PDE type 3, which is involved in cardiac contractility. Unlike alprostadil, which relaxes smooth muscle directly, *Viagra* does not cause an erection in the absence of arousal. In some men, alprostadil, because of its direct effect, produces a prolonged and painful erection called priapism. *Viagra* seems largely but not completely free of this problem.

The key clinical trial supporting the approval of *Viagra* was a 24-week comparison of oral sildenafil at daily doses ranging from 25 mg to 100 mg with placebo in more than 500 men with erectile dysfunction of organic, pyschogenic, or mixed origins [*N Engl J Med* 1998;338:1397–404]. The investigators found that increasing the dose of sildenafil progressively improves erectile function and that the therapeutic response to *Viagra* is similar in men with various causes of impotence. Study subjects receiving *Viagra* reported that 69% of all attempts at sexual intercourse were successful, compared with 22% of all attempts reported by men given placebo. The average number of successful attempts per month was 5.9 for men taking *Viagra* and 1.5 for those taking a placebo. Remarkably, no objective measures were used to evaluate the efficacy of sildenafil. The side effects of sildenafil are not a major concern for most men. Men taking nitrates, however, should not use *Viagra* because it may produce an alarming drop in blood pressure.

The emergence of sildenafil for impotence is the result of good fortune rather than astute molecular design. Originally conceived for the treatment of angina and hypertension, sildenafil was not very effective. Several subjects participating in the heart trials, however, reported improved and more frequent erections while using the drug. The rest is history.

Even before Pfizer received approval to market *Viagra*, financial analysts had lofty expectations. They were not disappointed. *Viagra* had the most successful debut in pharmaceutical history, even though Pfizer spent little money on promotion for the first few months after marketing the drug. Four weeks after introduction, *Viagra* had 98% of the sexual dysfunction market. In its first full month on the US market, a total of 570,000 new prescription for *Viagra* was dispensed. By comparison, 149,000 new prescriptions were written in the first month for the diet pill *Redux*. Pfizer launched a direct-to-consumer advertising campaign in mid-1998.

In July 1998, Pfizer reported a 37% increase in second-quarter net income driven largely by sales of *Viagra*. From April 10, when Viagra was launched, through June 26, a total of 2.7 million prescriptions were written for the impotence drug. Analysts noted that the rate of sales was starting to level off but the drug had not yet been officially launched internationally. Pfizer hopes to introduce the drug in 50 countries by the end of the year [*The Wall Street Journal,* July 10, 1998, p B5]. In September, a pharmaceutical market-research firm forecast that sales of *Viagra* will reach $1 billion by March 1999, despite lower than average third-party coverage.

Physicians were overwhelmed with requests to prescribe *Viagra* but were not complaining about the unexpected business. Fueling the initial demand was unprecedented media coverage. A still larger market looms. According to *The Wall Street Journal* [July 13, 1998, pp B1, B12], pharmaceutical companies are eager to expand to the women's market and at least six companies are already developing drugs aimed at women. Trying to ride the coattails of *Viagra* are vitamin and herbal products called *Viagro* and *Vaegra*. Pfizer is taking action against these firms, charging trademark infringement.

While initial media reports carried nothing but successful tales, later articles stressed limitations. For instance, *Viagra* only works in 4 of 5 men. Less likely to benefit are men with restricted tissue perfusion because of atherosclerosis. The highest failure rates are reported among men who have had prostate surgery and men with long-standing insulin-dependent diabetes. Men with coronary disease who, because of impotence, have not had sex for years should consult a physician before putting too much stress on an impaired heart.

As of May 26, 1998, six deaths were reported in men who had taken *Viagra,* prompting Pfizer to again warn that the drug must not be used in men taking nitroglycerin or other nitrates. The warning particularly targeted emergency room physicians, alerting them that men complaining of chest pain, perhaps due to heart disease, should be asked if they are taking *Viagra* before being given nitrates. Pfizer also warned people who engage in high-risk sex that *Viagra* should not be combined with "poppers" (amyl nitrate or butyl nitrate). On investigating the six cases, the company reported that they were probably due to cardiac stress during sexual intercourse by elderly men with heart disease, or to a combination of *Viagra* with nitrate medication. About 85% of men taking *Viagra* are over the age of 50. For a 50-year old man with a history of heart disease, sexual activity nearly triples the baseline risk of a heart attack although the absolute risk is small.

Also in May, ophthalmologists warned that the long-term implications of visual side effects reported by some men using *Viagra* are uncertain; some feared it could cause permanent loss of vision in patients who already have retinal dysfunction [*Scrip,* May 27, 1998, p 23]. Eye experts reminded everyone that older patients with macular degeneration and diabetics with retinopathy are likely to suffer from impotence. During the trials, about 10% of men taking the usual 50 mg dose of *Viagra* reported a blue cast to their vision. Half the men taking more than 100 mg reported the same experience.

At the end of June, nearly three months after approving *Viagra,* the FDA had received about 100 reports of men suffering serious adverse reactions, including 30 deaths, after taking *Viagra*. Most were elderly and had health problems. The FDA convened a group of experts to study the reports but the panel found no reason to question the safety of *Viagra*. While it is clear that men taking nitrates should not use the impotence drug, some clinicians think that *Viagra* is suspect in men taking any kind of antihypertensive medication [*The Wall Street Journal,* June 29, 1998, p B6].

Also troubled by the potential adverse effects of *Viagra* is Public Citizen's Health Research Group (HRG) [*Scrip,* July 8, 1998, p 24]. The consumer organization maintains in a July 1 letter to the FDA that labeling for *Viagra* should contain contraindications against use in men with diseases or conditions that were excluded from clinical trials, a move that would substantially decrease the size of the market for the drug. HRG also finds that labeling does not clearly warn against taking more than 100 mg a day, doses that may precipitate vision problems [*The Pink Sheet* 1998;60(No 27):6].

In August, the American College of Cardiology and the American Heart Association released interim recommendations for prescribing *Viagra* to patients at risk of cardiovascular events. The organizations reiterated early cautions and listed other medical profiles in which sildenafil may be particularly hazardous. These include patients with active coronary ischemia who are not taking nitrates, patients with low blood pressure, patients on complicated antihypertensive regimens, and patients taking drugs likely to prolong the half-life of *Viagra* [*Lancet* 1998;352:549]. Immediately following the recommendations, HRG demanded that the FDA convene a meeting of its cardiovascular drugs advisory committee. The advisory panel was not asked for an opinion on *Viagra* before the drug received FDA approval [*Scrip,* August 26, 1998, p 16].

Also in August, the FDA issued a safety update on *Viagra*. The agency reported that 51 of the 69 patients in the US who died after taking the drug had cardiovascular or cerebrovascular disease or had one or more risk factors. The average age of people who died was 64 years. Of the 41 patients for whom the time of ingestion was known, 25 died within four to five hours and 18 died during or immediately after sexual intercourse. *The Pink Sheet* [1998;60(No35):11] observes that although *Viagra* labeling cautions physicians to evaluate their patients' cardiovascular status prior to prescribing the drug, many men using the drug have a history of heart disease and/or diabetes because those conditions are associated with male erectile dysfunction.

In September, a research letter reported a 65-year old man who developed an acute MI 30 minutes after taking a single tablet of *Viagra* [*Lancet* 1998;352:957–58]. The authors hold that the close temporal relationship between ingesting sildenafil and onset of severe chest pains due to acute MI in a patient without a history of chest pain or risk factors for cardiovascular disease suggests that sildenafil was causally related to the AMI. They add that since chest pain occurred before any attempt at sexual intercourse was made, ". . . sexual exertion can not be regarded as a precipitating factor." The vasodilatory effects of sildenafil are not likely to be restricted to the corpus cavernosa. The authors suggest: "Redistribution of arterial blood flow may have undermined adequate coronary perfusion and led to [acute myocardial infarction] AMI."

A single dose of *Viagra* costs about $10 at retail. Product labeling limits use to once a day. Medical insurers, fearing huge payments to millions of American men, are adopting strict reimbursement policies for the drug. At best, insurers will reimburse only documented claims of men who suffer from physical ailments or diseases known to result in erectile dysfunction. Health plans are also limiting the number of doses of *Viagra* reimbursed each month. One plan reimburses for only six doses per month. A lawsuit is looming to force health insurers to improve reimbursement rates. The only law suit launched against Pfizer involves a man who drove into a tree shortly after taking *Viagra*.

By June, some of the nations biggest health insurers had announced that they would not reimburse for *Viagra*. The firms said that even providing 6 to 12 pills per month would be too expensive, adding hundreds of millions of dollars to annual costs. Kaiser Permanente, the nation's largest nonprofit health maintenance organization with nine million members, announced that *Viagra* would only be available as an extra benefit at an additional cost. Aetna U.S. Health Care announced a similar policy [*The New York Times,* June 20, 1998, p A6]. Prudential HealthCare and Humana have also decided to deny coverage for *Viagra,* on the grounds of a lack of clinical data to prove its safety in long-term use. An article in *The New York Times* [July 11, 1998, p B1, B2] observed that health plans cite many reasons for denying coverage of specific drugs or procedures, calling them cosmetic, medically unnecessary, experimental, or dangerous. But cost is one reason they almost never cite.

In July, to everyone's surprise, health officials in Washington notified states that their Medicaid programs must pay for *Viagra*. The administrator of the Health Care Financing Administration (HCFA) said that the law protecting the poor and disabled requires coverage of the costs of all approved drugs prescribed for legitimate medical reasons. Of the 37 million people enrolled in Medicaid, only about four million are men, and only a small subset would seek the drug. Medicare, the program for the 39 million elderly Americans, does not cover costs of medication [*The Wall Street Journal*, July 2, 1998, p B5].

On receiving the message from HCFA, state governors were in an uproar, and New York and Wisconsin announced that they intended to defy the directive to provide *Viagra* through Medicaid. The National Governors' Association said Medicaid coverage of *Viagra* should be a state option, not a Federal mandate. The governor of New York said: "The Federal Government should not be requiring New York or any other state to pay for *Viagra* until there is a better understanding of the impact this drug has on patients." A health official in Wisconsin observed: "We don't believe that *Viagra* is medically necessary." Not all states hold this view and 26 are reimbursing for *Viagra*. The contretemps could end up in court [*The New York Times*, July 3, 1998, p A10].

Advocates for the disabled expressed outrage that the Federal Government was requiring coverage of *Viagra* while allowing states to deny or cut back coverage of medical equipment needed by people with severe physical limitation. The fact that some insurers are covering *Viagra* but not contraception has angered the American College of Obstetrics and Gynecology and provoked charges of sex discrimination. The publicity given to the obvious double standard prompted an embarrassed Congress to develop legislation— the Lowey provision—to cover the cost of contraceptives for federal employees [*The Wall Street Journal*, September 4, 1993, p A4]. The omnibus budget bill, signed by the President in October, includes the provision. About 1.2 million women of childbearing age who are beneficiaries in the Federal Employees Health Benefits program are now eligible for prescription contraceptives [*Scrip*, October 21, 1998, p 16]. The mandate may have a ripple effect on the entire health-care industry. Other critics observe that our society is willing to pay for men's erections but not for infertility treatment.

Many patients are prepared to pay for their own prescriptions if their health insurers do not cover the drug. To reduce costs for their patients, some physicians are prescribing 100 mg tablets of *Viagra* and telling them to cut the tablet in half—a 50 mg dose works well in most men. *Viagra* must be taken between 30 minutes to one hour before sexual activity. Pfizer would like to have a more rapidly acting formulation and has entered into an agreement with RP Scherer, a manufacturer of novel dosage forms. The goal is to use Scherer's technology to make a freeze-dried porous wafer that contains the drug and dissolves rapidly on the tongue without water.

Other pharmaceutical companies are also developing selective PDE inhibitors and may soon have products to compete with *Viagra*. The next oral product to reach the market, however, is likely to be *Vasomax*. It is a reformulation of phentolamine, an old drug for lowering blood pressure. Even if approved, *Vasomax* is unlikely to be as effective as *Viagra*. Also in development is a cream formulation of alprostadil for application to the glans of the penis. Another company is evaluating sublingual apomorphine for impotence. Apomorphine acts centrally, stimulating nerve signals to increase blood flow and produce an erection. At a recent meeting of urologists, researchers told the participants that oral phentolamine and sublingual apomorphine will not be a serious challenge to *Viagra* [*Scrip,* June 5, 1998, p 20]. A summary of the meeting is available in *JAMA* [1998;280:119-20].

Like *Soma*—take a gram and not give a damn—from Huxley's "Brave New World," *Viagra* is a social phenomenon [*Scrip Magazine,* June/August 1998, pp 17–18]. Media coverage seems endless. A travel agency in Japan offers men a four-day tour of Hawaii, which includes a consultation with a physician and the cost of a prescription for 30 tablets of *Viagra. The New York Times* [June 23, 1998, p B9, B11] reports that experts on sexuality and therapists are finding that *Viagra* ". . . may actually throw into chaos [marital] relationships that have fallen into their own routine, sexual dysfunction and all." Large quantities of *Viagra* are finding their way to healthy men who seek "an extra helping" [*The Wall Street Journal,* June 15, 1998, p B1, B8]. Pfizer insists that *Viagra* has no effect in men who do not have erectile dysfunction and that testimonials from sexually active men are the result of a placebo effect.

In September, the European Commission cleared the way for *Viagra* to be sold in EU nations [*The Wall Street Journal,* September 15, 1998, p B4]. The label in Europe will note that priapism has been reported after taking *Viagra*. Patients are advised to seek medical help if such erections last for more than four hours.

While Pfizer can now market *Viagra* in Europe, each country in the union still must decide whether the drug will be paid for by its national health insurance. Observers expect the reimbursement controversy to be most heated in the UK and Germany. The UK National Health Service is advising doctors not to prescribe the drug until NHS decides whether it will provide reimbursement for the product. A flood of prescriptions for *Viagra* could leave the government without sufficient funds to pay for patients with more urgent conditions. The decision to approve *Viagra* was met with an entirely different response in Poland, a nation that aspires to membership in the EU [*The Wall Street Journal,* September 16, 1998, p A22]. A minister for family planning proposed subsidizing the drug, ". . . to boost births in our homeland."

A recent perspective in *JAMA* [1998;280:867–69] noted that Pfizer has produced a virtual library of guides to treat erectile dysfunction for urologists, psychiatrists, endocrinologists, cardiologists, and primary care physicians. Also readily available are brochures for patients. Primary care physicians have written the majority of prescriptions for *Viagra.*

In October, the Pentagon estimated that it would spend about $50 million in 1999 to provide *Viagra* to US troops and military retirees. According to *The New York Times* [October 4, 1998, p y21], the cost is equivalent to that of two Harrier jets or 45 Tomahawk cruise missiles. In a rare display of fiscal responsibility, Defense Department health officials told Congress that if the drug was given to everyone in the military who wanted it, the cost could top $100 million. They also assured Congress that no one will be allowed more than six tablets per month, and lost, stolen, or destroyed tablets will not be replaced.

For a time, the commercial success of *Viagra* seemed unstoppable. Some analysts predicted that sales could reach $10 billion to $20 billion a year world-wide, many times that of any other drug. In October, however, Pfizer reported sales of $141 million world-wide for the third quarter, including $115 million in the US. While nothing to sneeze at, the performance paled in comparison with US sales of $411 million in the second quarter. Prescription sales peaked at more than 300,000 per week in May 1998, an extraordinary rate, but progressively declined to about 160,000 per week in September. What changed? *The Wall Street Journal* [October 15, 1998, p B1,B15] points to a sharp decrease in media attention, fear of side effects, and managed-care restrictions on reimbursement. Yet another reason, expressed by some men, is unfulfilled expectations.

In the midst of slumping sales, future prospects for *Viagra* were further limited by the addition of new warnings. *The Wall Street Journal* [November 25, 1998, B7] reported that Pfizer and the FDA agreed to caution patients to use *Viagra* with care if they have a history of heart disease, hypertension, or retinitis pigmentosa, a degenerative disease of the retina. Following the lead of European regulators, the FDA has also directed that information on priapism be added to *Viagra's* labeling. Men are urged to seek medical treatment if their erections last longer than four hours. By November, 130 men had died while taking the impotence drug. The FDA said that 70% of them had one or more risk factors for cardiovascular disease.

Propecia for the Prevention and Restoration of Hair Loss in Men. FDA's approval of an oral product called *Propecia,* containing 1 mg of finasteride, set the stage for a marketing battle with topical *Rogaine* (minoxidil), which does not require a prescription, to determine which product will preserve the hair of 33 million American men with pattern baldness [*Med Letter* 1998;40:25–27]. Most of the potential customers view hair loss as a sign of aging and now spend nearly a billion dollars each year on hair products and treatments.

To make matters more interesting, a new formulation called *Rogaine Extra Strength for Men* is now available. It contains more minoxidil, 5% vs. 2% in the original product, and is said to be 45% more effective than the original product. Both *Rogaine* and *Propecia* contain ingredients found in other prescription products—oral minoxidil for hypertension and oral finasteride (*Proscar*) for the treatment of benign prostatic hyperplasia. Neither product has been very successful in the marketplace. The indication for baldness offers the opportunity for a commercial renaissance. The prospects for *Rogaine* are more limited because of generic competition for the original product, but Pharmacia and Upjohn hopes to receive marketing exclusivity for the new *Extra Strength* formulation. Because health insurance will not cover the cost of products aimed at preventing hair loss, both hair-restorers will be heavily promoted directly to consumers. Both *Propecia* and *Rogaine* require regular use for several months before results are evident and both must be taken over a lifetime to maintain benefit. Both work best in men with hair loss at the vertex of the head.

Finasteride works by inhibiting the conversion of testosterone to dihydrotestosterone. Dihydrotestosterone promotes both prostate growth and hair loss. Sexual dysfunction in 1–2% of users is a potential obstacle to the successful marketing of *Propecia.* Finasteride can cause a birth defect in male offspring—hypospadias—so *Propecia* is not approved for women. Clinical trials have recruited only men 18 to 41 years old, so effects of *Propecia* on older men are not known.

The cost to the pharmacist of a one-month supply of *Propecia* is about

$47. The cost to the pharmacist of a one-month supply of *Rogaine Extra Strength* is about $28. Merck's pricing strategy invites deceit. Five tablets of *Propecia,* each containing 1 mg finasteride, costs three times more than one tablet of *Proscar* containing 5 mg finasteride. Not only is the original product much cheaper per mg, substantial cost reimbursement is available for *Proscar* from most insurance plans.

OTHER INDICATIONS

Hydroxyurea in Sickle Cell Anemia
New Drugs for Bladder Control
Thalidomide (*Thalomid*) for Leprosy-Related Condition
Doxycycline for Periodontal Disease
Topical Brinzolamide for Glaucoma
Risedronate (*Actonell*) for Paget's Disease

Hydroxyurea in Sickle Cell Anemia. Sickle cell anemia is a rare, inherited blood disorder that affects more than 90,000 people in the US, mostly African-Americans. The disease is characterized by chronic anemia and periodic painful crises, in which the sickle-shaped red blood cells become stuck in narrow blood vessels. Treatment options are limited.

In 1998, the FDA approved the use of hydroxyurea (*Droxia*) to prevent painful crises and reduce the need for blood transfusions in adults with sickle cell anemia [*Scrip*, No 2316, p 21]. Hydroxyurea has been available as an antineoplastic agent for more than 30 years under the name *Hydrea*. The drug has been used off-label for years to treat sickle-cell anemia.

In the trials supporting approval, investigators found that hydroxyurea decreases the annual sickle cell crisis rate by nearly 50%, the number of patients requiring transfusion by 30%, and the number of transfusions by 37%. Patients with six or more crises per year at baseline seem to derive the greatest benefit in crisis reduction. Trial investigators reported that patients treated with hydroxyurea had a lower mortality rate than patents receiving placebo, but the difference did not reach statistical significance.

Hydroxyurea often precipitates neutropenia, and requires hematologic monitoring. A major concern is the potential carcinogenicity of the drug, which prompted FDA's oncological drugs advisory panel to limit its recommendation for approval to adults only. *Droxia's* label carries a black-box warning for potential carcinogenicity. Another concern is potential teratogenicity. A five-year follow-up study of the patients participating in the efficacy trials is planned to determine whether the incidence of cancer, birth defects, or other long-term adverse effects is higher than expected. FDA would like to see the prescribing of hydroxyurea limited to physicians experienced in the use of the drug for the new indication.

New Drugs for Bladder Control. Pharmacia and Upjohn has launched tolterodine (*Detrol*), a muscarinic receptor antagonist, for the treatment of patients with symptoms of urinary frequency, urgency, or urge incontinence because of an unstable or overactive bladder. *Detrol* inhibits bladder contractions and delays the desire to void. An estimated 17 million Americans, largely women, have symptoms of an overactive bladder but no more than 20% seek help. Many people are unaware that overactive bladder can be treated or are too embarrassed to discuss the condition. The company will promote the drug through direct-to-consumer advertising and educational material aimed at gynecologists, urologists, and primary care physicians. The World Health Organization (WHO) also wishes to inform people that poor bladder control is a treatable disease. Toward that end, WHO recently started the process of reclassifying urinary incontinence as a disease rather than a condition [*Scrip,* July 10, 1998, p 22].

Pharmacologically, tolterodine is similar to oxybutynin, which has been available for 20 years. The new drug seems no more effective than oxybutynin but is less likely to cause dry mouth, a common side effect of antimuscarinic drugs. In controlled trials, *Detrol* decreased the median number of urinations from ten per day to eight per day. There is no direct evidence, however, of an effect on continence (i.e., whether the patient has fewer accidents while on the drug). Patients receiving *Detrol* in three different trials had fewer incontinence episodes than patients assigned placebo, but differences were not statistically significant.

Physicians in Sweden, where the drug has been available for almost two years, say that tolterodine improves quality of life but is not a breakthrough therapy. *Detrol,* however, is much more expensive than generic oxybutynin and probably should be reserved for patients who do not tolerate the side effects of the older drug. More competition will come from a controlled-released, once-a-day formulation of oxybutynin, developed by Alza and called *Ditropan XL.* The product is under review at the FDA.

An open-label study of *Ditropan XL* shows pronounced reduction or elimination of weekly urge incontinence episodes and/or total incontinence episodes over 12 weeks. Only 2% of patients discontinued therapy because of dry mouth. Alza officials say that reducing incontinence episodes is far more important than reducing the frequency of urination. The first controlled phase III trial, involving 105 patients, indicates that *Ditropan XL* is as effective as conventional oxybutynin with an almost 50% lower incidence of moderate or severe dry mouth [*Scrip,* No 2349, July 3, 1998, p 19]. Both therapies reduce the number of weekly urge incontinence episodes by about 85%. The proportion of patients who achieve full continence, about 40%, is similar in each group. Analysts note that the incidence of dry mouth with *Ditropan XL* is about the same as that resulting from treatment with tolterodine.

More competition for *Detrol* will come from Schering-Plough's *Detrunorm* (propiverine), launched in the UK in September 1998. The drug is used to treat urge incontinence disorder and acts as a smooth muscle relaxant, combining antimuscarinic and calcium antagonist activity. *Detrunorm* increases bladder capacity and reduces the frequency of micturation. It appears to have less antimuscarinic activity than tolterodine and may have a more favorable safety profile [*Scrip,* September 30, 1998, p 22].

Thalidomide (Thalomid) for Leprosy-Related Condition. Thalidomide, the morning sickness drug that resulted in thousands of babies with severe limb defects, has been approved for use in the US for the first time. Forty years ago, much of the world (46 countries in all) witnessed the tragic effects of thalidomide. But pregnant women in the US were spared because at that time, the FDA reviewed new drugs so much more slowly than other regulatory bodies that thalidomide was condemned before it could reach the American market.

In 1998, the FDA was far better prepared to deal with thalidomide. A large measure of confidence was drawn from the agency's ability to minimize birth defects associated with isotretinoin (*Accutane),* a vitamin A analogue and potent teratogen used for severe forms of acne. Based on the *Accutane* experience, FDA approved thalidomide (*Thalomid*) relatively quickly for a narrow indication, erythema nodosum leprosum, a severe and debilitating complication of leprosy. Chronic therapy will usually be required. Mindful that once thalidomide was on the market, physicians were likely to prescribe the drug for a variety of other potential indications, the FDA imposed unprecedented restrictions on the distribution of thalidomide [*The New York Times,* July 17, 1998, pp A1, A13].

Celgene, the company that developed the drug for leprosy, has established a fetal exposure program called STEPS—System for Thalidomide Education and Prescription Safety. Only physicians who are registered in the STEPS program are able to prescribe thalidomide. Patients, after counseling on the risks and benefits of treatment, must comply with mandatory contraceptive measures, agree to registration, and respond to surveys. No more than four weeks of treatment may be prescribed and automatic refills are prohibited. Dispensing the product is prohibited without written confirmation of a negative pregnancy test within 24 hours of starting the drug. Testing is required weekly for the first month of use and then monthly in women with regular menstrual cycles. Patients must use two methods of contraception during treatment with thalidomide. Male patients receiving thalidomide must also agree to use condoms when engaging in sexual intercourse. Packaging for thalidomide will include a photograph of a baby deformed by the drug [*The Pink Sheet* 1998;60:3–4].

Celgene plans to submit applications for additional uses of thalidomide. At the top of the list are AIDS-related cachexia and a similar wasting syndrome in some patients with cancer [*Scrip*, July 22,1998, p 19]. Thalidomide selectively inhibits tumor necrosis factor, one of the cytokines implicated in the development of cachexia. An application for treatment of HIV-infected patients with aphthous ulcers is likely to follow. Celgene also plans to pursue a multiple myeloma indication. Other companies are exploring the use of thalidomide as an anti-angiogenic agent for the treatment of Kaposi's sarcoma and other cancers, and for the treatment and prevention of graft versus host disease in patients receiving bone marrow transplantation.

Doxycycline for Periodontal Disease. The first stage of periodontitis is a bacterial infection of the gums, which progresses by means of a build-up of plaque to the formation of pockets between the gums and teeth. Plaque can spread below the gumline causing teeth to loosen. It is estimated that 50 million Americans have periodontal disease, but only 7.5 million currently receive treatment.

In September, the FDA approved *Atridox* for treatment of chronic adult periodontitis [*The Pink Sheet* 1998;60(No37):4–5]. Atrix developed the product using its proprietary *Atrigel* drug delivery system combined with doxycycline. The product is applied as a gel to affected areas. On application, the gel conforms to the shape of the periodontal pocket and solidifies. A 50-mg dose of doxycycline diffuses out of the gel into surrounding tissue over seven days. Application of *Atridox* may be repeated four months after initial therapy. Atrix says that *Atridox* has a dual action—improving pocket depth and strengthening the attachment of the tooth. A related product, *Actisite*, contains tetracycline in a periodontal fiber.

Clinical trials enrolling 831 patients supported the approval of *Atridox*. Investigators demonstrated that the product is at least 75% as effective as scaling and root planing, the standard threshold for any product approved as stand alone therapy for periodontitis. However, there are no expectations at this time that *Atridox* will replace the traditional mechanical removal of bacterial buildup for treating periodontal disease. Other studies show a significant decrease in disease-causing bacteria at sites treated with *Atridox*, without an increase in resistance to doxycycline.

The agency has also approved a pill called *Periostat*—a matrix metallo-proteinase inhibitor—to treat periodontal disease. It contains a low dose of doxycycline, too low to kill bacteria but sufficient to inhibit the formation of collagenase in inflamed gums. Collagenase is formed in response to advanced disease. The enzyme attacks bacteria but it also breaks down tissues that hold teeth in place, and may reduce the need for frequent scaling and root planing. Approval was based a 190-patient controlled trial. After nine months of *Periostat* 20 mg twice daily as an adjunct to scaling and root planing, patients with varying severity of disease had significant decreases in pocket depth compared with mechanical removal alone. One study, in patients who took *Periostat* every day after a dentist had scraped away the plaque, found a 50% improvement in gum reattachment to teeth compared with patients who had plaque removal alone [*The Pink Sheet* 1998;60(No40):7].

A product containing the antibacterial agent chlorhexidine, called *Perio-Chip*, has also received FDA's approval for marketing. It is described as the first biodegradable delivery system to be available to reduce pocket depth in adult periodontitis. The product consists of a small chip that is inserted into infected periodontal pockets after standard therapy. If needed, the chip may be inserted every three months. It releases chlorhexidine over 7 to 10 days. Two large studies of the adjunctive use of *Periochip* with standard therapy reported a significant reduction in pocket depth compared with scaling and planing alone. Clinically important reductions of 2 mm or more were seen in 13.5% of patients on standard therapy alone compared with 30.3% of patients on combination therapy [*Scrip*, October 7, 1998, p 22].

Fueling interest in an aggressive medical approach to treat periodontal disease is the suspected linkage of gum disease to heart attacks and strokes [*The Wall Street Journal*, October 1, 1998, p B9]. A position paper prepared by the Research, Science, and Therapy Committee of the American Academy of Periodontology provides information on the role of periodontal disease in systemic diseases. Systemic diseases include bacteremia, infective endocarditis, cardiovascular disease and atherosclerosis, prosthetic device infection, diabetes mellitus, respiratory diseases, and adverse pregnancy outcomes [*J Periodontol* 1998;69:841–50].

Topical Brinzolamide for Glaucoma. Brinzolamide (*Azopt*), a carbonic anhydrase inhibitor like dorzolamide (*Trusopt*), is used topically in the form of an ophthalmic suspension for the treatment of elevated intraocular pressure due to ocular hypertension or open-angle glaucoma. A three-month well controlled trial shows that brinzolamide is as effective as usual doses of dorzolamide or timolol [*Timoptic*], a β-blocker, in decreasing intraocular pressure [*Am J Ophthamol* 1998;126:400-408]. Added to timolol, brinzolamide further reduces intraocular pressure. Transient blurring of vision and an unpleasant aftertaste have been the most common complaints of patients using the drug. According to *The Medical Letter* [1998;40:95-96]: "Brinzolamide appears to be as effective as dorzolamide in lowering intraocular pressure. For patients who complain of burning and stinging with dorzolamide, it may be worth trying."

Risedronate (Actonell) for Paget's Disease. Proctor & Gamble has launched an oral bisphosphonate, risedronate (*Actonell*), for the treatment of a bone disorder called Paget's disease, said to affect 3% of people over the age of 40 [*Scrip*, October 9, 1998, p 18]. Evidence indicates that risedronate benefits patients who have a level of serum alkaline phosphatase at least twice the upper limit of normal, the presence of symptoms, a risk for future complications, or who fail to respond to other therapies. The goal of treatment is to normalize serum alkaline phosphatase levels and reduce pain. *Actonell* will compete with another bisphosphonate etidronate (*Didronel*). Risedronate is also in development for osteoporosis.

LATE BREAKING REPORTS

Infectious Disease

FDA Approves Abacavir (Ziagen). Despite evidence of serious and sometimes fatal reactions, the FDA approved Glaxo's new nucleoside reverse transcriptase inhibitor. *Ziagen* is especially indicated for those patients who cannot tolerate protease inhibitors. Pharmacists will provide patients with a card that alerts them to possible development of allergic reaction symptoms, which can lead to fatally low blood pressure [*The Wall Street Journal*, December 21, 1998, p B2].

Sustiva: First-Line Therapy for HIV Infection. After only two months on the US market, *Sustiva* (efavirenz) is rapidly finding a place as a potential first-line therapy [*Scrip,* December 11, 1998, p 20]. *Sustiva* is the first NNRTI to be deemed equivalent to protease inhibitors in US guidelines for the treatment of established HIV infection. Like a protease inhibitor, *Sustiva* must be given with two nucleoside RTIs. DuPont Pharmaceuticals has noted that initial HIV therapy with *Sustiva* instead of a protease inhibitor allows patients to reserve protease inhibitors for later use.

Oncology

New Second-Line Agent for SCLC. At the end of November, topotecan (*Hycamtin*) received unconditional approval for the treatment of small-cell lung cancer (SCLC) after failure of first-line chemotherapy. The pivotal phase III trial in 211 relapsed patients showed a 24% response rate in those who received *Hycamtin* and an 18% response rate in those who received additional chemotherapy. Hematological toxicity will complicate treatment [*The Pink Sheet* 1998;60(No49):14].

Pain Management

FDA Approves COX-2 Selective NSAID. On December 31, 1998, the FDA announced the eagerly awaited approval of *Celebrex* for arthritis. Because the FDA stated that there was no proof that the new drug produces less gastrointestinal damage than older competitors such as naproxen and ibuprofen, Searle was not celebrating. The agency's warning raises the question of how many arthritis patients will switch from conventional NSAIDs to *Celebrex*.

Respiratory Disease

Montelukast (Singulair) Flagged for Rare Adverse Reaction. A "Dear Doctor" letter from Merck in December 1998 alerts physicians to rare cases of allergic granulomatous angiitis in patients receiving the leukotriene receptor antagonist for asthma. The reaction resembles Churg-Strauss syndrome, which is a form of systemic necrotizing vasculitis with prominent lung involvement. It generally manifests as an abnormally large number of eosinophils—granular leukocytes—in blood. A causal association between *Singulair* and the reaction, however, has not been established. Based on reports, Merck estimates the incidence to be less than 0.01%. The reaction has also been observed in patients receiving another leukotriene antagonist, zafirlukast (*Accolate*) [*The Pink Sheet* 1998;60(No49):11].

Women's Health

New Data Support Use of Raloxifene (Evista) for Breast Cancer Prevention. Clinical trial results show that regular use of Lilly's *Evista* (raloxifene) by healthy postmenopausal women results in a 55% reduction in the risk of breast cancer compared with placebo. The study involved 10,575 women who were followed for a median time of three years and four months. At that time, there were 3.8 cases of breast cancer per 1000 women who received placebo, compared with 1.7 cases per 1000 women who received *Evista* [*The Wall Street Journal,* December 11, 1998, pp A3,A8]. Lilly has negotiated with the FDA to make label changes that reflect the latest data on breast cancer risk. The new label will include data reflecting a risk reduction, but it will also state that the effectiveness of raloxifene to reduce the risk of breast cancer has not been established [*Ibid,* December 14, 1998, p B3].

Other Indications

FDA Approves Provigil for Narcolepsy. At the end of December, Cephalon received FDA approval to market *Provigil* (modafinil), the first new non-amphetamine narcolepsy drug in decades. More information about modafinil can be found in Chapter 4. The director of a sleep laboratory said that *Provigil,* " . . . is specific for promoting wakefulness, without causing the side effects of other drugs" [*The Wall Street Journal,* December 29, 1998, p B5]. *Provigil* should be available in early 1999.

2 Drug Evaluation
Controlled Clinical Studies

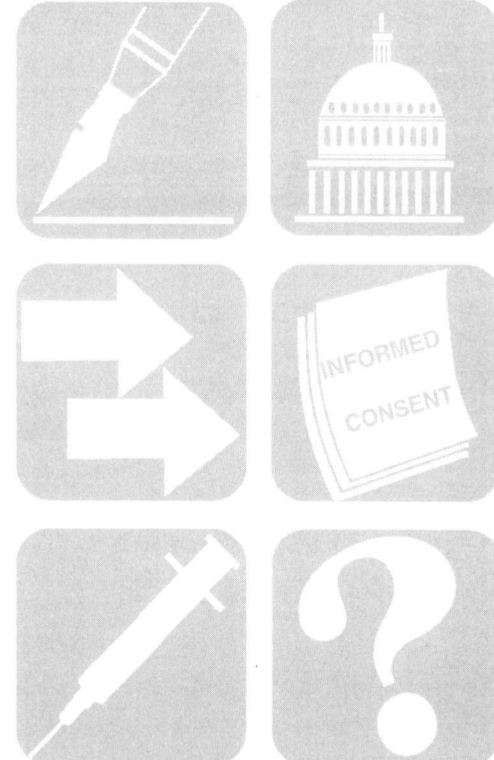

CARDIOVASCULAR DISEASE

Aspirin and Warfarin Prevent First Heart Attack. There is unequivocal evidence that low-dose aspirin reduces the risk of subsequent heart attacks in patients who have already had a myocardial infarction (MI). However, two trials evaluating low-dose aspirin for primary prevention in men, deemed to be at high risk of heart disease but who had not yet suffered a heart attack, have produced conflicting results. While there is uncertainty, it is likely that aspirin provides a benefit to high-risk but otherwise healthy men who take a small dose every day.

The anticoagulant warfarin has also been shown to benefit the secondary prevention population but is used infrequently because of fears about increased bleeding risk. There is also evidence in the primary prevention population that low-intensity anticoagulation with warfarin results in favorable changes in clotting factors that may decrease the risk of an ischemic event. Because both warfarin and aspirin can increase the risk of bleeding, they are not used ordinarily in combination.

A recent study—the Thrombosis Prevention Trial—in a primary prevention population (middle-aged men at high risk of ischemic heart disease) challenges that wisdom [*Lancet* 1998;351:233–41]. The results offer new and important insights to primary prevention. The investigators randomized the nearly 6,000 participants to one of four groups—aspirin alone, warfarin alone, the combination of the two, or placebo. Aspirin was given as one 75 mg *Bayer Aspirin* tablet each day and warfarin was titrated to an international normalized ratio (INR) of 1.5. INR is a widely used measurement of blood coagulation. This intensity of anticoagulation is less than that recommended to prevent deep vein thrombosis after surgery and is likely to cause less serious bleeding. Patients were followed for 8 to 13 years.

The investigators report that both warfarin and aspirin reduce the risk of a first MI and that the lowest rate of MI occurs in men receiving a combination of warfarin and aspirin. Warfarin reduced the risk of a heart attack by 21%, aspirin reduced the risk by 20%, and the combination by 34%. The combination, however, was also associated with a small increase in the rate of cerebral hemorrhage. Increased cranial bleeding was not observed with either drug alone. Cerebral bleeds occurred mostly in patients with high blood pressure; better patient selection may reduce the risk. Warfarin alone seemed more effective than aspirin in preventing fatal heart attacks, but aspirin was more effective in preventing non-fatal heart attacks. The results in patients receiving warfarin are intriguing. Apparently, inhibition of the coagulation cascade and fibrin deposition can protect high-risk men against a heart attack.

The researchers estimated that about five heart attacks would be avoided by treating 1000 men with combined warfarin and aspirin for one year and that three heart attacks would be avoided by treating 1,000 men with either warfarin or aspirin for one year. Taking into account the relative incidence of heart attack and hemorrhagic stroke, the investigators say that the combination prevents about 12 times as many heart attacks as it causes stroke.

What will be the impact of these findings on practice? The risk of cerebral bleeding in men who receive both warfarin and aspirin is worrisome. Asking a basically healthy population to take a small, but possibly disabling or even fatal, risk to achieve a benefit that will be realized in the future, is a questionable proposition. The evidence now shows that low-intensity anticoagulation with warfarin alone prevents a first heart attack. However, warfarin seems no more effective than aspirin, and the use of warfarin is complicated by the need to monitor blood coagulation. Therefore, low intensity anticoagulation is unlikely to find adherents, except for prevention in patients who do not tolerate aspirin. Hence, the most important clinical finding of the Thrombosis Prevention Trial is an affirmation of the beneficial role of low-dose aspirin to prevent a first MI in high-risk men.

Long-Term Oral Anticoagulant Therapy for Acute Coronary Syndromes. Patients with acute coronary syndromes—unstable angina and/or non-Q wave myocardial infarction (MI)—have high rates of recurrent ischemic events despite treatment with aspirin. The addition of long-term warfarin therapy may reduce this risk. The effects of warfarin, at two intensities of anticoagulation, in patients with acute coronary syndromes are described in a recent report [*Circulation* 1998;98:1064–70]. In the first phase of the study, 309 patients were randomized to receive a fixed low-dose—3 mg daily—of warfarin for six months or standard therapy. The fixed-dose strategy resulted in a modestly elevated mean INR of 1.5. Eighty-seven percent of patients in both groups received aspirin. In the second phase, the protocol was modified so that 97 patients were allocated to receive standard therapy or warfarin at a dose adjusted to produce an INR of 2.3. Eighty-five percent of patients in both groups received aspirin.

In the first phase, outcomes were worse in those treated with low-intensity warfarin than in those receiving standard therapy. Although differences did not reach statistical significance, low-dose warfarin seemed to worsen the situation and increase the risk of bleeding. In phase two, however, the rates of cardiovascular death, new MI, and refractory angina at three months were 5.1% in the adjusted-dose warfarin group and 12.1% in the standard group. The rates of all death, new MI, and stroke were 5.1% in the warfarin group and 13.1% in the standard therapy group. Significantly fewer patients were hospitalized for unstable angina in the warfarin group, 7.1%, than in the control group, 17.2%. There was a significant excess of minor but not major bleeds in the warfarin group compared with the control group—28.6% vs. 12.1%.

The authors conclude that for patients with acute coronary syndromes, "Long-term therapy with moderate-intensity warfarin (INR, 2.0 to 2.5) plus aspirin but not low-intensity warfarin (INR, 1.5) plus aspirin appears to reduce the rate of recurrent ischemic event. . . ."

Computer-Guided Dosing of Warfarin Outperforms Traditional Dosing. As a result of a worldwide increase in the use of oral anticoagulant treatment, the responsibility for dosing has devolved to health care professionals with little specific training in the management of anticoagulation. A possible way of maintaining the current standards for safety and efficacy in specialty clinics is by computerization of anticoagulant dosing. To this end, investigators compared the performance of computer-based anticoagulant dosing with traditional dosing guided by experienced medical staff [*Lancet* 1998;352:1505–09].

The program [DAWN AC anticoagulant therapy management system (version 407)] has two main modules—the induction module for starting warfarin therapy over the first four days to reach a dose within 1 mg of the eventual maintenance dose, and the maintenance module for fine-tuning the dose to the therapeutic range and sustaining it.

Investigators randomized 258 patients to a computer-generated dose group or a traditional dose group. The principal endpoint was time spent in the therapeutic anticoagulation range, as measured by the INR. The results were encouraging. The proportion of dose changes was lower in the computer dose group than in the traditional dose group and there were fewer INR values outside the therapeutic range. The authors conclude that the computer program gave better INR control than the experienced medical staff, but clinical outcome and cost effectiveness remain to be evaluated.

Ticlopidine (Ticlid) Effective for Angioplasty but Adverse Effects Limit Use. Both ticlopidine (*Ticlid*) and the recently approved clopidogrel (*Plavix*) inhibit ADP-induced human fibrinogen binding to the glycoprotein IIb/IIIa platelet receptor. They thereby interfere with platelet-to-platelet interaction and platelet aggregation, and result in reduced formation of thrombi. *Ticlid* is probably as effective as aspirin in a wide range of indications and possibly more effective in the treatment of stroke and transient ischemic episodes [*N Engl J Med* 1989;321:501–07] but it has more serious side effects than aspirin and costs much more.

Recent reports focus on the use of ticlopidine to prevent complications following angioplasty and stent implantation. One study documents a clear superiority of the combination of ticlopidine and aspirin over oral anticoagulant plus aspirin to prevent death, acute MI, and the need for urgent revascularization over a 30-day period following the procedure [*N Engl J Med* 1996;334:1084–89]. Another study shows that the antiplatelet activity of ticlopidine plus aspirin in patients with coronary artery disease following successful coronary stent placement is significantly better than the antiplatelet activity of aspirin alone [*J Am Coll Cardiol* 1997;29:1515–19]. A more recent report indicates that the combination of ticlopidine and aspirin inhibits platelet activity more effectively than either drug alone [*Circulation* 1998;97:1046–52]. Data from a small clinical trial suggest that the combination reduces stent-thrombosis rate and MI to a greater extent than does aspirin alone [*Circulation* 1996;93:215–22].

Unfortunately, *Ticlid* has an unfavorable side effect profile. The most serious complication is neutropenia, which occurs in about one patient in forty. While generally reversible, ticlopidine-related neutropenia can be severe and life-threatening. Blood counts are needed every two weeks for the first three months of treatment. Cardiologists usually prescribe the drug for no more than four weeks but long-term use is not unusual for stroke prevention.

Further complicating the use of ticlopidine is a recent report of 60 cases of thrombotic thrombocytopenic purpura (TTP) in patients taking the drug. TTP is a life-threatening condition thought to be a rare side effect of ticlopidine [*Ann Intern Med* 1998;128;128:541–44]. About one-third of the cases cited in the report did not recover. Plasmapheresis reduced mortality by 50%. The authors say that TTP is underdiagnosed and undertreated. Moreover, compliance with monitoring guidelines may not aid early detection of TTP because most patients' platelet counts are within normal limits shortly before onset. The authors call for labeling changes and a "Dear Doctor" letter to alert physicians to this unrecognized problem. Clopidogrel (*Plavix)* has been suggested as a replacement for *Ticlid* because it does not pose the risk of neutropenia and, so far, there are no reports of TTP resulting from clopidogrel therapy.

Abciximab (ReoPro) Shines in Angioplasty Trial. Centocor/Lilly's antiplatelet monoclonal antibody abciximab (*ReoPro*) was the first glycoprotein IIb/

IIIa receptor inhibitor to receive approval from the FDA to prevent complications (e.g., restenosis of the treated artery) following coronary angioplasty. Initially, the approved use was limited to high-risk patients because of concerns about excess bleeding. Some time later, investigators determined that by reducing the dose of co-administered heparin, abciximab was safe and effective for almost all patients undergoing a revascularization procedure.

The pivotal clinical trials supporting these indications were carried out before stent usage became common in patients undergoing revascularization. Stents are small metal scaffolds that prop open arteries. Today, stents are used in up to 70% of patients undergoing revascularization in the US. Worldwide, coronary stenting along with administration of heparin, aspirin, and ticlopidine or clopidogrel to prevent the formation of thrombi, is performed in more than 500,000 patients each year.

Trials show that stenting is superior to balloon angioplasty because it reduces the need for additional revascularization procedures. Some cardiologists even suggested that the effectiveness of stents might eliminate the need for abciximab. However, a presentation at the March American College of Cardiology meeting demonstrated that *ReoPro* is effective for patients with ischemic heart disease undergoing coronary stenting [*Scrip*, No 2322, April 1, 1998, p 22].

The EPISTENT trial involved 63 hospitals in the US and Canada. The investigators randomized 2400 patients with ischemic heart disease who needed coronary revascularization to one of three groups—stenting plus placebo, stenting plus abciximab, or balloon angioplasty plus abciximab. The composite primary endpoint—death, heart attack, or urgent revascularization at 30 days—occurred in 10.8% of those receiving stent plus placebo, 6.9% of the patients assigned to angioplasty plus abciximab, and 5.3% of those randomized to stent plus abciximab [*Lancet* 1998;352:87–92]. Most of the observed benefit in the trial resulted from reduction in heart attacks during or soon after the revascularization procedure. Among the 600 women in the study, 11.7% of those in the stent-placebo group had a heart attack or died within 24 hours after the procedure, compared with 8.7% in the stent-abciximab group, and 5.1% in the angioplasty-abciximab group. The comparable outcomes in men were 10.5%, 4.2%, and 7.6%, respectively. Stents may be less effective in women than in men because women have smaller arteries and commercially available stents may be too large.

According to a report presented at the August meeting of the European Society of Cardiology, the combination of a stent and abciximab, compared with stents alone, decreased the incidence of the composite primary endpoint from 11.4% to 5.6% six months after randomization. Incidence in the balloon angioplasty plus abciximab group was 7.8%. The six-month results were especially striking in patients with diabetes, who made up about 20% of all patients undergoing coronary revascularization. Among these patients, the composite primary endpoint occurred in 13% of patients given a stent and abciximab, 25.2% in the stent alone group, and 23.4% assigned to angioplasty plus abciximab. The data indicate that the combination of a stent and abciximab eliminates the excess risk of restenosis among patients with diabetes compared with patients who do not have diabetes. The overall findings suggest that for every 1000 patients treated with a stent and abciximab, 7 deaths, 51 heart attacks, and 10 urgent revascularizations can be prevented [*Lancet* 1998;352:711].

The researchers conclude that blocking platelet glycoprotein-IIb/IIIa with abciximab substantially improves the safety of coronary stenting procedures. *ReoPro* prevents complications of revascularization procedures whether or not stenting is used. Indeed, balloon angioplasty with abciximab seems safer than stenting without abciximab. The results are likely to increase the use of *ReoPro,* but universal use is constrained by the cost of the drug. A careful cost-effectiveness analysis may overcome that problem. Centocor and Eli Lilly hope to extend sales of *ReoPro* still further by seeking new indications, such as unstable angina, stroke, and use with a thrombolytic agent for patients with emergent MI.

Hirudin and Enoxaparin Show Benefit in Unstable Angina. Unstable angina is the result of a rupture of an atherosclerotic plaque in the artery wall with formation of a clot restricting blood flow to the heart. It is the most common reason for admission to coronary care units. The clot only partially or intermittently blocks the artery, but the patient is placed at high risk of having a heart attack if the clot completely blocks the artery. There are two targets for the treatment of unstable angina—thrombin and platelets. Today, standard therapy is the antithrombin agent heparin and the antiplatelet drug aspirin. Newly introduced gpIIb/IIIa inhibitors, however, are more potent antiplatelet agents than aspirin. Low molecular weight heparins (LMWHs), such as enoxaparin (*Lovenox*), and direct acting antithrombin agents, such as hirudin, may have advantages over unfractionated heparin. LMWHs, unlike unfractionated heparin, do not need regular monitoring of clotting time and have the advantage of more convenient administration than heparin—subcutaneous injection rather than continuous intravenous infusion. Hirudin and related agents have the potential advantage of targeting clot-bound thrombin as well as circulating thrombin.

Two recent trials show the advantages of newer therapies over standard therapy [*Scrip*, September 2, 1998, p 22]. The findings were presented at the European Society of Cardiology Meeting in August. Both the OASIS-2 trial with hirudin and the TIMI-11b trial with enoxaparin demonstrated small benefits of the study drugs compared with heparin in patients with acute coronary syndromes (i.e., unstable angina/non-Q wave MI). A third study, FRAXIS, however, with another LMWH, nadroparin (*Fraxiparine*), showed no benefit in a similar population.

The OASIS-2 results show that for every 1000 patients treated, the use of hirudin instead of heparin will at day seven prevent 14 cardiovascular events, including death, acute MI and refractory ischemia, at the cost of two blood transfusions. Whether there is a significantly different outcome between hirudin and heparin at 30 days after treatment is not known. The results of the TIMI-11b study show that for every 1000 patients treated, the use of enoxaparin instead of heparin will prevent 24 events at day 14 after treatment. In the FRAXIS trial, which compared nadroparin with heparin, the primary endpoint was not significantly different between groups at 6 days, 14 days, or 3 months.

The reports provoked a great deal of confusion. An earlier report with a slightly different form of hirudin had results similar to those reported from OASIS-2. At that time, the additional benefits were considered trivial in light of the cost of hirudin, and the manufacturer abandoned efforts to develop the drug. Now, Hoechst Marion Roussel concludes that the results of OASIS-2 with their form of hirudin are strongly positive and says it would definitely apply for approval for this indication. Participants at the meeting also pondered why one LMWH shows benefits while others have not, and how physicians would choose among hirudin, LMWHs, and the gpIIb/IIIa inhibitors. According to leading cardiologists in Europe, the gpIIb/IIIa inhibitors are currently recommended in combination with heparin. Hirudin and LMWHs are both viewed as alternatives to heparin.

Addition of Enoxaparin Prevents Venous Thromboembolism after Surgery.
Deep vein thrombosis (DVT), which may lead to pulmonary embolism, is a life-threatening complication that develops in about one in four untreated patients undergoing elective neurosurgery. To reduce the prevalence of this

complication, surgeons have favored compression stockings over anticoagulants because of concern about intracranial bleeding. Now, investigators have compared the use of compression stockings alone with the use of compression stockings plus the administration of the low molecular weight heparin enoxaparin (*Lovenex*) for the prevention of DVT when applied within 24 hours after the surgical procedure [*N Engl J Med* 1998;339:80–85]. In their study, enoxaparin, 40 mg once daily, or placebo was given subcutaneously for not less than seven days.

The investigators found that DVT developed in 32% of those who used stockings, but in only 17% of those who wore stockings and received enoxaparin. The rates of proximal DVT were 13% for patients receiving placebo and 5% for patients receiving enoxaparin. The rate of intracranial bleeding was about 3% in each group. The investigators conclude that enoxaparin combined with compression stockings is more effective than compression stockings alone for prevention of venous thromboembolism after elective neurosurgery and does not cause excessive bleeding.

Limited Role for Drugs in Cardiac Arrest. The results of two clinical studies presented at the American College of Cardiology meeting in March 1998, show once more that defibrillators are preferable to drug therapy for the prevention of sudden death in patients with lethal arrhythmias [*Scrip*, No 2325, April 10, 1998, p 19]. The CASH trial compared amiodarone (*Cordarone*), metoprolol, and propafenone (*Rythmol*) with an implantable defibrillator in 300 patients resuscitated from sudden cardiac death. The propafenone arm was stopped early because of increased mortality compared with the defibrillator arm (30% vs. 11%). After 24 months, mortality in the remaining drug arms was about 20% compared with 12% in the defibrillator group.

The CIDS trial compared an implantable defibrillator with amiodarone in 650 patients who recovered from cardiac arrest or a life-threatening episode of sustained ventricular tachycardia. The results show a 20% reduction in death in the defibrillator group compared with the amiodarone group after a mean follow-up of three years. One expert observed that amiodarone may still be appropriate for patients who continue to have tachycardia despite having received a defibrillator. Amiodarone may also reduce the occurrence of atrial fibrillation after cardiac by-pass surgery.

Lower Limit of LDL-Cholesterol Reduction Unresolved. HMG CoA reductase inhibitors (statins) lower blood levels of low-density lipoprotein (LDL) cholesterol and reduce the risk of heart attacks. To what level LDL-cholesterol should be lowered, however, is the subject of debate. Some cardiologists think that the goal should be a level below 100 mg/dl, a target that is difficult to achieve with a single drug. Three reports in a recent issue of *Circulation* confirm the correlation between reduction of LDL-cholesterol and risk reduction, but differ in their conclusions on whether it is worthwhile to reduce LDL-cholesterol values from low to very low.

In the Cholesterol and Recurrent Events (CARE) trial, more than 4,000 patients who had had a heart attack received pravastatin (*Pravachol*) or placebo. At baseline, participants' LDL-cholesterol levels ranged from 115 to 174 mg/dl and total cholesterol levels were elevated but less than 240 mg/dl. Pravastatin reduced the combined end point of coronary death or recurrent MI by 24%. The LDL-cholesterol concentrations achieved during treatment were a significant predictor of the coronary event rate, whereas the extent of their reduction was not. The coronary event rate declined as LDL-cholesterol decreased from 174 to 125 mg/dl, but no further decline was seen in the LDL-cholesterol range from 125 to 71 mg/dl. The authors conclude that physicians should use statins to reduce LDL-cholesterol to a low level (125 mg/dl) in as many at-risk patients as possible rather than trying to drive LDL-cholesterol to a very low level (less than 100 mg/dl) which may require multiple drugs and high doses [*Circulation* 1998;97: 1446–52].

The second paper reports a new analysis from 4S, the Scandinavian Simvastatin Survival Study. The placebo-controlled trial enrolled nearly 4,500 patients with coronary heart disease (CHD) and total cholesterol levels ranging from 213 to 310 mg/dL. Simvastatin (*Zocor*) reduced coronary events by 34%, but there was no total or LDL-cholesterol threshold value below which there was no further risk reduction. The investigators estimate that for each additional 1% reduction in LDL-cholesterol, the risk of a major coronary event decreases by 1.7% [*Circulation* 1998;97:1453–60].

The third report presents results from WOSCOPS, the West of Scotland Coronary Prevention Study. WOSCOPS examined the use of a statin for primary prevention of CHD. Subjects with LDL-cholesterol values of at least 155 mg/dl but less than 232 mg/dl and at high risk for CHD received pravastatin or placebo. The rate of coronary morbidity or mortality was substantially reduced in those taking pravastatin. However, the average LDL-cholesterol value during treatment was reduced to only 137 mg/dl, which left unresolved the threshold question [*Circulation* 1998;97:1440–45]. Trials are underway to specifically address the issue of lower limits, but the results will not be available for several years.

Simvastatin versus Atorvastatin. There is now evidence that Merck's *Zocor* (simvastatin) increases levels of high-density lipoprotein (HDL) cholesterol more effectively than a competing product, Warner-Lambert/ Pfizer's *Lipitor* (atorvastatin) [*Scrip,* September 11, 1998]. *Lipitor* has rapidly gained market share because of its potency in reducing low-density lipoprotein (LDL) cholesterol. Patients with heart disease who take simvastatin usually require titration up to higher-than-usual doses to achieve very low LDL-cholesterol levels. Such levels can usually be reached on the lowest dose of atorvastatin. Therefore, patients taking *Lipitor* (atorvastatin) can make a single visit to their physician and do not require dosage adjustments. *Lipitor* is also the drug of choice for people with very high triglyceride levels.

As virtually everyone knows, HDL-cholesterol is thought to be protective. In the past, some have speculated that for women with dyslipidemia, increasing HDL-cholesterol may be more beneficial in the long run than lowering LDL-cholesterol. Differing effects of simvastatin and atorvastatin on HDL-cholesterol levels have been shown in two studies. The first—the CURVES study—was supported by Warner-Lambert and published in March 1998 in the *Journal of the American College of Cardiology* [1998;81:582–87]. This study compared the effects of five different statins and showed the superiority of atorvastatin over the other agents to lower LDL-cholesterol. Effects on HDL-cholesterol were not different among the agents, except for simvastatin 40 mg, which produced a greater increase in HDL-cholesterol than did atorvastatin at the same dose.

In a more recent, yet unpublished, study, investigators supported by Merck randomized 842 patients with dyslipidemia to four different groups—40 mg or 80 mg simvastatin, or 20 mg or 40 mg atorvastatin. Simvastatin 40 mg and atorvastatin 20 mg worked about equally well to lower LDL-cholesterol and triglycerides. Simvastatin 80 mg and atorvastatin 40 mg were also comparable in this regard. Each dose of simvastatin, however, was more effective than either dose of atorvastatin in increasing the levels of HDL-cholesterol. Differences in efficacy were particularly notable in patients with low levels of HDL-cholesterol at baseline—less than 35 mg/dl. Simvastatin 80 mg increased HDL-cholesterol by 17% compared with an increase of 6.6% for atorvastatin 40 mg. It will be interesting to see how Merck uses the new information to promote *Zocor.*

Primary Prevention of Acute Coronary Events with a Statin. HMG-CoA reductase inhibitors (statins) reduce the incidence of fatal and nonfatal events in patients with coronary artery disease (CAD) and high levels of LDL-cholesterol as well as in patients with CAD and average levels of LDL-cholesterol. These agents also benefit patients who have never had a heart attack, but are at risk because of their elevated levels of LDL-cholesterol and other factors. A new study, AFCAPS/TexCAPS, extends these finding to men and women who not only have no evidence of vascular disease, but also have average LDL-cholesterol levels [*JAMA* 1998;279:1615–22]. The participants were at higher risk for CAD than the general population, but mainly because of low levels of HDL-cholesterol. Nevertheless, most of the subjects in this study were not eligible for drug treatment according to current National Cholesterol Education Program guidelines.

The investigators randomized 5068 men and 997 women. Their mean baseline level of total cholesterol was 221 mg/dl, their mean LDL-cholesterol level was 150 mg/dl, and their mean HDL-cholesterol level was 36 mg/dl for men and 40 mg/dl for women. Their HDL-cholesterol levels placed the men and women participants in the 25th and 16th percentiles, respectively. The men ranged in age from 45 to 73 years, and the women from 55 to 73 years. Each patient received either lovastatin or placebo. The major measured outcome was the first acute major coronary event defined as fatal or nonfatal heart attack, unstable angina, or sudden cardiac death.

After an average of 5.2 years, lovastatin reduced LDL-cholesterol level by 25%, the incidence of the composite end point by 37%, the incidence of acute MI by 40%, the incidence of unstable angina events by 32%, and the need for a revascularization procedure by 33%. These findings support the inclusion of HDL-cholesterol in risk-factor assessment for CAD. Survey data suggest that approximately eight million Americans without documented cardiovascular disease meet the age and lipid criteria of AFCAPS/TexCAPS

There is now substantial evidence to suggest that the benefits of statins are not entirely the result of lipid lowering. Clinical trials of these agents show that baseline or treated levels of LDL-cholesterol are only weakly associated with cardiovascular events. Statins may also modify endothelial function, inflammatory response, plaque stability, and thrombus formation. These properties of statins may help to explain the early and significant reduction in cardiovascular events reported in clinical trials of statin therapy [*JAMA* 1998;279:1643–50].

Pravastatin Prevents Morbidity and Mortality in All Patients with Coronary Heart Disease. Most patients with CHD have cholesterol levels that are not markedly elevated. Most controlled trials of cholesterol-lowering therapy, however, have enrolled patients with at least moderate hypercholesterolemia. The Long-Term Intervention with Pravastatin in Ischaemic Disease (LIPID) trial was initiated about ten years ago. The aim was to investigate the effects of lowering cholesterol with pravastatin (*Pravachol*) on death from CHD among patients with a history of MI or unstable angina and a broad range of initial cholesterol levels (155 to 271 mg/dl).

In the double-blind, randomized study, about 9000 patients who were 31 to 75 years old received pravastatin (40 mg daily) or placebo over a mean follow-up period of about six years. Study participants were representative of those patients seen in current medical practice.

Death from CHD occurred in 8.3% of the patients in the placebo group and 6.4% of those in the pravastatin group. This a relative risk (RR) reduction of 24%. Overall mortality was 14.1% in the placebo group and 11.0% in the pravastatin group (RR reduction 22%). The incidence of each cardiovascular outcome—MI, death from CHD or nonfatal MI, stroke, and coronary revascularization—was consistently lower among patients assigned to receive pravastatin.

The investigators estimated that 30 deaths, 28 nonfatal MIs, and 9 nonfatal strokes were avoided for every 1000 patients treated with pravastatin. Twenty-three coronary artery bypass graft procedures, 20 coronary angioplasty procedures, and 82 hospital admissions for unstable angina were also avoided per 1000 study patients treated.

During the course of the LIPID trial, the results of two other large-scale, secondary prevention studies of HMG-CoA reductase inhibitors were reported–the Scandinavian Simvastatin Survival Study (4S) and the Cholesterol Recurrent Events (CARE) trial. The 4S [*Lancet* 1994; 344:1383–89] demonstrated that simvastatin significantly reduced mortality from CHD and overall mortality in patients with cholesterol levels of 213 to 309 mg/dl. Mean baseline cholesterol level in the LIPID trial was 44 mg/dl lower than in the 4S (217 compared with 261 mg/dl). Another difference is that far more people had undergone coronary revascularization in the LIPID trial (41%) than in the 4S (8%).

The CARE trial [*N Engl J Med* 1996;335:1001–09], which enrolled patients with cholesterol levels below 240 mg/dl (similar to levels in patients enrolled in the LIPID trial), showed that pravastatin significantly reduced the occurrence of a composite outcome of death due to CHD and nonfatal MI. The LIPID trial extended the findings of the CARE study by providing evidence of benefit in terms of both mortality from CHD and total mortality.

The LIPID investigators say that because of these findings, cholesterol-lowering therapy should be considered for virtually all patients presenting with CHD. They argue that the current low rate of cholesterol-lowering therapy among patients with CHD is no longer acceptable.

A subset analysis derived from the CARE trial focused on a group at very high risk of experiencing another heart attack—patients 65 to 75 years old with MI and average cholesterol levels [*Ann Intern Med* 1998;129:681–89]. The participants had total cholesterol levels less than 240 mg/dl and LDL-cholesterol levels ranging from 115 to 174 mg/dl. Over five years, major coronary events occurred in 28% of patients receiving placebo and 20% of patients assigned to pravastatin. Coronary death occurred in 10.3% of patients given placebo and 5.8% of those taking pravastatin. Pravastatin also significantly reduced the incidence stroke.

The investigators estimated that 11 older patients must be treated for five years to prevent a major coronary event and 22 to prevent a coronary death. They also observe: "For every 1000 older patients treated, 225 cardiovascular hospitalizations would be prevented compared with 121 hospitalizations in 1000 younger patients." The potential for benefit in older patients is substantial.

Atorvastatin (Lipitor) May Reduce Need for Coronary Revascularization. In less than two years on the US market, atorvastatin (*Lipitor*) has become America's most frequently prescribed cholesterol-lowering agent. However, unlike the case for its competitors, pravastatin and simvastatin, there has been little evidence of the clinical benefits of atorvastatin. Nevertheless, physicians prescribe atorvastatin because of its profound ability to lower cholesterol, its ability to reduce elevated levels of triglyceride, and the belief that all HMG-CoA reductase inhibitors (statins) provide the same benefits.

At the annual scientific meeting of the American Heart Association in November 1998, investigators reported the results of an important study that sought to determine whether aggressive lipid lowering therapy reduces the need for coronary revascularization procedures [*The Wall Street Journal*, November 12, 1998, B6]. They randomized 341 patients who had mild symptoms and stenoses in just one or two arteries to high doses of atorvastatin or to coronary angioplasty. The group receiving drug therapy had a decrease in LDL-cholesterol of 63 mg/dl, from 140 mg/dl before treatment to 77 mg/dl. Over the next 18 months, 13% of those treated with atorvastatin had a coronary event, compared with 21% of those undergoing angioplasty.

Although mean anginal pain relief was greater for those assigned to mechanical revascularization, more of them required hospitalization because of an ischemic episode or needed to undergo another angioplasty procedure.

The study was not large enough nor were the participants at sufficient risk to demonstrate a reduction in death or heart attacks. Atorvastatin's benefit derived largely from reduced hospital admissions for severe chest pain. Some experts think that in the future the first signs of angina may be treated with aggressive lipid-lowering therapy rather than coronary angioplasty.

ACE Inhibitors for Heart Failure: Dosing Issues. The key role of ACE inhibitors in the treatment of heart failure is well established. Some argue that in the absence of a compelling contraindication, physicians should prescribe them to all patients with left ventricular dysfunction, whether they are symptomatic or not. Given this recommendation, only 30–40% of eligible patients receive these drugs. Physicians may avoid ACE inhibitors for patients with mildly impaired renal function or low blood pressure or discontinue therapy after an asymptomatic decline in blood pressure or renal function. Evidence suggests that many of these patients can safely use and benefit from ACE inhibitors when careful dose titration and monitoring are provided.

Another issue of concern to cardiologists is that ACE inhibitors are often prescribed in doses lower than those found to be beneficial in clinical trials. Some physicians assume that the dose-response curve is flat beyond low doses and higher doses only lead to more side effects with little benefit. Data suggest, however, that while the dose-response curve for symptomatic improvement is indeed rather flat, increases in dose decrease mortality. Some physicians also believe that they can judge ACE inhibitors' effects on survival by evaluating drug effects on symptoms. The mechanisms underlying symptomatic improvement and mortality reduction, however, may be different. Symptomatic improvement may not reflect the mortality benefit.

The results of a large clinical trial—the ATLAS Study—presented at the annual meeting of the American College of Cardiology may resolve the dosing debate. The study enrolled more than 3,000 patients with moderate to severe heart failure and compared low-dose lisinopril (2.5 to 5 mg daily) with high doses (32.5 to 35 mg daily). The investigators report a trend toward improved survival for patients receiving the higher doses—on average they lived three months longer. High doses of lisinopril, compared to low doses, significantly decreased the combined end point of all-cause mortality and hospitalization as well as the combined end point of cardiovascular mortality and hospitalization. Although the high doses marginally increase the risk of side effects—hypotension and worsening renal function—they were, on average, pretty well tolerated. These findings support the idea that the effect of ACE inhibitors on survival is related to dose and should prompt a reconsideration of prescribing patterns [*Prescriber's Letter* 1998;5:26–27].

Spironolactone (Aldactone) Benefits Patients with Heart Failure. Those attending the American Heart Association meeting in November learned that a placebo-controlled trial of Searle's *Aldactone* (spironolactone)—RALES—was stopped early because of a significant reduction in mortality. More than 1,600 patients had received treatment for up to 3.5 years at the time the study was terminated [*Scrip*, September 9, 1998, p 29].

Spironolactone has been available as a potassium-sparing diuretic for many years. It produces only mild diuresis and, for that reason, is not ordinarily given to patients with heart failure. Cardiologists favor loop diuretics such as furosemide. The aldosterone-antagonist action of spironolactone, however, has stimulated new interest in its possible application for heart failure. Recent work has shown that aldosterone does more than regulate sodium and potassium homeostasis in the kidneys. It also acts on other tissue, particularly the heart, where some think aldosterone potentiates fibrosis. The report in *Scrip* notes that aldosterone levels are increased in heart failure and are predictive of mortality. ACE inhibitors suppress the hormone but seem to lose their effect over time and aldosterone levels begin to rise. At this point patients may benefit from an effective, direct antagonist.

Spironolactone is burdened with poor specificity and serious side effects. A new generation of selective aldosterone receptor antagonists is now in development with the hope of increasing anti-aldosterone activity and doing away with harmful effects.

Bisoprolol: A β-Blocker for Heart Failure. For many years, β-blockers were contraindicated for patients with heart failure because of their negative inotropic effects. The pendulum, however, is swinging in the other direction. The FDA has approved carvedilol (*Coreg*), a nonselective β-blocker, to be used with other drugs for the treatment of heart failure. Now, according to the final results of the placebo-controlled CIBIS-2 trial, presented at the European Cardiology Meeting in August, another β-blocker, bisoprolol (*Zebeta*), is showing promise [*Scrip*, August 28, 1998, p 15]. Unlike carvedilol, bisoprolol acts only at the β-1 receptor and has no effect on α-receptors.

CIBIS-2 enrolled 2647 ambulatory patients with chronic heart failure. Patients had a left ventricular ejection fraction of less than 35% and were receiving a diuretic and an ACE inhibitor. Mean follow-up was only 1.4 years because a mortality reduction in favor of bisoprolol, gleaned from an interim analysis, prompted the investigators to stop the study. CIBIS-2 is the first clinical trial of β-blocker treatment in patients with congestive heart failure to have the power to detect a benefit on mortality.

The interim analysis showed that bisoprolol significantly reduced overall mortality when compared with placebo. Mortality rates were 11.8% and 17.3%, respectively. The main effect was on sudden death. According to the findings, treatment of 100 patients with bisoprolol for one year would save four lives. Hospital admission rates were also significantly lower in the bisoprolol group than in the placebo group—33.6% vs. 39.8%. CIBIS-2 provides the most convincing evidence to date to support the use of β-blockers in heart failure. The lead investigator said that all patients with symptomatic heart failure should now receive a β-blocker in addition to an ACE inhibitor and a diuretic. One expert, however, urges caution. "Prescribing β-blockers must follow the start low, go slow principle." The findings of CIBIS-2 raise yet another thorny issue. Are placebo-controlled trials of β-blockers in heart failure still ethical? [*Lancet* 1998;352:793].

New Studies May Change Treatment Guidelines for Hypertension. Investigators at a meeting of the International Society for Hypertension presented the results of two important studies addressing the question: What is the most effective way to help patients manage high blood pressure? The HOT study [*Lancet* 1998;351:1755–62] shows that aggressive treatment of elevated blood pressure significantly reduces their chance of a heart attack. The CAPP study demonstrates that ACE inhibitors are at least as effective as treatment with diuretics and β-blockers in reducing deaths, heart attacks, and strokes among people with hypertension [*Scrip,* June 17, 1998, p 24–25].

The American Heart Association estimates that more than 50 million Americans have high blood pressure, a leading risk factor for stroke and coronary heart disease [*The Wall Street Journal,* June 10, 1998, p B2]. The pharmaceutical industry markets diuretics, β-blockers, calcium channel blockers, ACE inhibitors, and angiotensin II receptor inhibitors for the treatment of hypertension. The drugs in each of these five classes reduce blood pressure, but few studies have documented that specific treatments reduce serious complications of hypertension or mortality.

The multicenter HOT trial randomized 17,790 patients with hypertension (diastolic blood pressure between 100 and 115 mm Hg) to one of three treatment goals—target diastolic blood pressures of less than or equal to 90 mm Hg, less than or equal to 85 mm Hg, and less than or equal to 80 mm Hg. Felodipine (*Plendil*), a long-acting calcium antagonist, was selected as initial therapy, with the successive addition of an ACE inhibitor, β-blocker, and diuretic, if needed, to achieve treatment goal. In addition, half the patients were randomly assigned to 75 mg aspirin per day while the other half received placebo. Average blood pressure at baseline was 170/105 mm Hg.

After six years of treatment, 92% of the patients had diastolic pressures of less than 90 mm Hg. The investigators confirmed that the lower the treatment target, the greater was the fall in diastolic pressure. Diastolic pressures were reduced by 22 mg Hg, 24 mm Hg, and 26 mm Hg, respectively, in the three target groups. The lowest incidence of major cardiovascular events occurred at a mean achieved diastolic blood pressure of 82.6 mm Hg; the lowest risk of cardiovascular mortality occurred at 86.5 mm Hg. Pushing blood pressure still lower had no additional benefit, but caused no harm. In patients with diabetes, there was a 51% reduction in major cardiovascular events in the 80 mm Hg or less group compared with the 90 mm Hg or less group. Aspirin reduced major cardiovascular events by 15% and fatal or nonfatal MIs by 36%, but increased nonfatal major bleeds.

The number of heart attacks for the roughly six thousand patients in each group was 84 in those with a treatment target of 90 mm Hg or less, 64 in those with a target of 85 mm Hg or less, and 61 in those with a target of 80 mm Hg or less. There were too few deaths among patients over the course of the study to determine whether lower blood pressure improved survival.

The CAPP trial, which compared captopril (*Captopen*) with either a diuretic or β-blocker in 11,000 patients with hypertension, concluded that ACE inhibitors should join diuretics and β-blockers as first-line agents for high blood pressure treatment. Diuretics and β-blockers were the only classes of antihypertensive drugs that had been proven to reduce cardiovascular events in the general hypertensive population.

After six years of follow-up, the CAPP investigators found there was no difference in the primary endpoint—stroke, acute MI, or cardiovascular death—between the two groups. Captopril had a better effect than the diuretic or β-blocker in 575 patients with diabetes, significantly reducing the primary endpoint by 41%. This outcome was driven primarily by a 66% reduction in acute MI. Many physicians already use ACE inhibitors as the first-choice antihypertensive agent in diabetes because they are thought to preserve renal function.

Selecting the Right Antihypertensive Agent. Which one of the array of agents available for the treatment of hypertension is best for the patient? In the general population, about 90% of patients with an elevated diastolic blood pressure (DBP) have stage 1 (DBP 90 to 99 mm Hg) or stage 2 (DBP 100 to 109 mm Hg) hypertension. These patients are the most likely to benefit from single-drug therapy. The several antihypertensive drug classes, however, elicit widely varying blood pressure responses among equally hypertensive people.

There is evidence that the estimation of renin level is useful to evaluate the pathophysiology of hypertension and to plan treatment. An algorithm developed using this information suggests that diuretic therapy would be most effective in low-renin hypertension and least effective when renin levels are high. On the other hand, ACE inhibitors and β-blockers are expected to be effective in patients with high renin levels and less effective in low-renin hypertension. This model, however, has never been tested.

Another strategy for selecting the "right" drug is by age-race subgroup. This approach is based on the results obtained in a 1300-patient trial on the efficacy of antihypertensive agents—the Department of Veterans Affairs Cooperative Study on Antihypertensive Agents.

Using the data from the Veterans Affairs Cooperative Study, researchers have recently reported the result of a study initiated to determine whether renin profiles or age-race subgroups best identify the antihypertensive agent most likely to be effective monotherapy [*JAMA* 1998;280:1168–72].

The investigators focused on 1105 ambulatory patients with entry diastolic blood pressure of 95 to 109 mm Hg. The patients were randomized to hydrochlorothiazide, atenolol, captopril, clonidine, sustained-release diltiazem, or prazosin. The main outcome measure was efficacy determined by the percentage of patients achieving goal diastolic blood pressure (<90 mm Hg) in response to a single drug selected using patients' renin profile or age-race subgroup.

The researchers found that clonidine and diltiazem had consistent response rates regardless of renin profile. Hydrochlorothiazide and prazosin were best in low- and medium-renin profiles; captopril and atenolol were best in medium- and high-renin profiles. Response rates by age-race subgroup ranged in younger black men from 70% for hydrochlorothiazide to 90% for prazosin, in older black men from 50% for captopril to 97% for diltiazem, in younger white men from 70% for hydrochlorothiazide to 92% for atenolol, and in older white men from 84% for hydrochlorothiazide to 95% for diltiazem.

Patients with a correct treatment for their renin profile but incorrect for age-race subgroup had a response rate of 59%; patients with an incorrect treatment for their renin profile but a correct one for age-race subgroup had a response rate of 63%. After controlling for diastolic blood pressure and other factors, age-profile significantly predicted response to single-drug therapy, whereas the predictive power of the renin profile was of borderline significance. Renin profile had no additional predictive benefit after age-race subgroup was considered. This cost-free method for the selection of an initial single drug for treatment of stage 1 and stage 2 hypertension is fully consistent with current national guidelines for the treatment of hypertension.

DIABETES

Troglitazone (*Rezulin*) in Patients with Type 2 Diabetes
 Mellitus
Multiple Benefits of ACE Inhibitors in Patients with Diabetes
Early, Intensive Insulin Therapy Preserves Islet Function in
 Type 1 Diabetics
Intensive Glucose Control for Type 2 Diabetes
Tight Control of Blood Pressure for Type 2 Diabetes
Improved Glucose Control with Glipizide Realizes Short-
 Term Benefits

Troglitazone in Patients with Type 2 Diabetes Mellitus. Troglitazone
(*Rezulin*) is the first agent in a new class of drugs called thiazolidinediones
to reach the US market. These agents work in a novel way. They reduce
blood glucose level by increasing insulin-mediated glucose disposal. Unlike
sulfonylureas (e.g., glyburide and glipizide), which increase pancreatic secretion of insulin, *Rezulin* does not cause hypoglycemia. Support for FDA
approval of *Rezulin* included the results of two well controlled clinical trials.

In one study, researchers recruited patients with poorly controlled type-
2 diabetes despite daily injections of insulin [*N Engl J Med* 1998;338:861–66].
At the start of the study patients had glycosylated hemoglobin values of 8% to
12%. Glycosylated hemoglobin (HbA_{1c}) is a marker for the average blood glucose level during the past month. Values of 4.3% to 6.1% are considered normal.

The patients were randomized to receive 200 or 600 mg *Rezulin* or
placebo daily for 26 weeks. Insulin doses were maintained or decreased when
necessary to prevent hypoglycemia. During the course of the study mean
glycosylated hemoglobin values decreased by 0.8% in those receiving the
lower dose of *Rezulin* and by 1.4% in those receiving the higher dose, despite
concurrent lowering of the insulin dose by 11% and 20%, respectively. Compared with baseline, no changes in glycosylated glucose or insulin occurred
in patients assigned to placebo.

The 1.4% absolute decline in glycosylated hemoglobin values in the
group given 600 mg of *Rezulin* represents a decline of about 15% from the
baseline values. In type-1 diabetics, a 15% decrease in glycosylated hemoglobin
leads to a 60% reduction in the risk of diabetic retinopathy progression.

In a second trial, 29 patients with type-2 diabetes discontinued their
medication and received either metformin (*Glucophage*) or *Rezulin* 400 mg

daily for three months, after which they received both drugs for another three months [*N Engl J Med* 1998;338:867–72]. Mean glycosylated hemoglobin at screening was about 9.5%. Fasting plasma glucose concentrations decreased by 20% during *Glucophage* therapy and to the same degree during monotherapy with *Rezulin*. Endogenous glucose production decreased by 19% during *Glucophage* therapy, whereas it was unchanged in those taking *Rezulin*. The mean rate of glucose disposal increased by 54% during therapy with *Rezulin* and 13% during therapy with *Glucophage*. In combination, *Rezulin* and *Glucophage* further lowered fasting glucose levels by 18% and mean glycosylated hemoglobin value by 1.4%.

The investigators conclude that *Glucophage* and *Rezulin* have equal and additive beneficial effects on glycemic control in patients with type-2 diabetes. The results also support the understanding that *Glucophage* acts primarily by decreasing endogenous glucose production and *Rezulin* by increasing the rate of peripheral glucose disposal.

Unfortunately, *Rezulin* can cause liver dysfunction, which in some cases has been fatal or required a liver transplant. A survey of North American clinical trials of *Rezulin* shows that 1.9% of patients receiving the drug had liver enzyme levels more than three times the upper limit of normal, compared with 0.6% of patients who received placebo. The changes were reversible in all the patients. Patients who are taking Rezulin need to have liver enzymes monitored frequently [*N Engl J Med* 1998;338:916–17].

Some experts think that *Rezulin* should be a first-line drug for patients with mild type-2 diabetes, especially obese patients with marked insulin resistance. *Rezulin* can be combined with other oral antidiabetic drugs for patients with more severe hyperglycemia. In light of the toxicity of *Rezulin*, however, its use should be limited to patients who can be evaluated frequently for signs of hepatic dysfunction [*N Engl J Med* 1998;338:908–09].

Multiple Benefits of ACE Inhibitors in Patients with Diabetes. About 30% to 40% of patients with diabetes mellitus develop clinical evidence of diabetic nephropathy. Renal function declines progressively and leads to end-stage renal failure. Hypertension is often a culprit and antihypertensive agents slow the decline. Recent studies show that ACE inhibitors, probably independent of their antihypertensive activity, decrease efferent arteriolar resistance and glomerular capillary pressure and are effective for treating nephropathy in diabetics. Investigators have demonstrated a benefit in both hypertensive and normotensive diabetics. Captopril and lisinopril are the most extensively studied agents. There is also evidence to support the suggestion that physicians consider the use of ACE inhibitors in all patients with hypertension and/or chronic renal insufficiency and significant proteinuria.

A recent study provides still another reason to consider an ACE inhibitor as part of the treatment of diabetes. A multinational trial has shown that lisinopril (*Zestril*) significantly decreases the progression of retinopathy in normotensive patients with type 1 diabetes [*Lancet* 1998;351:28-31]. More than 70% of patients with type 1 diabetes develop retinopathy after 20 years, and 10% become blind. Until now, treatment has been limited to good control of blood glucose.

Over a two-year period, retinopathy progressed by at least one grade on a standard scale in 13% of patients on lisinopril and 23% of patients on placebo. Lisinopril also reduced the risk of progression by two or more grades by nearly 70% and greatly reduced the risk of progression to proliferative retinopathy. The authors believe that physicians should consider an ACE inhibitor for all patients with type 1 diabetes who have some degree of retinopathy. Clinicians are cautiously optimistic that the results will apply to the far larger number of people with type 2 diabetes.

Cardiovascular disease is the leading cause of death among people with type 2 diabetes. Poorly controlled hypertension intensifies the problem. An increasing number of patients with diabetes and hypertension are receiving an ACE inhibitor. ACE inhibitors have been shown to increase survival after an acute MI and in patients with congestive heart failure. Many physicians, however, still rely on calcium channel blockers. They too are indicated for the treatment of a variety of cardiovascular diseases. Recently, however, concerns have been aroused about the safety of these drugs, particularly the short-acting dihydropyridine derivatives such as nifedipine.

Interim results of the first direct comparison of an ACE inhibitor and a calcium antagonist on cardiovascular outcomes in patients with type 2 diabetes and hypertension were reported recently [*N Engl J Med* 1998;338:645–52]. Four hundred seventy patients participated in the trial and an equal number received enalapril (*Vasotec*) or nisoldipine (*Sular*). Analysis after a five-year follow-up showed similar control of blood pressure, blood glucose, and lipid levels. There was, however, a significantly higher incidence of fatal and nonfatal MIs among those assigned to therapy with nisoldipine (a total of 25 events) than among those assigned to receive enalapril (a total of five events). Compared with patients who received *Vasotec*, patients taking *Sular* had a RR of 9.5 with a 95% confidence interval of 2.3

to 21.4. Although the study design does not allow one to distinguish among a deleterious effect of *Sular,* a protective effect of *Vasotec,* or a combination of both as the reason for the observed difference, the ACE inhibitor is clearly the better choice.

Early, Intensive Insulin Therapy Preserves Islet Function in Type 1 Diabetics. Many people in the early stages of type 1 diabetes retain residual islet function and insulin secretion. These people find it easier to achieve near-normal glucose control at this early stage than they do later in the absence of islet function. Some experts believe that aggressive insulin therapy immediately after diagnosis of type 1 diabetes for patients who have islet function can modify the natural history of the disease.

A recent report from the Diabetes Control and Complications Trial (DCCT) shows that intensive therapy directed at maintaining glucose levels as close to normal as possible delays the onset and slows the progression of microvascular complications in patients with type 1 diabetes [*JAMA* 1998;280:140–46]. At base line, 855 of the DCCT participants had had diabetes for less than five years. Of those, 303 had residual islet function. They were assigned to receive intensive therapy—three or more insulin injections daily or continuous subcutaneous infusions of insulin, guided by four or more glucose tests per day—or conventional therapy with one or two injections daily and minimal monitoring. Patients were followed for up to six years.

Those treated intensively had greater insulin secretion during the first five years than those given conventional therapy. Islet function was extended about two years. Residual capacity to secrete insulin allowed patients to more effectively manage their condition than could those with no islet function at baseline. Patients with residual islet function had before and during treatment a lower glycosylated hemoglobin level, a 50% reduced risk for progression of retinopathy, and a 65% lower risk for severe hypoglycemia with seizure or coma. In light of their findings, the researchers stress the importance of initiating intensive diabetic management as early as possible after diagnosis of type 1 diabetes for patients who have residual islet function.

Intensive Glucose Control for Type 2 Diabetes. In September, eagerly awaited reports from the United Kingdom Prospective Diabetes Study (UK-PDS) on intensive blood-glucose control in type 2 diabetics appeared in *The Lancet.* The UKPDS was an extraordinary effort, spanning more than 20 years. The trial was initiated in the mid-1970s. A commentary on the new reports [*Lancet*1998;352:832–33] provides a perspective of the prevailing medical and scientific environment at the time, which is important for an understanding of the study and its complex design.

In 1970, researchers and clinicians learned the results of the University Group Diabetes Program (UGDP) study. The UGDP involved 1000 patients with type 2 diabetes and compared five different treatments—diet with placebo; fixed insulin doses based on bodyweight; variable doses of insulin adjusted according to glucose levels; tolbutamide, the most widely used sulfonylurea at the time; and phenformin, a biguanide. To everyone's disappointment, the variable dose insulin regimen was no more effective than the fixed dose strategy in decreasing microvascular or cardiovascular outcomes, even though the group assigned variable doses had lower fasting blood glucose concentrations. Moreover, tolbutamide and phenformin increased the risk of cardiovascular mortality. Phenformin was later withdrawn from the market because of the attendant risk of cardiac events and the risk of potentially fatal lactic acidosis. Twenty years passed until another biguanide, metformin, reached the US market.

Pharmaceutical manufacturers of anti-diabetic sulfonylureas roundly criticized the UGDP trial and a great deal of controversy ensued. The commentary in *The Lancet* observes: "The UKPDS was born amidst this tremendous uncertainty about the appropriate metabolic goals for type 2 diabetes, and the relative merits of the available therapies." The aim of UKPDS was to find out once and for all whether intensive management of blood glucose produces a better long-term outcome than a more conventional, less intensive strategy.

One phase of the study (UKPDS 33) involved 3867 patients with newly diagnosed type 2 diabetes. They were randomly assigned to intensive treatment with either a sulfonylurea—chlorpropamide, glibenclamide, or glipizide—or insulin, or to conventional treatment with a diabetes-specific diet. The goal for the intensive group was a fasting plasma glucose of less than 6 mmol/L. For the conventional group, the aim was the best achievable fasting glucose level.

Over ten years, glycosylated hemoglobin was 7.0% in the intensive group compared with 7.9% in the conventional group. There were no differnces in glycosylated hemoglobin among agents in the intensive group. Compared with the conventional group, a 12% lower risk was found in the intensive treatment group for any diabetes-related endpoint, a 10% lower risk for any diabetes-related death, and a 6% lower risk for all-cause mortality. The improvements in diabetes-related mortality and total mortality, however, were not statistically significant. Most of the risk reduction in diabetes-related endpoints was due to a 25% reduction in the risk of retinopathy. Patients in the intensive group, particularly those receiving insulin, had more hypoglycemic episodes and weight gain.

The investigators conclude: "Intensive blood-glucose control by either sulphonylureas or insulin substantially decreases the risk of microvascular complication, but not macrovascular disease, in patients with type 2 diabetes." Intensive control had little effect on heart disease or stroke. On the other hand, none of the individual drugs had an adverse effect on cardiovascular outcomes [*Lancet* 1998;352:837–53].

UKPSD 34 involved 753 overweight patients with newly diagnosed type 2 diabetes. Individuals had fasting plasma glucose levels ranging from 6.1 to 15.0 mmol/L. Over a period of 10.7 years, they received conventional treatment, which was primarily diet-based, or intensive treatment with metformin. A secondary analysis compared the 343 patients randomized to metformin with 951 overweight patients allocated to intensive control with chlorpropamide, glibenclamide, or insulin.

Median glycosylated hemoglobin was 7.4% in the metformin group compared with 8.0% in the conventional treatment group. Compared to those treated with conventional therapy, patients receiving metformin had a risk reduction of 32% for any diabetes-related endpoint, 42% for diabetes-related death, and 36% for all cause mortality. Among the drugs used by patients randomized to intensive treatment, metformin had a greater effect than chlorpropamide, glibenclamide, or insulin for any diabetes-related endpoint, all cause mortality, and stroke. The authors conclude: "Since intensive glucose control with metformin appears to decrease the risk of diabetes-related endpoints in overweight diabetic patients, and is associated with less weight gain and fewer hypoglycemic attacks than are insulin and sulphonylureas, it may be the first-line pharmacological therapy of choice in these patients" [*Lancet* 1998;352:854–65].

A commentary in *The Lancet* [1998;352:832–33] observes that professional organizations will now scramble to decide how to translate the UKPDS results. The main message is that intensive therapy of type 2 diabetes is beneficial. Findings that tight glucose control reduces long-term adverse outcomes in patients with type 1 diabetes also seem to apply to patients with type 2 diabetes. The lack of adverse effects of sulfonylureas on cardiovascular outcomes, which refutes the findings of UGDP, is reassuring. Metformin (*Glucophage*) seems to have a distinct clinical advantage over sulfonylureas or insulin for overweight patients. Whether metformin should be selected over troglitazone (*Rezulin*) or other recently marketed agents for type 2 diabetes remains to be determined. A recent study suggests that metformin and troglitazone are equally effective in controlling blood glucose levels [*N Engl J Med* 1998;338:861–66].

Tight Control of Blood Pressure for Type 2 Diabetes. The UKPDS not only investigated the benefits of intensive glucose control for patients with type 2 diabetes, but also evaluated the effects of tight blood pressure control [*Br Med J* 1998;317:703–13, 713–20]. Untreated or undertreated hypertension is a major risk factor for macrovascular complications in type 2 diabetics.

The investigators compared tight control with relaxed control using captopril, an angiotensin converting enzyme inhibitor, or atenolol, a β-blocker. Target blood pressures were <150/85 mm Hg and <180/105 mm Hg, respectively. Mean baseline blood pressure was 160/94 mm Hg.

At the end of the study, mean blood pressure was 144/82 mm Hg in the tight-control group and 154/87 mm Hg in the relaxed-control group. Compared with relaxed control, tight control reduced diabetes-related end points by 24%, deaths related to diabetes by 32%, strokes by 44%, and micro-vascular end points by 37%. There was also a reduced risk of all-cause mortality, but the impact was not statistical significant. After nine years of follow up, those assigned to tight control also had a 34% reduced risk of significant deterioration of retinopathy, and a 47% reduced risk of clinically important deterioration of visual acuity.

More patients in the captopril group than in the atenolol group took the allocated treatment (78% vs. 65%). Nevertheless, the two drugs were equally effective in reducing blood pressure. Captopril and atenolol were also equally effective in reducing the risk of macrovascular end points. Similar proportions of patients in the two groups showed deterioration in retinopathy and renal function. According to the investigators: "This study provided no evidence that either drug has any specific beneficial or deleterious effect, suggesting that blood pressure reduction in itself may be more important than the treatment used."

Improved Glucose Control with Glipizide Realizes Short-Term Benefits. A recent randomized study in 569 patients with type 2 diabetes shows that improvements in the control of blood glucose can lead to greater well-being and work productivity [*JAMA* 1998;280:1490–96]. In the study, 377 patients were told to follow an assigned diet and also received daily doses of extended-release glipizide (*Glucatrol XL*) for 12 weeks. The rest of the patients were assigned to diet alone.

At the conclusion of the study, the group of patients on both drug and diet had significantly lower levels of glycosylated hemoglobin (HbA$_{1c}$)—7.3% vs. 9.3%—and better control of serum glucose levels—126 mg/dl vs. 168 mg/dl. Quality of life measures—symptom distress, perceived health, cognitive functioning, and overall well-being—were consistently greater in the active treatment group. Hypoglycemia did not detract from quality of life because the number of episodes were few. The group that did not receive glipizide was far more likely to be absent from work.

According to *The Wall Street Journal* [November 4, 1998, p B9], the findings are likely to give impetus to a recent initiative launched by the American Diabetes Association and the American Association of Health Plans, which represents the managed care industry. The organizations seek to develop a systematic approach to the treatment of people with diabetes. The head of one health plan said that only one-third of physicians who treat diabetic patients strive to maintain tight control.

GASTROINTESTINAL DISEASE

Prilosec versus *Cytotec* for NSAID-Induced GI Ulcers
H Pylori Eradication of No Benefit for NSAID-Induced GI Ulcers

Prilosec versus Cytotec for NSAID-Induced GI Ulcers. Nonsteroidal anti-inflammatory drugs (NSAIDs) are widely used, particularly in the elderly, but have substantial gastroduodenal toxicity. Endoscopic studies show that the prevalence of peptic ulcers is 20% to 30% among regular users of NSAIDs. Misoprostol (*Cytotec*), a synthetic prostaglandin, has mucosal protective properties and is the only drug approved in the US for the prevention of NSAID-induced ulcers. A combination product called *Athrotec* that contains both the NSAID diclofenac and misoprostol is also marketed. *Cytotec* replenishes the cytoprotective prostaglandins that NSAIDs deplete from the gastroduodenal mucosa. Not infrequently, however, patients taking *Cytotec* complain of diarrhea and abdominal pains.

An alternative approach to protect the mucosa is by suppressing acid secretion. H_2-receptor antagonists (e.g., cimetidine and ranitidine) are not very effective for healing or preventing NSAID-related gastric ulcers, but they do accelerate healing and help prevent duodenal ulcers. Omeprazole (*Prilosec*), a proton pump inhibitor, has a more profound effect on gastric acid secretion than do H_2-receptor antagonists. Might omeprazole be an effective alternative to *Cytotec*?

Indeed, a recent study shows that *Prilosec* may be a safer and more effective choice for both the treatment and prevention of gastroduodenal ulcers associated with the use of NSAIDs [*N Engl J Med* 1998;338:727–34]. The study panel consisted of 935 patients who required continuous NSAID therapy and who had ulcers or erosions (at least 10) in the stomach or duodenum. While continuing treatment with NSAIDs, they received either *Prilosec* 20 mg once daily or *Cytotec* 200 μg four times a day for up to eight weeks. During the course of the study, the rates of treatment success—the absence of ulcers and the presence of less than five erosions—were similar for both drugs. *Prilosec* was more effective in healing gastric and duodenal ulcers and *Cytotec* more effective in healing erosions.

After the healing phase of the study, the investigators assigned 732 patients in whom treatment was successful to maintenance therapy with *Prilosec, Cytotec,* or placebo for six months. More patients remained in remission during maintenance treatment with *Prilosec* than with *Cytotec* (61% vs. 48%). In both phases of the investigation, *Prilosec* was tolerated better than was *Cytotec* and fewer patients on *Prilosec* dropped out because of adverse effects. The availability of *Prilosec* as a better-tolerated alternative to *Cytotec* may increase the use of prophylactic therapy in patients taking NSAIDs.

In a closely related study that was reported at the same time, other investigators found that omeprazole heals and prevents ulcers more effectively in patients who use NSAIDs regularly than does ranitidine [*N Engl J Med* 1998;338:719–26]. At the end of the study's healing phase, treatment was successful in 80% of patients in the omeprazole group and 63% of those in the ranitidine group. At the end of the maintenance phase, 72% of the patients receiving omeprazole were in remission compared with 59% of those receiving ranitidine.

H Pylori Eradication of no Benefit for NSAID-Induced GI Ulcers. Infection with *Helicobacter pylori* or the regular use of nonsteroidal anti-inflammatory drugs (NSAIDs) account for nearly all gastroduodenal ulcers. Eradication of *H pylori* in patients not taking NSAIDs heals and substantially decreases the rate of recurrence of gastric and duodenal ulcers. There is confusion, however, as to the role of the organism and its eradication in the development and healing of NSAID-induced ulcers. To this end, investigators have recently reported the results of a controlled trial designed to investigate the hypothesis that *H pylori* eradication would have no effect on ulcer recurrence [*Lancet* 1998;352:1016–21].

The research team enrolled adult men and women who required continuous treatment with NSAIDs and had *H pylori* infection as well as a current ulcer or one in the recent past, and/or moderate to severe dyspepsia. The patients were randomized to receive omeprazole plus placebo or omeprazole and antibiotics—amoxicillin and clarithromycin. Two-thirds of patients who received eradication treatment were free of *H pylori* by the end of the six-month study, compared with 14% of the control group. After four weeks, 75% of the eradication group with ulcers at the start of the study were ulcer-free, compared with 86% of the control group. The comparable rates after eight weeks were 86% and 100%. The difference was related to slower healing of gastric ulcers in patients on eradication treatment (50% vs. 88% at four weeks and 72% vs. 100% at eight weeks). The estimated probability of being ulcer-free at six-months, however, was about the same for each group—0.56 for eradication treatment and 0.53 for control treatment.

The researchers conclude that *H pylori* eradication in long-term users of NSAIDs leads to impaired healing of gastric ulcers but does not affect the outcome in terms of recurrence of peptic ulcers or dyspepsia over six months. The work does not support recommendations to test for and eradicate *H pylori* in patients already taking NSAIDs who have developed ulcers. On the other hand, eradication of the organism before the initiation of NSAID therapy may provide a benefit [*Lancet* 1997;352:1001–03].

INFECTIOUS DISEASE

Zinc Not Effective for Common Cold in Children. Although the common cold is ordinarily a benign, self-limited viral infection, it does cause discomfort and substantial economic loss. Investigations of oral zinc to ameliorate the symptoms of the common cold have yielded mixed results—five positive trials and five negative trials. The most recent and most compelling trial reports that zinc lozenges reduce the symptoms of a cold in adults [*Ann Intern Med* 125:81–88]. Those findings prompted a study in children [*JAMA* 1998;279:1962–67].

A total of 249 children in grades 1 through 12 were enrolled within 24 hours of onset of at least two symptoms of the common cold. They received either zinc lozenges or placebo lozenges. Main outcome measures were the resolution of symptoms based on subjective daily symptom scores for cough, nasal congestion, and sore throat, among others. The median time to resolution of all cold symptoms was nine days in each group. The time to resolution of any one of nine symptoms of a cold was also similar in each group. Children receiving active treatment had more adverse events, including bad taste, nausea, oral discomfort, and diarrhea than did those receiving placebo.

Zinc, like vitamin C, which has received extraordinary attention as a putative treatment for the common cold, enhances the immune system, but only in deficient individuals. In developing countries, zinc has an important role in children's health. Demonstrating an effect of zinc lozenges on the common cold in children who are nutritionally replete may be quite difficult. Physicians, however, will be challenged to explain to a parent of a "sick" child that neither antibiotics nor zinc lozenges will do much good in shortening the duration of active infection and turn them away empty-handed [*JAMA* 1998;29:2000–01].

Vitamin Supplements Decrease Adverse Pregnancy Outcomes in HIV-Infected Women. At the end of 1997, 30 million people worldwide were infected with HIV. About 90% were in developing countries, mostly in sub-Sahara Africa. Large numbers of HIV-infected pregnant women are found in these nations. HIV-positive pregnant women have a higher risk of losing a fetus or suffering a preterm birth and face the grim prospect of vertical transmission of the virus. Poor nutrition may exacerbate an already bad situation. Observational studies suggest that improved nutrition may reduce some of the problems. Now, investigators have carried out a placebo-controlled trial to investigate the effects of supplements of vitamin A, multivitamins, or both on birth outcomes among pregnant HIV-infected women living in Tanzania [*Lancet* 1998;351:1477–82.

More than 1000 HIV-seropositive pregnant women between 12 and 27 weeks of gestation received placebo, vitamin A, multivitamins excluding vitamin A, or multivitamins including vitamin A. Supplementation with multivitamins decreased the risk of fetal death by 39%, of low birth weight by 44%, of severe preterm birth by 39%, and of small for gestational age by 43%. Vitamin A supplementation had no effect on these variables. Multivitamins, but not vitamin A, also increased CD4 T-cell counts in the mother.

The investigators speculate that the beneficial effect of multivitamins is mediated through improved fetal nutritional status, enhanced fetal immunity, and decreased risk of infection. They also suggest that a more compelling potential mechanism of action of the multivitamins is through improvement of mothers' hematological status. Low hemoglobin concentrations are associated with higher risks of miscarriages, preterm birth and low birth weight. The authors conclude that multivitamin supplementation is a low-cost way of decreasing adverse pregnancy outcomes and increasing T-cell counts in HIV-infected women.

Short-Term AZT Reduces Vertical Transmission of HIV. Transmission of HIV from mother to infant can occur in utero, during labor and vaginal delivery, and after birth through breast feeding. Researchers estimate that 25% to 30% of HIV transmission occurs in utero, and up to 70% to 75% occurs at the time of delivery. Possible mechanisms for the transmission of HIV during labor and delivery are direct exposure to maternal body fluids and transplacental microtransfusions [*JAMA* 1998;280:17–18].

In the US and other developed nations, pregnant HIV-infected women are treated with oral zidovudine (AZT, *Retrovir*) five times daily for the last 26 weeks of pregnancy, followed by intravenous zidovudine during labor and delivery. The newborn then receives zidovudine for six weeks. Mothers are cautioned not to breast-feed. This regimen reduces transmission by up to two-thirds, from about 25% to 8%, but is expensive and too complex to be useful in developing countries where more than one million children have been infected with HIV and millions more will be infected before the turn of the century.

Preliminary results from a placebo-controlled study in Thailand show that an abbreviated course of *Retrovir* given by mouth late in pregnancy— twice daily for only the last three or four weeks, and during delivery—reduces HIV transmission by 50%. The protocol used in the study is the first practical and cost-effective therapy for patients in indigent nations [*Scrip*, No 2312, February 25, 1998, p 26]. Based on these findings, placebo arms of several studies in developing countries were stopped and the women offered *Retrovir*. Whether the short-course of treatment is effective for the offspring of women who do not present until delivery or women who breast-feed remains to be seen.

While short-term therapy slashes drug costs, they remain beyond the means of some nations. Two weeks after the termination of the landmark study, Glaxo Wellcome, the manufacturer of *Retrovir*, announced that it would cut the price of the drug by as much as 75% to ensure that the estimated three million infected pregnant women in impoverished nations have the opportunity to receive therapy [*The Wall Street Journal*, March 5, 1998, p B1, B2]. Glaxo's announcement marks the first time a major pharmaceutical company has agreed to cut the price of HIV medication so that it may be introduced in regions where the infection is epidemic. Glaxo's generosity prompted Bristol-Myers Squibb, Abbott Laboratories, and Roche Holdings to come forward and make HIV medication available to underdeveloped countries at steep discounts.

Shortly after the news of increased accessibility to *Retrovir*, the United Nations announced it will start a pilot program to treat 30,000 pregnant women infected with HIV in 11 countries where the infection is spreading rapidly [*The New York Times,* June 29, 1998, p A15]. This action, however, was strongly attacked by French advocacy groups who criticized the program for not providing therapy for the mother after pregnancy. They accused the UN of creating an orphan factory.

Initial Therapy of HIV Infection: Conservative or Aggressive? Limited federal and state funds to purchase anti-HIV medication for the indigent has led to conservative initial treatment of HIV infection to reduce costs. These strategies delay medication until viral load has exceeded a threshold and initiate therapy with only two reverse transcriptase inhibitors (RTIs) or a protease inhibitor. A clinical trial, initiated a few years ago, compared triple therapy with the combination of indinavir (*Crixivan*), zidovudine (*Retrovir*), and lamivudine (*Epivir*) with indinavir monotherapy or a combination of zidovudine and lamivudine [*N Engl J Med* 1997;337:734–39]. All patients were offered open-label triple therapy when this regimen proved to be superior in a preliminary analysis. Patients initially randomized to indinavir monotherapy or the two RTIs received assigned medication for 24 to 52 weeks before receiving open-label triple therapy. All patients were followed for a total of 100 weeks. The natural course of this trial provided an opportunity to compare triple therapy regimes, either started immediately or after less aggressive therapy failed.

In a new report, investigators describe the effects on viral load of initiating triple therapy at once compared with initiating therapy with a less aggressive strategy. At baseline, patients had HIV RNA levels of 20,000 copies/ml or more. Initiation of treatment with triple therapy suppressed the virus to less than 500 copies in 78% of participating patients. Only 30% of patients who received combination zidovudine and lamivudine and 45% of the patients in the indinavir monotherapy group achieved this level of viral load reduction [*JAMA* 1998;280:35–41].

Genotypic analysis of viral resistance helps explain the mechanisms of failure of sequential antiretroviral therapy. At the time of open-label crossover, 94% of the patients assigned to zidovudine/lamivudine had developed a form of the virus associated with lamivudine resistance, which dampened the effects of adding indinavir to the RTIs. Similarly, at the time of crossover to open-label triple therapy, 64% of patients originally treated with indinavir monotherapy had developed virus associated with indinavir resistance. Initiating treatment with triple therapy inhibits HIV replication more effectively than indinavir alone or the combination of zidovudine and lamivudine and thereby inhibits emergence of drug-resistant mutant viruses, increasing the likelihood that the antiretroviral effect is maintained for a prolonged period of time.

Maintenance Therapy Fails to Maintain Suppression of HIV Load. Some diseases such as leukemia are initially attacked aggressively with medication, a treatment called induction therapy, and then kept under control with maintenance therapy that uses fewer medications or more modest doses. Would this strategy apply to the treatment of HIV infection? Two research teams set out to evaluate that possibility and their findings are reported in the October 29, 1998 issue of *The New England Journal of Medicine* [1998; 339:1261–68, 1269–76]. The hope was that highly active antiretroviral therapy at the outset might reduce viral load to such a low level that some of the drugs could be stopped, and the virus kept in check by the patient's immune system and a less intense "maintenance therapy." Efforts, however, to reduce the number of medications after "induction therapy" failed, allowing the virus to re-emerge.

In both studies, patients initially received three drugs, achieved suppression of the virus in blood, and then after several months of treatment stopped one or two of the drugs. Virus levels rebounded quickly in a significant number of patients, and the studies were halted so that triple therapy could be reinstated. The director of one study said the findings underscore warnings already given to patients that combination therapy is a long-term proposition, and that failure to comply may allow the virus to rebound and possibly develop resistant strains.

In one study, patients received the protease inhibitor indinavir and two NRTIs, zidovudine and lamivudine. At the end of six months, one-third of the patients continued the three drugs, one-third took indinavir alone, and one-third took zidovudine and lamivudine. Among patients who continued triple therapy, only 4% had viral rebound. In each of the other two groups, however, 23% of the patients relapsed within two months. The second study involved the same drugs given for three months. Study subjects then stayed on triple therapy or switched to a combination of zidovudine and lamivudine or zidovudine and indinavir. About 9% of the patients who continued aggressive therapy had viral rebound compared with 31% in the zidovudine/lamivudine group and 22% in the zidovudine/indinavir group. These findings confirm those in an earlier report [*Lancet* 1998;352:185–90].

While the results are disappointing, the hope remains that keeping patients on induction therapy for a longer period of time might allow less intensive therapy thereafter. The National Institute of Allergy and Infectious Disease is planning such a study. Fifty patients receiving triple therapy whose virus levels have been undetectable for a year or more will stop all medication to see if their immune systems have recovered sufficiently to control the infection [*The New York Times,* October 29, 1998, pp A1,A17].

A commentary accompanying the new reports reminds us that while a significant number of patients had viral rebound when intensive therapy was stopped, the majority did not [*N Engl J Med* 1998;339;1319–20]. There are patients for whom this strategy is useful. Whether such patients are likely to relapse in the longer term is unknown. The author observes: "Given the limited follow-up in these studies, it would be premature to stop investigating the efficacy of induction therapy followed by maintenance therapy for HIV-1 infection, especially in light of new data showing that the duration of remission is related to the length of induction therapy and the potency of the therapeutic regimen."

Earlier in 1998, investigators studying untreated patients with HIV infection reported that a five drug regimen including zidovudine, lamivudine, abacavir, indinavir, and nevirapine was more effective in eliminating viral RNA from the plasma than was a three drug regimen—zidovudine, lamivudine, and ritonavir [*AIDS* 1998 (July 30);12:F117–22]. With the five drug regimen, the median time to reach a level of less than 50 copies HIV RNA per ml was eight weeks shorter than with the three-drug regimen. The results suggest that suppression of viral load in HIV-infected patients by standard triple-drug therapy can be improved upon.

It's Not "Just the Virus Stupid." For years, HIV treatment has been based on the dogma "it's the virus stupid." However, as the struggle to find a cure for HIV infection advances, most people now agree that it isn't "just the virus."

The dogma has served us well and led to highly active antiretroviral therapy (HAART), which is still evolving as new drugs emerge. HAART has revolutionized HIV disease treatment because it drives viral load in blood to undetectable levels, increases CD4 cell count, banishes symptoms, and stalls disease progression. If HIV-infected patients are treated with HAART early after exposure, when the immune system is not irreversibly damaged, the system will probably recover. But few people receive treatment that early. In those who do not, the ability to control the virus is not restored by HAART. The virus continues to smolder in reservoir cells that harbor it from antiretroviral therapy.

Among the reservoir cells are long-lived, quiescent CD4 memory cells. If drug therapy is stopped or compromised, the virus in these cells may re-ignite. This set of circumstances suggests that combining HAART with strategies to boost immunity and enhance specific anti-HIV responses may improve outcomes [*Lancet* 199;352:1686].

HIV-infected patients do not have symptoms until their CD4 T-cell counts fall below a critical level. The only treatment known to directly expand the CD4 T-cell pool is the natural immune system regulator interleukin-2 (IL-2). Preliminary evidence suggests that IL-2 also has antiviral activity. The mechanism may be related to improved efficacy of CD8 cells. Whether IL-2 improves clinical outcome is not known.

Because IL-2 induces proinflammatory cytokines, there is concern that it might enhance HIV expression by activating latently infected cells. This action, however, turns out to be beneficial. Researchers presenting at the Annual Meeting of the Infectious Disease Society of American in November 1998 suggested that when reservoir cells are activated, the virus is also activated and destroys the cells. When IL-2 is given with HAART, the potent regimen stops the released virions from infecting other cells. Given repeatedly, dual therapy with HAART and IL-2 may progressively reduce the reservoir of latently infected cells and cure the infection [*Ibid*].

Research scientists presented preliminary evidence of the efficacy of this new strategy at the International Congress of Immunology, also held in November, in New Delhi [*Science* 1998;282:1394–95]. The research team studied 26 HIV-infected patients. Twelve of the participants received HAART for 1 to 3 years and fourteen received the same antiretroviral therapy plus IL-2 given repeatedly but with a minimum of 8 weeks between treatments. After treatment, all 26 patients had undetectable levels of HIV in their blood. Consistent with the researchers' hopes and hypothesis, they found no HIV capable of replication in resting T-cells cultured from peripheral blood of 6 of the 14 subjects who had received IL-2. In contrast, the team found live HIV in the resting T-cells from all of the 12 patients who received HAART alone. A lymph node biopsy on one of the patients who showed no sign of virus in their T-cells also showed no HIV capable of replication in lymph node tissue. The new findings raise hopes that eradication of the virus may be a possibility, but the work is not yet definitive. HIV may still lurk in other known reservoirs. The final test requires that all therapy be stopped and that long-term observation shows no re-emergence of the infection.

Infusion of antibodies or histocompatible lymphocytes may be another way to enhance immunity. One research group is studying whether intensive lymphocyte transfers from a healthy twin can restore immunity in an HIV-infected twin [*Lancet* 199;352:1686].

Lamivudine for Chronic Hepatitis B. More than 300 million people throughout the world have chronic infection with hepatitis B virus (HBV). More than 75% of cases occur in people of Asian origin. The human and medical costs of chronic infection are enormous because it causes cirrhosis, liver cancer, and death. Interferon alfa, given by injection, is the only agent specifically approved for chronic HBV infection. Its effects are variable and the drug may produce potentially dose-limiting adverse events. Interferon alfa is least effective in Asian patients.

Lamivudine's ability to inhibit viral DNA replication holds promise for HBV treatment. Studies have shown that up to six months of treatment with lamivudine markedly reduces serum HBV DNA levels in Asians and whites. For patients taking at least 100 mg per day, the median suppression of serum HBV DNA is greater than 98% in most patients. However, when treatment is stopped, HBV DNA levels return to pretreatment levels. Now, investigators have conducted a study to determine whether a one-year duration of viral suppression results in improved outcomes [*N Engl J Med* 1998;339:61–68].

The investigators randomly assigned 358 Chinese patients with chronic HBV infection to receive 25 mg of lamivudine, 100 mg of lamivudine, or placebo orally once daily. The primary endpoint was a two-point improvement in the overall Knodell score, which is the sum of the scores for necrosis, inflammation, intralobular degeneration, and fibrosis, determined by histologic examination of liver biopsies.

They found that hepatic necroinflammatory activity improved by two points or more in 56% of patients in the 100 mg lamivudine group, 49% of the 25 mg lamivudine group, and 25% of the placebo group. Necroinflammatory activity worsened in about 8% of those receiving either dose of lamivudine and in 26% of those receiving placebo. The 100 mg dose of lamivudine also prevented the progression of fibrosis. In contrast, treatment with interferon shows histologic improvements in only a few patients.

Lamivudine therapy also induced sustained normalization of liver enzymes. Both doses of lamivudine reduced serum HBV levels, but the degree of suppression was significantly greater with the higher dose. Patients receiving the higher dose of lamivudine were significantly more likely to have lost hepatitis B e antigen than patients receiving placebo. The rate of HBeAg seroconversion, however, was only 16% in the higher-dose group, which is about the same as or somewhat lower than rates seen with patients treated with interferon. The incidence of adverse events was similar in all groups. Interferon is associated with flu-like symptoms, neutropenia, prolonged fatigue, and depression in some patients. Lamivudine's safety profile is better.

An editorial published with the report emphasizes that the mechanism of action of lamivudine does not allow for the elimination of the source of viral replication, and hepatitis B may flare up after the drug is stopped [*N Engl J Med* 1998;339114–15]. The author notes that had investigators performed liver biopsies several weeks or months after discontinuing treatment, rather than at week 52, the percentage of patients who had improvement in necroinflammatory activity might have been much less. He also stresses that seroconversion is simply a sign of the quiescence of hepatitis B and is not tantamount to eradication of the virus or cure. The greatest benefit of lamivudine may be its ability to reverse or arrest fibrotic changes in the liver, thereby blocking the architectural distortion that leads to cirrhosis.

Acyclovir for Prevention of Ocular Herpes Infection. Herpes simplex virus (HSV) infection is a leading cause of corneal opacification and loss of vision and affects some 400,000 Americans, with new cases occurring at a rate of 50,000 per year. Laboratory studies suggest that systemic acyclovir (*Zovirax*) can suppress experimental reactivation of ocular HSV disease. Prompted by these findings, investigators set out to determine whether treatment with oral acyclovir for one year would prevent ocular recurrences in immunocompetent persons who had had an episode of ocular HSV within the preceding year [*N Engl J Med* 1998;339:300–06].

They randomly assigned 703 patients to acyclovir or placebo, twice daily. Study outcomes were the development rates of ocular or non-ocular HSV disease during a 12-month treatment period followed by a six-month observation period. During the treatment period, ocular HSV disease recurred in 19% of the acyclovir group and 32% of the placebo group. Among 337 patients with a more serious form of ocular HSV disease—stromal keratitis—recurrence was seen in 14% of the acyclovir group and 28% in the placebo group. The probability of a recurrence of non-ocular HSV disease was also lower in the acyclovir group than in the placebo group. No benefit was seen beyond the treatment period; during observation, the rate or recurrence was similar in the acyclovir group and the placebo group.

The authors conclude: "Long-term antiviral prophylaxis is most important for patients with a history of HSV stromal keratitis, since it can prevent additional episodes and potential loss of vision." The effectiveness of oral acyclovir to prevent recurrence of stromal keratitis suggests that viral replication does have a role in this form of the disease. This is contrary to the previously-held view that stromal keratitis reflects an immune response to viral antigen rather than active viral replication [*New Engl J Med* 1998; 339:340–41].

Oral Famciclovir for Suppression of Recurrent Genital Herpes. Genital herpes simplex virus (HSV) is among the most common sexually transmitted diseases, with a prevalence of about 20% in adults in the US. Symptomatic recurrent infection is seen in the majority of patients who acquire the virus, with almost half experiencing at least six painful recurrences a year. Episodic treatment with an antiviral agent is usually sufficient to effectively manage recurrences. Acyclovir, valacyclovir (a prodrug of acyclovir), and famciclovir (a prodrug of penciclovir) are approved for the acute treatment of recurrent genital herpes. For some patients, however, preventive treatment to suppress recurrences may provide more benefit than acute treatment. Given a choice, far more patients opt for suppressive therapy over acute treatment. Acyclovir (*Zovirax*) and valacyclovir (*Valtrex*) both have this indication but famciclovir (*Famvir*) does not.

A placebo-controlled dose-ranging study was the first to demonstrate the efficacy of famciclovir in the suppression of recurrent genital herpes [*Arch Intern Med* 1997;157:343–49]. Results from that study showed that 90% of patients remained free of HSV when given 250 mg famciclovir twice daily for four months. Once-daily dosing, however, produced less complete suppression, with only 60% to 70% of patients remaining free of recurrences. The objective of a more recent, multicenter center study involving 455 patients was to confirm the earlier results with famciclovir and to determine if giving the drug three times a day was a more effective strategy [*JAMA* 1998; 280;887–92].

Patients were at least 18 years old with a history of six or more episodes of genital herpes during the past year. They were assigned to receive 125 mg or 250 mg famciclovir three times daily, 250 mg twice daily, or placebo for 52 weeks. The main outcome measures were the time to the first recurrence of genital HSV infection, the proportion of patients remaining free of HSV recurrence at six months, and the frequency of adverse events.

Famciclovir delayed the time to the first recurrence of genital herpes without regard to dosing regimen. Median time to recurrence for famciclovir recipients was 222 to 336 days compared with 47 days for placebo recipients.

At six months, the proportion of patients remaining free of HSV recurrence ranged from 79% to 86% in the active treatment groups compared with 27% in the placebo group. There were no important differences in the efficacy of oral famciclovir 125 mg or 250 mg three times a day or 250 mg twice daily. The drug was well tolerated at all doses.

An accompanying editorial notes that for long-term suppression of genital herpes famciclovir is more effective than acyclovir or valacyclovir, but the cost of therapy with famciclovir is considerably greater. The author also cautions physicians to counsel patients receiving suppressive antiviral medication that they might still transmit HSV to their sexual partners [*JAMA* 1998;280;928–29].

Inflammatory Disease

Budesonide and Mesalamine for Active Crohn's Disease. Inflammatory bowel diseases—Crohn's disease, ulcerative colitis, and others—are second only to rheumatoid arthritis among the most common chronic inflammatory disorders. Their cause is unknown. Prednisolone and other glucocorticoids are commonly used to treat the acute phase of Crohn's disease but these agents have serious side effects. The introduction of budesonide, a poorly absorbed and rapidly metabolized glucocorticoid, is an important advance. Oral budesonide is as effective as prednisolone in inducing remission and causes less adrenal suppression and fewer side effects. Although it is less effective than steroids, delayed-release mesalamine, an aminosalicylate with anti-inflammatory activity, is better tolerated and often used as first-line therapy for patients with mild to moderately active Crohn's disease. The delayed-release formulation offers the opportunity of drug delivery to the disease site—the small bowel and ascending colon.

A recent report concerns a study that compared delayed-release forms of budesonide and mesalamine for the treatment of active Crohn's disease affecting the ileum, the ascending colon, or both [*N Engl J Med* 1998; 339:370–04]. The investigators enrolled 182 patients with active disease—a Crohn's Disease Activity Index of 200 to 400. They were assigned to receive budesonide once daily or mesalamine twice daily for 16 weeks. The primary endpoint was clinical remission, defined as a score of 150 or less.

The rates of remission after eight weeks of treatment were 69% in the budesonide group and 45% in the mesalamine group. Corresponding rates after 16 weeks were 62% and 36%. The number of patients with an adverse event was similar in the two groups. Among patients completing treatment, the morning plasma cortisol levels (an index of adrenal suppression), were normal in 67% of those receiving budesonide and 83% of those assigned to mesalamine. The typical glucocorticoid-related side effects of moon face, hirsutisim, and acne were infrequent in both groups. The results are promising but long-term studies are needed. Oral budesonide is not yet available in the US.

Mental Health

Old Versus New Antidepressants for Patients with Heart Disease
Paroxetine (*Paxil*) for the Treatment of Social Anxiety Disorder
Long-Term Sertraline (*Zoloft*) of Benefit for Chronic Depression

Old Versus New Antidepressants for Patients with Heart Disease. The first breakthrough in the treatment of depression was the introduction of a class of drugs called tricyclic antidepressants (TCAs). The class includes imipramine, nortriptyline, and many other agents. These drugs are very effective but burdened with adverse effects. Some years later, the pharmaceutical industry developed a new class of agents called selective serotonin reuptake inhibitors (SSRIs). Fluoxetine (*Prozac*) was the first SSRI to receive approval in the US. Whether or not SSRIs are more effective than TCAs is debated, but they do have a better safety profile and are better tolerated.

Recently, attention has focused on depression in patients with heart disease. There is compelling evidence that patients who develop depression following a heart attack are at much greater risk of death than medically comparable post-MI patients who are not depressed. It is not known whether treatment of the depressive episode will safely reduce the associated increase in cardiac mortality. Nevertheless, physicians treat patients with heart disease for depression and mostly use TCAs. Is there a difference in safety and efficacy between treatment of such patients with a TCA or an SSRI?

To answer that question a team of psychiatrists and cardiologists enrolled 81 patients who met the *Diagnostic and Statistical Manual of Mental Disorders, Fourth Edition* (DSM IV) criteria for major depressive disorder and who had documented ischemic heart disease. They randomized the patients to treatment with either paroxetine (*Paxil*) or nortriptyline for six weeks. Both drugs were effective. About 60% of the patients improved significantly on *Paxil* and 55% on nortriptyline. The drugs did differ, however, in their effects on the heart and in their tolerability.

Paxil had no significant effect on any of the cardiac parameters selected for evaluation, whereas nortriptyline produced a sustained 11% increase in heart rate. In patients with ischemic heart disease there is a positive correlation between heart rate and mortality. Adverse cardiac events occurred in 2% of patients receiving *Paxil* and 18% of patients receiving nortriptyline. Ninety percent of *Paxil*-treatment patients completed the medication trial compared with only 65% of nortriptyline-treated patients. Although the two classes of antidepressants seem to be equally effective, the trial argues persuasively for the use of SSRIs rather than TCAs to treat patients with heart disease and depression.

Paroxetine (Paxil) for the Treatment of Social Anxiety Disorder. Social anxiety disorder, also called social phobia, is said to affect 5% to 10% of the US population. Characterizing the disorder is a pathologic fear of saying or doing something to embarrass or humiliate oneself. Consequently, people who have social phobia endure scrutiny with intense distress and avoid such situations. People with social phobia are more likely than the general population to develop other anxiety disorders and mood disorders, and more likely to abuse alcohol and other substances. Psychiatrists say that social phobia is the most prevalent anxiety disorder in the US, and also say that the condition often goes unrecognized. Both cognitive-behavior therapy and pharmacologic treatment benefit those with social phobia, but only about 25% of people with the disorder receive treatment [*JAMA* 1998;280:685–86].

Selective serotonin reuptake inhibitors (SSRIs) seem to be effective in people with social phobia. Up until now, however, the evidence has been scant. A new report shows that a relatively short course of paroxetine (*Paxil*) results in substantial and clinically meaningful reductions in symptoms and disability of social anxiety disorder.

To evaluate the effects of paroxetine, investigators recruited 187 people meeting the criteria for generalized social phobia. They were randomly assigned to receive an 11-week course of either paroxetine or placebo. At the end of the trial, more than half (55%) of the 91 persons taking the SSRI and 22 (24%) of the 92 persons taking placebo were much improved or very much improved as judged by a before and after global rating scale. Anxiety scores, according to another standardized scale, decreased by an average of nearly 40% among those receiving paroxetine but by only 17% among those receiving placebo.

This is the first multicenter, double-blind randomized study of an SSRI in social phobia. The results clearly show that paroxetine, and possibly related drugs, is effective in reducing the symptoms and avoidance associated with the social phobia. The UK Medicines Control Agency cleared the supplemental indication for paroxetine—called *Seroxat* in Europe—in October. SmithKline Beecham submitted an application for the indication to FDA in May 1998, and awaits a decision. In the US, *Paxil* is indicated for depression, panic disorder, and obsessive-compulsive disorder.

Long-Term Sertraline of Benefit for Chronic Depression. Successful treatment of the acute phase of depression is usually followed by a continuation phase of therapy for four months or more to prevent early relapse. This approach is now a standard of care. Patients with chronic depression, however, may need further treatment. There is little information on the efficacy of maintenance therapy with an antidepressant. A recent report describes the first well-controlled evaluation of the safety and sustained prophylactic efficacy of maintenance treatment with an SSRI [_JAMA_ 1998;280:1665–72].

The investigators enrolled 161 outpatients with chronic depression who had responded to sertraline (_Zoloft_) in a 12-week acute-phase treatment trial and continued to have a satisfactory response during a subsequent four-month continuation phase. They randomly assigned the patients to receive sertraline in a flexible dose up to 200 mg/day or placebo, for 76 weeks.

Sertraline provided significantly greater prophylaxis against recurrence of depression than did placebo. Only 6% of 77 patients in the sertraline group compared with 23% of 84 patients in the placebo group relapsed. Clinically important depressive symptoms re-emerged in 26% of patients in the active drug group and in 50% of those in the placebo group. Patients who received placebo were four times more likely to experience recurrence of depression.

Neurological Disease

Excedrin-Extra Strength to Treat Migraine Headache
Riboflavin to Prevent Migraine Headache
Best Treatment for Status Epilepticus
New Dosage Forms to Treat Acute Repetitive Seizures
Selegiline-Levodopa Combination Increases Mortality
    for Patients with Parkinson's Disease
Dopamine Agonist—Pramipexole—Reduces Tremor
    in Parkinson's Disease
Donepezil (*Aricept*) Improves Cognition and
    Function in Alzheimer Disease
Drug Therapy for Multiple Sclerosis

Excedrin-Extra Strength to Treat Migraine Headache. About eighteen million Americans are intermittently disabled from migraine headaches. The large majority is undiagnosed and most sufferers have not even consulted a physician. Most patients with migraine use nonprescription medications (e.g., aspirin, acetaminophen, ibuprofen, ketoprofen, and naproxen). Some use herbal products such as feverfew. The only nonprescription medication approved by the FDA for the treatment of mild to moderate pain associated with migraine headache is a commercially available combination of acetaminophen, aspirin, and caffeine (*Excedrin Extra-Strength*). In three separate trials, investigators have shown that two tablets of this pain reliever significantly hasten recovery from a migraine attack and may decrease nausea, vomiting, and sensitivity to light and sound [*Arch Neurol* 1998;55:210–17].

The trials supporting the approval of *Excedrin Extra-Strength* enrolled patients with moderate or severe headache pain. The investigators excluded the most severely disabled patients, including patients whose attacks usually required bed rest, or who vomited frequently. The 1,200 patients participating in the study took either the drug combination or placebo as a single-dose treatment of an acute migraine attack. Pain intensity was reduced to mild or none two hours after the dose in 50% of drug-treated patients compared with 33% of placebo-treated patients. By six hours after the dose, 51% of the drug-treated group were free of pain compared with 24% of the placebo-treated group.

In approving *Excedrin Extra-Strength* for the treatment of migraine, the FDA asked Bristol-Myers Squibb not only to formulate new labeling but also to come up with a new package and a new name. The FDA reasoned that patients with migraine headaches require specific warnings and directions for use. *Excedrin Migraine,* containing the same ingredients and sold at the same price as *Excedrin Extra-Strength,* is the result of those requests. The currently recommended "Step Approach" to migraine treatment that starts with simple analgesics and adds more powerful and more costly drugs as needed, receives a considerable boost from this study.

Riboflavin to Prevent Migraine Headache. Several classes of drugs can prevent migraine headaches and should be considered when the frequency of headache is more than two to three times a month or when a single headache is severely disabling. The list of drugs is long and a recent report suggests that we may need to add riboflavin [*Neurology* 1998;50:466–70].

Fifty-five patients who regularly had two to eight attacks per month were given either 400 mg of riboflavin or placebo daily and followed for four months. Riboflavin decreased the frequency of attacks but the benefit was evident after only one month. The vitamin also decreased the number of days with headache, headache severity, duration of headache, and days with nausea and vomiting. The authors conclude that riboflavin deserves comparison with better established agents.

Best Treatment for Status Epilepticus. Status epilepticus is a life-threatening emergency. Generalized convulsive status epilepticus is the most common form. An array of anticonvulsant medications has been advocated for initial treatment and each has a large number of adherents. The choices, however, are not based on convincing evidence. Recognizing the need for more information, the Veterans Affairs Status Epilepticus Cooperative Study Group designed a five-year study to comparatively evaluate four intravenous regimens—diazepam followed by phenytoin, lorazepam, phenobarbital, and phenytoin [*N Engl J Med* 1998;339:792–98]. The 384 patients had either overt status, defined as visible generalized convulsions, or more serious subtle status, indicated by coma and ictal discharges on the electroencephalogram.

Lorazepam successfully resolved the episode in 65% of those assigned to receive it, phenobarbital in 58%, diazepam and phenytoin in 56%, and phenytoin in 44%. Lorazepam was significantly more effective than phenytoin but differences between lorazepam and the other two treatments did not reach the 0.05 level of statistical significance. There were no differences among the treatments in protecting against recurrence. Although three treatment options are roughly equivalent, the researchers lean toward the use of lorazepam because it requires the least amount of time to administer an effective dose. The authors conclude: "Because even the best treatments were successful in only about two thirds of the patients with overt status epilepticus and one fourth of the patients with subtle status epilepticus, our study underscores the need for better methods of treating generalized convulsive status epilepticus and its underling causes."

New Dosage Forms to Treat Acute Repetitive Seizures. Epilepsy affects about two million people in the US. Some patients periodically have acute repetitive seizures, sometimes called serial seizures. If left untreated, acute repetitive seizures can evolve into status epilepticus. Oral benzodiazepines are effective, but administration is frequently difficult when the patient is actively convulsing. Benzodiazepine injection is also effective, but requires trained personnel. Except for intravenous administration, rectal diazepam solutions seem to have the fastest onset of action to stop acute repetitive seizures and can be administered safely by trained caregivers. Rectal suppositories are an alternative but absorption is slow. A rectal gel may be an advantageous compromise and one such preparation, *Diastat* Rectal Delivery System, is available by prescription in the US.

In a recent study, investigators studied 47 children and 44 adults with a history of acute repetitive seizures who were treated at home during an exacerbation with either diazepam gel or a placebo gel [*N Engl J Med* 1998;338:1869–75]. Children were given one dose at the onset of acute repetitive seizures and a second dose four hours later. The same applied to adults but they also received a third dose at 12 hours after onset. Treatment outcomes were frequency and severity of symptoms. As rated by care givers, outcomes were significantly better among those who received diazepam gel than in those assigned placebo. Diazepam was significantly more effective than placebo in reducing seizure frequency in both children and adults. Caregiver's global outcome score was superior in children receiving diazepam, but the difference in the adult group was not statistically significant. No patient given diazepam and 13% of patients in the placebo group required emergency medical care. Sleepiness, seen in one-third of patients in the diazepam group and 11% of patients in the placebo group, was the most common side effect.

An expert commenting on the work described the strategy as an, ". . . extremely useful way to treat children with malignant epilepsy syndromes such as Lennox-Gastaut syndrome, because immediate treatment may rapidly abort an attack" [*Lancet* 1998;352:41]. He stressed, however, that dose titration is essential to avoid respiratory depression. Editorial comments accompanying the report note that diazepam gel is very expensive, costing $70 to $90 for a 10 mg dose. The author suggests that in most cases pediatric neurologists will continue to give the parenteral solution of diazepam, which costs only $6, when they wish to abort seizures rapidly [*N Engl J Med* 1998;338:1916–18].

Another strategy to rapidly abort pediatric seizures is the intranasal administration of midazolam. An application to practice was reported recently. Over a three-month period, 20 eligible children from one month to 16 years old who presented at a pediatric emergency department with generalized motor seizures were treated with intranasal midazolam. Each child received a solution of midazolam at a dose of 0.2 mg/kg total body weight delivered by dropper into each nostril. Intranasal midazolam aborted the seizure within five minutes of administration in all but one child. There were no recurrences of seizures within 60 minutes after treatment. The child who did not respond to midazolam also failed to respond to intravenous diazepam and was finally controlled with intravenous phenytoin. The authors comment that intranasal midazolam could be a useful first aid technique for parents of epileptic children who receive appropriate instructions [*Lancet* 1998;352:620].

Selegiline-Levodopa Combination Increases Mortality for Patients with Parkinson's Disease. The place of selegiline (*Eldepryl*) in the treatment of Parkinson's disease is not entirely clear. The drug is thought to protect against nigral cell death, to slow disease progression, and to reduce mortality. In 1995, however, interim results from the Parkinson's Disease Research Group of the United Kingdom suggested a 60% increase in mortality in patients with early Parkinson's disease who were randomized to receive treatment with combined selegiline and levodopa compared with levodopa alone. Moreover, the addition of selegiline to levodopa was no more effective than levodopa alone [*BMJ* 1995;311:1602–07]. Since the report, the number of selegiline prescriptions has decreased by nearly half in the UK.

Because the study was criticized and the conclusions considered dubious by some experts, the research group analyzed updated data from that study [*BMJ* 1998;316:1191–96]. The new report includes an additional 21 months of follow up and a total follow up of nearly seven years. For all patients, the mortality rate was 33% greater in the combined therapy group than in the monotherapy group (95% CI, 1.02 to 1.74). The excess mortality in the combination therapy group is equivalent to one excess death for every 75 patients treated for one year.

Despite methodological uncertainties in the trial, the authors argue that there are clear clinical implications of their results. Most important, there is no evidence that combined treatment with levodopa and selegiline confers advantages over levodopa treatment alone for patients with newly diagnosed and mild disease. The results, however, do not gainsay the strategy of starting a new patient on selegiline and withdrawing it when symptoms become more troublesome and levodopa is indicated. A physician considering the addition of selegiline for a patient with advanced disease, however, should carefully determine whether the combined treatment really provides an additional benefit.

Dopamine Agonist—Pramipexole—Reduces Tremor in Parkinson's Disease.

A new study, presented at the International Congress of Movement Disorders in October 1998, shows that pramipexole (*Mirapex*), unlike other agents in its class, significantly reduces rest tremor in patients with Parkinson's disease [*Scrip*, October 23, 1998, p 18]. Pramipexole acts on the dopamine D3 receptor, whereas other dopamine agonists used in Parkinson's disease act on D2 receptors.

Three main symptoms characterize Parkinson's disease—akinesia (slowness of movement), rigidity, and tremor. Akinesia is considered the most disabling. Tremor is less disabling but causes psychosocial problems because it is so visible. Tremor can also affect eating and drinking. Up until now, drugs to ameliorate the symptoms of the disease have relieved akinesia and rigidity, but have had little effect on tremor.

In the new study, 84 patients with significant tremor were assigned to either pramipexole or placebo. After three weeks, there was a significant difference in tremor score in favor of pramipexole. This advantage persisted over the remaining four weeks of the treatment period. Nearly three-quarters of patients on pramipexole had a 30% or greater improvement in tremor score compared with 26% of those on placebo.

Donepezil (Aricept) Improves Cognition and Function in Alzheimer Disease.

About 5% to 10% of Americans older than 65 years and as many as 50% of those older than 85 years are estimated to have Alzheimer disease. Many of the symptoms of the common dementia are related to a cholinergic deficit in certain areas of the brain. The only treatment available in the US is a cholinesterase inhibitor called donepezil (*Aricept*). Tacrine, an earlier cholinesterase inhibitor, was withdrawn from the market on approval of *Aricept*. These agents, by inhibiting acetylcholinesterase in the central nervous system, reduce the hydrolysis of the neurotransmitter acetylcholine and promote cholinergic activity. Donepezil is more selective for acetylcholinesterase than tacrine and produces fewer adverse effects at therapeutic doses.

A key study that supported the approval of *Aricept* by the FDA is a 12-week placebo-controlled trial in 468 patients with a probable diagnosis of Alzheimer disease [*Arch Intern Med* 1998;158:1021–31]. Donepezil, taken once daily, enhances cognition as measured by a standardized disease-specific psychometric test and improves clinician-rated global function in patients with mild to moderately severe Alzheimer disease. Improvement was seen as early as three weeks after initiation of therapy. No significant effects were seen in patients assigned to placebo. Based on the changes in the rating scales, physicians should see significant improvement in cognitive and global functions in 35% to 60% of patients and achieve stabilization in an additional 20% to 45%. Also important, the rate of patient withdrawal was much lower for donepezil than rates reported for tacrine and other cholinesterase inhibitors over a similar period.

Drug Therapy for Multiple Sclerosis. Multiple sclerosis (MS) is an inflammatory disease of the central nervous system (CNS) and affects about 300,000 people in the US and more than one million worldwide. About 40% of patients first experience a relapsing-remitting clinical course. Patients are clinically stable between relapses. After repeated attacks, however, the disease course becomes progressive. This stage is called secondary progressive disease. Approximately 15% of all MS patients have primary progressive disease with no distinct relapses and remissions. MS is thought to be triggered by CD4+ T-lymphocytes and therapies aimed at MS have focused on suppressing T-cell activity [*Scrip Magazine*, November 1998, pp 60–64].

In the past few years, new therapeutic options have become available for patients in the relapsing-remitting stage of the disease. They include interferon beta-1b (*Betaseron*), interferon beta-1a (*Avonex*), and glatiramer (*Copaxone*). Glatiramer is a synthetic polypeptide designed to induce tolerance to myelin basic protein (MBP). MBP is thought to be an important auto-antigen in MS, responsible for triggering T-cell attack.

The results of phase III trials of interferon beta-1a and interferon beta-1b for MS were reported recently in *The Lancet*. The PRISMS trial confirms that interferon beta-1a reduces clinical relapse rate, delays time to onset of sustained progression, and reduces the number of CNS lesions detected by MRI in patients with relapsing-remitting MS [*Lancet* 1998;352:1498–504]. The European SP trial of interferon beta-1b in secondary progressive disease shows that treatment significantly delays time to onset of sustained progression of disease and significantly reduces relapse rate and the number of new MRI lesions [*Ibid*, pp 1491-97]. A commentary on these reports says that these findings justify expanding the indications for interferon beta-1b to patients with secondary progressive MS [*Ibid*, pp 1486–87].

A new study from Denmark shows that oral methylprednisolone is effective for the treatment of flare-ups in MS patients [*Neurol* 1998;51:529–34]. This is the first demonstration of the effectiveness of high-dose methyl-prednisolone and adds great weight to the limited evidence supporting any role for the corticosteroid in the amelioration of acute attacks.

The researchers compared the effects of oral high-dose methylpredniso-lone—500 mg once a day for five days with a ten-day tapering period—with placebo in 51 patients who had a MS episode of no longer than four weeks' duration. Patients taking active drug fared consistently better than those taking placebo. At eight weeks after initiating therapy, one-third of patients in the placebo group improved by one point on a disability status scale, whereas two-thirds of patients taking methylprednisolone had a similar im-provement. Resolution of a flare-up, however, seemed to require a longer duration of treatment with oral rather than intravenous methylprednisolone, and oral administration was associated with gastric side effects.

A medical expert in the UK observed: "I tend to favor intravenous methylprednisolone because it enforces bed rest, which by itself may improve the outcome of flare-ups. However, with the present shortage of beds in the UK, it is undoubtedly more cost-effective to give oral preparations." [*Lancet* 1998;352:712].

Obesity

Olestra and Gastrointestinal Symptoms. Olestra (*Olean*) is a mixture of hexa-, hepta-, and octa-esters of sucrose formed from long-chain fatty acids derived from an edible vegetable oil. Olestra is not hydrolyzed after ingestion, is not absorbed, and provides no dietary energy or fat. Although olestra is not a drug, its use as a fat replacement in the diet has the therapeutic intention of reducing the risk of obesity and heart disease. The American Heart Association recommends a diet in which fat contributes 30% or less of total energy.

Critics of technological advances have widely publicized anecdotal reports of people experiencing gastrointestinal (GI) symptoms after consuming products containing olestra. To evaluate the validity of those claims, investigators determined whether *ad libitum* consumption of potato chips with the fat substitute results in more frequent or more intense GI adverse events than do regular chips made with triglyceride [*JAMA* 1998;279:150–52].

More than a thousand subjects were given a beverage and an unlabeled 13-oz bag of potato chips made with olestra or triglyceride during a free movie screening. Among the subjects in the olestra chip group, 15.8% reported one or more GI symptoms, compared with 17.6% of the subjects in the regular chip group. Furthermore, there were no significant differences between the two groups in specific GI symptoms (gas, diarrhea, abdominal cramping). Gourmands will note that significantly fewer olestra chips were consumed than regular chips, with olestra chips receiving lower taste scores. Consumption levels, however, did not correlate with reported symptoms in either group. Although an expert panel recently confirmed the safety of olestra, the FDA will continue to require products that contain olestra to carry a warning label concerning possible gastrointestinal distress.

Oncology

Tamoxifen Reduces the Incidence of Breast Cancer
Aspirin and Colon Cancer
Optimizing Chemotherapy for Childhood Acute
    Lymphoblastic Leukemia
Palliative for Prostate Cancer Offers No Benefit
Carboplatin Monotherapy as Effective as
    Combination Therapy in Ovarian Cancer

Tamoxifen Reduces the Incidence of Breast Cancer. Earlier this year, the front page of *The New York Times* [April 7, 1998, A1] reported: "Researchers Find the First Drug Known to Prevent Breast Cancer." The drug is tamoxifen, a novel molecule with both estrogenic and anti-estrogenic activity. Tamoxifen has been widely used in the treatment of breast cancer since 1978, under the brand name *Nolvadex*. The report in the *Times* relates that an interim analysis of the data from a large, US/Canadian, multicenter study that began in 1992, revealed that a group of women at high risk for breast cancer who took tamoxifen had 45% fewer cases than a similar group of women who took a placebo. Tamoxifen users also had fewer bone fractures of the hip, wrist, and spine than the women who received placebo. The results were so striking that the study's directors stopped the trial 14 months before its scheduled conclusion so that women receiving placebo could consider taking the drug.

Among the more than 13,000 high-risk participants in the study, called the Breast Cancer Prevention Trial (BCPT), were about 4,000 women 60 years old or older. They qualified as high-risk candidates on the basis of age alone. Breast cancer risk increases with age and by age 60, about 17 of every 1,000 women develop the disease within five years. Women as young as 35 years also participated in the study if their risk reached the same threshold. Risk assessment was based on such factors as whether a woman had a mother, sister, or daughter with breast cancer, had a condition that called for a breast biopsy, started menstruating at an early age, and had no children or had pregnancy later in life. Tamoxifen benefited women across all age groups. Women aged 50 years and older, however, derived a greater benefit from tamoxifen than did younger women, but they also had more serious adverse effects. There were no differences in the frequency or severity of adverse events in women younger than 50 years receiving either placebo or tamoxifen.

The full report of BCPT, including three months of data not previously presented, was published in the September 16, 1998, issue of the *Journal of the National Cancer Institute* [1998;90:1371–88]. The update shows a 49% reduction in the incidence of breast cancer among the 13,388 participants. The cumulative incidence of breast cancer through 69 months was 43.4 per 1000 women receiving placebo and 22.0 per 1000 women receiving tamoxifen. A decreased risk occurred in women aged 49 years or younger (44%), 50 to 59 years (51%), and 60 years or older (55%). Tamoxifen administration reduced the occurrence of estrogen-positive tumors by 69%. No benefit was seen in women with estrogen-negative tumors.

The results emerging from BCPT were not a complete surprise to interested scientists and clinicians. Studies have shown that administration of tamoxifen after successful treatment of breast cancer significantly reduces the incidence of cancer in the contralateral breast [*N Engl J Med* 1988;319:1681–92]. Researchers, however, were surprised by the magnitude of the benefit. Federal health officials described the findings as historic because the trial not only demonstrated the effectiveness of tamoxifen for primary prevention but it also offered evidence that its benefits outweigh its risks. The National Cancer Institute estimates that 29 million American women meet the risk eligibility criteria for BCPT and are candidates for tamoxifen prophylaxis.

Tamoxifen, like the pure agonist, estrogen, carries risks. While tamoxifen is an estrogen antagonist in breast tissue, it displays estrogenic activity in uterine tissue. This may lead to endometriosis and endometrial cancer [*J Clin Oncol* 199;16:779–92]. The BCPT reported 36 cases of endometrial cancer in the tamoxifen group compared with 15 in the placebo group. The risk of endometrial cancer associated with tamoxifen remains the largest hurdle to its expanded use for primary prevention. Evidence that the use of progestins with tamoxifen reduces the risk of endometrial stimulation is still preliminary. Whether a progestin-containing intrauterine device applied at the start of tamoxifen treatment will protect the endometrium is under investigation.

Tamoxifen also increases the risk of deep vein thrombosis (DVT) and pulmonary embolism (PE). The crude data from BCPT suggest that tamoxifen compared with placebo increases the risk of DVT by a factor of 1.6, the risk of PE by a factor of 2.8, and the risk of uterine cancer by a factor of 2.4. Another concern is that tamoxifen's benefits may wane after four or five years.

Zeneca, the firm that markets *Nolvadex,* plans to work with the FDA to have tamoxifen approved as quickly as possible for the prevention of breast cancer. Until then, physicians may prescribe tamoxifen for cancer prevention, but Zeneca may not promote the drug for that purpose. Whether or not to prescribe tamoxifen to a patient for primary prevention calls for a careful weighing of her risks of breast cancer and osteoporosis against her risks of endometrial cancer and blood clots. Some experts are urging general practitioners to wait for the guidelines being developed by the National Cancer Institute before prescribing the drug for this purpose.

While deliberating the new indication for tamoxifen, the FDA considered interim results of two trials in Europe, published after the announced findings of BCPT. Neither of the two tamoxifen chemoprevention trials shows the positive result reported by BCPT. One trial, involving only 2471 British women with a median follow-up of 70 months, shows no difference in the incidence of breast cancer (RR, 1.06) between the tamoxifen and placebo groups [*Lancet* 1998;352:98–101]. The second trial, enrolling 5408 Italian women with a median follow-up of 46 months, also finds no difference in the incidence of breast cancer between the tamoxifen and placebo groups [*Lancet* 1998;352:93–97]. Taken together these studies suggest either no effect of tamoxifen on breast cancer or at best a much smaller effect than that found in BCPT.

A commentary in *The Lancet* [1998;352:80–81] asks: Do differences among the three trials account for these contradictory outcomes? The power of BCPT to detect differences was greater than the European studies. Taken together, the two smaller trials provide only about two-thirds of the women-years of follow-up in BCPT. The women enrolled in the Italian trial had a much lower risk for breast cancer that did those in BCPT. The Italian trial also had compliance problems; nearly one-quarter of the women dropped out in the first year of the study. This may be important because the trial shows a preventive effect approaching significance among women who took assigned treatment for more than one year. The Italian trial also had considerably fewer women aged 60 years or older than BCPT. This may also be important because BCPT found a greater benefit of tamoxifen among older women than among younger women, and because the preventive effect in BCPT was confined to estrogen-receptor-positive tumors, which are more common in older women.

The British study enrolled considerably more women under the age of 50 than did BCPT or the Italian trial. The British study also had a longer exposure of women to tamoxifen than did BCPT. There is the possibility that the use of tamoxifen for more than five years may have reduced its protective benefits. Another explanation is that the striking effect seen in

BCPT with its relatively short follow-up is actually a treatment effect on early occult breast cancer; it may disappear with longer follow-up.

The commentary accompanying the European reports concludes that the findings of BCPT seem robust, internally consistent, and consistent with the 47% preventive effect of five years of tamoxifen in an overview of secondary prevention trials. The different results presented in the new reports may be largely due to a younger population in both trials compared with BCPT, to poor compliance in the Italian study, and to differences in the study populations' risk level and family history. "The failure of these trials to confirm the results of the US study, however, casts doubt on the wisdom of the rush . . . to prescribe tamoxifen widely for prevention." The author believes that longer follow-up is required to clarify benefits and risks and to confirm the BCPT results. The International Breast Cancer Prevention Study (IBIS) has now enrolled over 4000 of a target 7000 women and the investigators have determined that they will not stop the study because of reported benefits. The results of this trial, along with additional follow-up data from BCPT, the British study, and the Italian study, will be very important to those deciding how to advise women about breast cancer prevention.

In September, a FDA advisory panel advised the agency that it supported the approval of tamoxifen as a means to reduce the incidence of breast cancer in women at increased risk of the disease. The panel also urged the agency to work with Zeneca to develop a tamoxifen registry system to track outcomes in healthy women using the drug. A registry would also ensure against women receiving tamoxifen without educational material and long-term monitoring [*The Pink Sheet* 1998;60(No36):23–24].

The panel's decision is a boon to both Zeneca and Barr Laboratories, the maker of a generic version of tamoxifen. The recommendation also prompted Eli Lilly to review its marketing strategy for raloxifene (*Evista*), a selective estrogen receptor modulator approved for the treatment of osteoporosis. Lilly is seeking permission to promote the drug for prevention of breast cancer [*The New York Times,* September 3, 1998, p C7].

The advisory committee stopped short of recommending tamoxifen to prevent breast cancer but did agree that it reduced the risk of breast cancer. The panel also warned that it did not yet have enough information to determine which women were at high enough risk of breast cancer to make the drug's adverse effects worth its benefits. Some observers fear that tamoxifen will be over promoted and have an unfavorable benefit to risk ratio in low-risk women. A spokesperson for Zeneca said that the company planned to advertise the drug directly to women in 1999, after first educating general practitioners about its use. The director of the American tamoxifen trial pointed out that the National Cancer Institute has developed a computer program to permit women and their physicians to calculate an individual's risk of developing breast cancer as well compare her risk to that of women in the study. The information is available at the NCI Web site: *http://cancertrials.nci.nih.gov* [*The New York Times,* September 3, 1998, pp A1, A18].

The FDA cleared tamoxifen for marketing in late October [*The Wall Street Journal,* October 30, 1998, p B9]. The agency urged that the drug be prescribed only for women at high risk for developing the disease. Risk factors include women over age 50, those with at least two direct-line relatives with breast cancer, women with atypical breast biopsies, women who had their first child at 30 or older, and those who started menstruating at 11 or younger. Prophylaxis is recommended if a woman has two or more risk factors.

Zeneca will provide materials to physicians to help them determine the risk of individual women and maintain a toll-free hotline (1-800-34 LIFE 4). The recommended course of therapy is five years. Zeneca also announced that it had reached an agreement with Roche Laboratories to co-promote *Novaldex* in the US. A prevention study of tamoxifen in BRCA 1 and BRCA 2 carriers was initiated in the last quarter of 1998. The genetic study, using blood samples from BCPT, will examine whether tamoxifen reduces the risk of breast cancer in these very high-risk women.

Also of interest, the National Cancer Institute plans to launch the largest ever breast cancer clinical trial early in 1999—the Study of Tamoxifen and Raloxifene (STAR) [*Scrip,* October 28, 1998, p 27]. The five-year trial aims to enroll 22,000 postmenopausal women with a significant risk of breast cancer. The primary purpose of the trial is to determine whether raloxifene (*Evista*), which seems safer than tamoxifen, is also effective in reducing the risk of developing breast cancer in women who have not had the disease. Preliminary results from raloxifene trials show no increase in endometrial cancer.

In November 1998, the approval process for the new indication hit a snag because Zeneca and the FDA could not agree on the appropriate wording for a breast cancer prophylaxis indication. Zeneca wishes to use the word "prevention" to describe the benefits of tamoxifen. The FDA advisory group favors wording that describes closely the results of the trial, which would read, ". . . tamoxifen reduces the short-term incidence of breast cancer in women at high risk of developing the disease." Zeneca, however, wishes to see labeling that extrapolates on the results, which would read, ". . . tamoxifen is a preventative agent for the reduction of breast cancer in women at high risk of developing the disease."

Aspirin and Colon Cancer. Molecular evidence suggests that an isoform of cyclooxygenase (COX-2), a mediator of pain and inflammation, plays an important role in colorectal carcinogenesis. Aspirin and currently available nonsteroidal antiinflammatory drugs (NSAIDs) predominantly inhibit COX-1, but also have activity against COX-2. Researchers now think that COX-2 causes colon cancer cells to become resistant to apoptosis—naturally programmed cell death. NSAIDs, to the extent that they inhibit COX-2, restore the cell's ability to die, and cause tumor regression.

Patients with familial adenomatous polyposis (FAP) develop hundreds of intestinal polyps, some of which progress to cancer. Mutations in *APC* (*adenomatous polyposis coli*), the gene affected in FAP, occur in about 90% of colorectal cancers. Investigators have mimicked the phenotype in *APC*-deficient mice, which develop an extraordinary number of polyps within weeks of birth. By deleting one COX-2 gene in these mice, the investigators found that the number of polyps fell by 65%; by deleting both genes the number fell by 85%.

Because of the adverse effects of current NSAIDs on the gastrointestinal tract, presumably a consequence of COX-1 inhibition, colon-cancer prevention trials requiring years of prophylaxis and observation are not feasible. However, drugs that selectively inhibit COX-2 are in development and may be safer and more practical for prophylaxis. While waiting, some physicians may wish to consider prescribing prophylactic treatment with aspirin or another NSAID to high-risk patients. Limiting this option, however, is the question of what dose of aspirin to use.

We know that low-dose aspirin, which protects against coronary artery disease, is not effective for colon cancer prevention. In contrast to most observational studies, the well-controlled Physicians' Health Study (PHS) of men receiving 325 mg aspirin every other day or placebo found no association between aspirin use and colorectal cancer after five years. Although PHS investigators planned a 12-year trial, the aspirin arm of the study was stopped after six years because of very favorable findings. Participants then chose to receive or continue to receive either aspirin or placebo for the rest of the study.

Now, PHS Investigators have revisited the database to determine the effect of randomly assigned aspirin treatment and self-selected aspirin use on the incidence of colorectal cancer after 12 years [*Ann Intern Med* 1998; 128:713–20]. The researchers found no difference in colorectal cancer risk among participants not regularly taking aspirin, those who stopped regular use when the aspirin arm of the trial ended, those who started taking aspirin after the aspirin arm of the trial ended, and those who took aspirin throughout the 12-year study period. The authors suggest that the, ". . . low dose of aspirin used and the short treatment period could account for the null findings." One expert noted that, despite these results, ". . . the potential rewards of reducing a substantial number of deaths through understanding NSAID action remain" [*Lancet* 1998;351:'1334]. Intervention studies are now underway.

Optimizing Chemotherapy for Childhood Acute Lymphoblastic Leukemia.
About 70% of children with acute lymphoblastic leukemia (ALL) recover. Presenting characteristics of those who fail to respond to chemotherapy, however, are similar to those who do respond. One variable that may account in part for the difference in treatment outcome is the child's ability to eliminate anti-leukemic drugs from the body. A greater drug clearance means less exposure to the drug. Those with rapid drug clearance may benefit less than those with slower clearance, if the dose is determined only according to body-surface area. The clearance of anticancer drugs differs by a factor of three to ten among patients.

Previous work shows that outcome is significantly worse among children with ALL who clear methotrexate rapidly and thus have lower plasma levels of the drug than among those with slower clearance and higher sustained plasma levels. On the basis of these findings, researchers carried out a prospective study in newly diagnosed patients. Participants were four months to 19 years old and randomly assigned to receive doses of methotrexate, teniposide, and cytarabine. Dosage was based on either body-surface area or the measured clearance of the drugs in each patient [*N Engl J Med* 1998;338:400–505].

Patients who received individualized doses based on measured clearance had significantly fewer courses of treatment with systemic exposures below the target ranges than did patients who received doses based on body-surface area. Among the 170 patients, the 143 with B-lineage leukemia who received clearance-based therapies had a significantly better outcome than those given body-surface area-based therapies. Rates of continuous complete remission at five years were 76% and 66%, respectively. The risk of relapse for these patients was significantly related to the average systemic exposure to methotrexate, but not to the systemic exposure to teniposide or cytarabine. Methotrexate may be the critical drug for dose adjustments in treatment regimens similar to the one used in this study. The investigators found that individualization provided no benefit for patients with T-lineage leukemia. They conclude that individualizing the dose of methotrexate to account for differences in clearance among patients can improve the outcome in children with B-lineage ALL.

Palliative for Prostate Cancer Offers No Benefit. Patients with metastatic prostate cancer treated with the anti-androgen flutamide (*Eulexin*) after orchiectomy report a lower quality of life than do patients treated with a placebo after surgery [*J Natl Cancer Inst* 1998;90:1537–44]. The 737 participants in the study were drawn from a larger group of patients with prostate cancer enrolled in a study that compared orchiectomy plus flutamide with orchiectomy plus placebo. In the efficacy trial, there were no significant differences in survival or progression-free survival between the two groups [*N Engl J Med* 1998;339:1036–42]. Patients receiving flutamide reported having more diarrhea and worse emotional functioning. The investigators speculate that flutamide's ability to block androgen receptors in the brain may explain the emotional effects of the drug.

Carboplatin Monotherapy as Effective as Combination Therapy in Ovarian Cancer. Ovarian cancer is the leading cause of death from gynecological malignant disease. Surgery generally precedes chemotherapy. Meta-analyses incorporating data from nearly 10,000 patients from 45 randomized trials suggest that, in terms of survival, platinum-based therapy is more effective than a regimen that does not contain a platinum drug. Furthermore, platinum in combination is better than platinum monotherapy, and carboplatin and cisplatin are about equally effective. These results led many to conclude that combination chemotherapy consisting of cyclophosphamide, doxorubicin, and cisplatin (CAP) was probably the most effective treatment for women with ovarian cancer. Platinum, however, continues to be the single most active agent against ovarian cancer, and combination therapy requires a reduction in the dose of platinum to decrease toxicity. For this reason, some practitioners favor treatment with single-agent platinum at the highest tolerated dose.

To resolve the debate over the most effective treatment, researchers undertook a large international trial in 1526 patients that compared CAP with single-agent carboplatin. Carboplatin was chosen for the single-agent group because at optimal doses, it is less toxic than single-agent cisplatin. During the course of the study mortality was the same in the two treatment groups. The results indicate a median survival of 33 months and a two-year survival of 60% for both groups. The investigators found no evidence that CAP or carboplatin was more effective in any subgroup. On the other hand, CAP was considerably more toxic than carboplatin. The authors conclude that single-agent carboplatin is a safe, effective, and appropriate standard treatment for women with advanced ovarian cancer [*Lancet* 1998;352: 1571–76].

Pain Management

Preemptive Analgesia Gives Mixed Results. Despite advances in the management of pain, up to 60% of patients report moderate to severe discomfort after surgery. Current thinking is that tissue damage and pain during surgery sensitizes the central nervous system (CNS) sufficiently to enable subsequent, ordinarily painless, stimuli to be experienced as pain. Preemptive analgesia is a strategy to decrease pain perception and postoperative analgesic needs by using drugs before surgery to prevent sensitization. Preemptive analgesia has been validated in animal studies, but efforts to establish its clinical relevance have yielded mixed results.

A successful application of this strategy is described in a recent report that compared epidural bupivicaine, epidural fentanyl, or no epidural drug given before and during lower abdominal surgery, followed by aggressive postoperative epidural analgesia for all patients. On examining pain scores after surgery, the investigators found that epidural analgesia with bupivicaine or fentanyl significantly decreases postoperative pain during hospitalization and for several weeks after. The researchers believe that the success of their efforts was due, at least in part, to careful attention to postoperative analgesia and its role in preserving the benefits produced by the administration of pain therapy prior to surgery [*JAMA* 1998;279:1076–82].

An unsuccessful application of preemptive analgesia is found in another recent study, this one in patients undergoing lower-limb amputation. The investigators compared epidural bupivicaine and morphine given before, during, and after surgery with postoperative treatment alone. They found, contrary to other studies of phantom limb pain, that preemptive analgesia does not reduce pain intensity nor opioid consumption after surgery.

Differences in the intensity of postoperative pain in the conflicting studies may contribute to the different outcomes. Another confounding element in the amputation study is that, despite randomization, the daily opioid consumption before hospitalization was two-thirds greater in the preemptive analgesia group than in the control group [*Lancet* 1997;350:1353–57]. The jury is still out as to whether this intriguing strategy really works and, if so, under what conditions.

RESPIRATORY DISEASE

Inhaled Corticosteroids and COPD

Prolonged Corticosteroid Therapy Improves Acute
Respiratory Distress Syndrome

Montelukast (*Singulair*) and Salmeterol (*Serevent*)
for Exercise-Induced Asthma

Zafirlukast (*Accolate*) and Montelukast (*Singulair*)
Show Promise in Asthma

Nebulized Budesonide Compared with
Intramuscular Dexamethasone for Croup

Inhaled Corticosteroids and COPD. Chronic obstructive pulmonary disease
(COPD) describes a heterogeneous group of smoking-related lung disorders
such as chronic bronchitis, emphysema, and small-airways disease. Patients
with COPD have progressive deterioration of pulmonary function and quality
of life, and die early as a result of respiratory failure. Current treatment has
limited effectiveness. Pharmaceutical companies view patients with COPD as
a potentially lucrative and untapped market. In societies with large numbers
of smokers, deaths due to COPD far exceed deaths resulting from asthma.
In terms of hospital admissions for adults, COPD is a much greater burden
on health services than is asthma. The incidence of COPD is predicted to
increase threefold in the next decade.

Current treatment for mild to moderate COPD consists of bronchodilators–beta agonists and anticholinergics. Oral theophylline is added for patients
with more severe disease. Oral steroids are used routinely to treat exacerbations, but the place of inhaled steroids in a treatment plan has not been clear.

To address this uncertainty, a group of international researchers initiated
a trial comparing high-dose inhaled fluticasone (*Flovent*), twice daily, with
placebo over a six-month treatment period [*Lancet* 1998;351:773–80]. Participants were 281 current or former smokers between 50 and 75 years old
with a history of chronic bronchitis.

Approximately the same number of people in each group had at least
one exacerbation by the end of treatment. Those who received fluticasone,
however, had significantly fewer moderate or severe exacerbations than those
assigned to placebo. The investigators also observed small but clinically sig-

nificant improvements in peak expiratory flow rate, median symptom scores for daily cough, and sputum volume in those receiving fluticasone, but not in those receiving placebo. Patients on fluticasone were also able to increase their walking distance.

A commentary on this work takes a conservative position and suggests that only patients who show a striking response to oral or inhaled corticosteroids—a significant improvement in peak flow or a decrease in the number or severity of exacerbations—should be treated with inhaled steroids for more than six months. The author does not consider the findings sufficient to jettison current thinking that steroids have little effect on inflammation in COPD [*Lancet* 1998;351:766–67].

More recently, investigators at the European Respiratory Society meeting in September 1998 presented new information on both fluticasone and budesonide (*Pulmicort*), another inhaled steroid, in patients with COPD. Both products showed promising results in long-term studies. Both are already marketed for asthma. The new work suggests that inhaled steroids have an added benefit when used with bronchodilators [*Scrip*, October 7, 1998, p 21].

Data on fluticasone are derived from the three-year Inhaled Steroids in Chronic Obstructive Lung Disease in Europe (ISOLDE) study that involved 990 patients with moderate to severe COPD. After two weeks on oral prednisone, patients received inhaled fluticasone or placebo, and could use albuterol (salbutamol) and ipratropium when required for relief of symptoms. At the end of the study, significantly less deterioration in lung function was seen in the active treatment group than in the placebo group. Differences were evident after three months of therapy and were maintained over the entire study. Fluticasone reduced the exacerbation rate by 25%, and the rate of decline of health status by 35%. The investigators define "health status" as a measure of the effects of COPD on daily life, health, and well being.

Data on budesonide were presented by investigators participating in the European Respiratory Society Study on Inhaled Steroids in COPD (EUROSCOP), which showed a benefit in patients with mild to moderate COPD, and from the Copenhagen City Lung study, which showed no benefit in patients with mild disease. In the EUROSCOP study, the researchers found that at three months, budesonide, like fluticasone, significantly improved lung function, compared with placebo, and that this benefit was maintained for three years.

Prolonged Corticosteroid Therapy Improves Acute Respiratory Distress Syndrome. Acute respiratory distress syndrome (ARDS) is a devastating condition that affects 150,000 people in the US each year. The hallmark of the syndrome is severe hypoxemia. There is no medical treatment for ARDS and mortality is greater than 50%. Although intense inflammatory activity characterizes the syndrome in its first week, meta-analyses of randomized trials investigating a short course of 48 hours or less of high-dose corticosteroid find no evidence of a beneficial effect. Some investigators, however, who examined preliminary data, do report significant improvement in lung function during prolonged administration of corticosteroid.

Researchers have now completed a placebo-controlled trial of 24 patients evaluating the efficacy and safety of prolonged methylprednisolone therapy [*JAMA* 1998;280:159–65]. All participants had severe ARDS and showed no improvement in lung injury score by the seventh day of respiratory failure. Sixteen patients received corticosteroid and eight patients received placebo; assigned treatments were continued for 32 days. Four patients, later determined to be in the placebo group, failed to measurably improve lung injury score after ten days of treatment and were blindly crossed over to the alternative treatment. Primary outcome measures were improvement in lung function and mortality.

At day 10, methylprednisolone, compared with placebo, significantly improved lung injury score (primary outcome measure) and decreased multiple organ dysfunction syndrome score (secondary outcome measure). During the stay in the intensive care unit, all 16 patients treated with prolonged methylprednisolone therapy survived, compared with 5 of 8 patients assigned to placebo. Two additional patients in the treatment group died while in the hospital. On the downside, the rate of infection in methylprednisolone recipients was almost twice as high as in placebo recipients. The small size of the study demands that the beneficial effects of steroids be interpreted with caution. These results should be confirmed in a larger trial before late and prolonged administration of corticosteroid therapy gains widespread acceptance in the treatment of unresolving ARDS [*JAMA* 1998;280:182–83].

Montelukast (Singulair) and Salmeterol (Serevent) for Exercise-Induced Asthma. Exercise-induced bronchoconstriction is now recognized as an integral component of asthma rather than a variant form of the disease. Nearly all people with asthma experience bronchoconstriction when exercising rigorously, particularly in cold, dry air. Inflammatory substances, including cysteinyl leukotrienes, appear to mediate the reduction in airway caliber on cessation of rigorous exercise. Inhaled steroids substantially alleviate exercise-associated symptoms of asthma when taken over long periods. When steroids are not enough, physicians recommend that patients also inhale albuterol, cromolyn, or nedocromil 15 minutes before exercise. Although more effective than placebo, these agents are often less than optimal in children and adult athletes [*N Engl J Med* 1998;339:192–93].

For patients facing this physical challenge, there are new therapeutic options. These advances are highlighted in two recent reports. In one study, investigators evaluated the long-term effects of administering salmeterol, a long-acting beta agonist, to 20 patients with exercise-induced bronchoconstriction [*N Engl J Med* 1998;339:141–46]. The question they addressed is timely because there is concern that patients on long-term therapy with beta agonists may develop tachyphylaxis—a gradual loss of therapeutic benefit with continuous administration. Some think extended use of these agents may even worsen the disease.

Each patient received inhaled salmeterol (*Serevent*) or placebo twice daily for one month and then, after a one-week washout, crossed over to the other treatment for another month. On several occasions during each month of treatment, patients were asked to undergo a brief but vigorous period of stationary cycling while breathing cold air one-half hour after a morning dose and again at nine hours after the dose. The primary endpoint was the measure of the decrease in forced expiratory volume in one second (FEV_1) ten minutes after exertion.

The investigators found that salmeterol offers considerable protection against bronchoconstriction after exercise. They also noted no loss of benefit after a full month of treatment. The duration of protection after the inhalation of salmeterol, however, decreased sharply over time. On the first day of dosing, protection at nine hours after the dose was about the same as protection at 30 minutes. By day 14, however, the protective effect of salmeterol at nine hours was much less than at 30 minutes, and by day 29, there was no protection at nine hours. Nevertheless, the effectiveness of salmeterol is maintained for at least 30 minutes after inhalation during regular use for at least 30 days. This duration of protection on long-term therapy with salmeterol is probably greater than that offered by albuterol. An editorial on the work suggests that, ". . . clinicians may want to recommend salmeterol in preference to albuterol for the prevention of exercise-induced symptoms in patients with asthma who are physically active. . . ."

Another report in the same issue of *The New England Journal of Medicine* [1998;339:147–52] evaluated the ability of montelukast, a new leukotriene-receptor antagonist, to protect patients with mild asthma against exercise-induced bronchoconstriction. Clinical studies show that inhibitors of the synthesis of leukotriene and leukotriene-receptor antagonists are effective against exercise-induced bronchoconstriction.

The investigators randomized 110 patients with mild asthma who required only an inhaled short-acting beta agonist to receive 10 mg of montelukast (*Singulair*) or placebo once daily at bedtime for 12 weeks. Exercise challenges were performed on several occasions during treatment. At 12 weeks, montelukast inhibited exercise-induced bronchoconstriction by an average of almost 50%. Nearly one-quarter of the patients had complete protection—a decrease in FEV_1 of less than 10% after exercise. In the 75% of patients who responded to montelukast, protective effect persisted for at least 20 hours during long-term administration. Therefore, differentiating montelukast from a long-acting beta agonist is its ability to maintain the initial protective effect against exercise-induced bronchoconstriction after long-term therapy.

While the findings in these reports are important, we must be mindful of limitations. The studies compare the agents with placebo and not with a recommended medication such as an inhaled steroid. They include only patients with readily-controlled, stable asthma. Extending the research findings to patients with more severe asthma is, at this time, a leap of faith. Surely, however, a course of salmeterol or montelukast for patients who do not derive sufficient protection against exercise-induced bronchoconstriction from inhaled steroids seems to be a reasonable strategy.

Zafirlukast (Accolate) and Montelukast (Singulair) Show Promise in Asthma. New data on two leukotriene antagonists, zafirlukast and montelukast, were presented at the European Respiratory Society meeting in September 1998. These reports will increase interest in this new class of drugs for the treatment of asthma [*Scrip,* October 7, 1998, p 24]. The most recent guidelines from the National Heart, Lung, and Blood Institute suggest that leukotriene inhibitors may be used as an alternative to low-dose inhaled steroids in mild, persistent asthma. These agents are now the second most prescribed drugs for controlling asthma, behind inhaled corticosteroids but ahead of cromoglycate and nedocromil. In practice, leukotriene inhibitors are used both as first-line maintenance therapy in place of inhaled steroids in new patients, and as add-on therapy for patients already receiving inhaled steroids.

In a four-week crossover study, 70% of adolescents with asthma reported that they preferred *Accolate* tablets over inhaled beclomethasone (*Beclovent*). This suggests that the use of *Accolate* may result in improved compliance with prescribed therapy. Another study showed that adding *Accolate* to inhaled beclomethasone in patients who were symptomatic despite treatment produced improvements similar to those achieved by doubling the dose of the steroid. A large 12-week study comparing *Singulair* once daily with inhaled beclomethasone twice daily demonstrated that the leukotriene antagonist results in a larger initial response and a more rapid onset of action than the steroid. Overall, however, inhaled beclomethasone produced a larger average treatment response than did *Singulair*.

Nebulized Budesonide Compared with Intramuscular Dexamethasone for Croup. Croup is a syndrome of upper-airway obstruction, usually of viral origin, with characteristic symptoms. Each year, it is diagnosed in about 3% of all children under six years of age. Treatment consists of dexamethasone, given orally or by injection. There is preliminary evidence that inhaled budesonide may also be effective. To determine if budesonide is effective and how it compares with dexamethasone given by intramuscular (IM) injection, investigators recruited 144 children with croup and randomly assigned them to nebulized budesonide, IM dexamethasone, or placebo. All children also received racepinephrine. The children were assessed before treatment and then hourly for five hours. The investigators were particularly eager to learn whether active treatment reduced hospitalization rates.

Hospitalization was required for 71% of the children assigned placebo, 38% in the budesonide group, and 23% in the dexamethasone group. Children treated with budesonide or dexamethasone also had a significant improvement in croup scores, compared with children who were given placebo. Those treated with dexamethasone, however, had a greater improvement than those treated with budesonide.

The investigators conclude: "In children with moderately severe croup, treatment with intramuscular dexamethasone or nebulized budesonide resulted in more rapid clinical improvement that did the administration of placebo, with dexamethasone offering the greater improvement" [*N Engl J Med* 1998;339:498–503]. Another recent study reports that the clinical effect of nebulized budesonide is similar to that of oral dexamethasone [*JAMA* 1998;279:1629–32].

TRANSPLANTATION

Risk of Cancer in Kidney-Allograft Recipients. The introduction of cyclosporine (*Sandimmune*) was essential for the development of organ transplant surgery. Cyclosporine, however, is not a magic bullet and is potentially toxic to various tissues. To minimize these adverse effects, clinicians adjust the dose of cyclosporine to keep blood levels in a fairly narrow range. Clinicians strive to keep end-of-dose (trough) levels between 150 to 250 ng/ml. The degree of immunosuppression resulting from this range of blood levels, however, significantly increases the risk of infections and tumors. This dilemma is especially difficult in the management of kidney transplant recipients. A side-effect profile that is acceptable for heart, lung, and liver transplant recipients, for whom there is no life-sustaining option, is less so for kidney recipients, for whom dialysis is available. The weight of side effects, however, must be tempered by the results of studies that find renal-transplant recipients have a better quality of life and live longer than do patients maintained on dialysis [*Lancet* 1998;351:610–611].

Some experts think that the risk of cancer varies with the intensity of immunosuppression. To assess this variable risk, researchers studied more than 200 recipients of a first kidney allograft. All patients received cyclosporine and most received azathioprine. One year after transplantation, the investigators randomized half the patients to receive cyclosporine doses adjusted to yield trough blood concentrations of 75–125 ng/ml (low-dose group); the others received doses that yielded trough levels of 150–250 ng/ml (usual-dose group) [*Lancet* 1998;351:623–28]. Both groups were followed for about six years.

Mean trough blood concentrations after three months of therapy were about 200 ng/ml in the usual-dose group and 100 ng/ml in the low-dose group, and remained stable throughout the study. Despite the twofold difference in trough levels, there were no differences between the groups in renal function, graft survival, or overall survival. Episodes of graft rejection were uncommon but seen more frequently in the low-dose group. Sixty patients developed at least one cancer, 37 in the usual-dose group and 23 in the low-dose group. Two thirds of the 65 malignancies were skin cancers.

Sunlight, by causing DNA damage and by inducing immunological unrespon-siveness, strongly influences the pathogenesis of skin cancer. In light of these findings, physicians need to consider the optimal intensity of immunosup-pression and to persuade post-transplant patients to treat sunshine as radiation.

Women's Health

Fosamax Prevents Bone Loss in Postmenopausal Women
Estrogen/Bisphosphonate Combination for
    Osteoporosis
Fluoride Decreases Vertebral Fracture Rates
Parathyroid Hormone Prevents Bone Loss in Women
    Treated for Endometriosis
Aspirin Does Not Prevent Preeclampsia
Isosorbide Mononitrate for Cervical Ripening before
    Abortion
Benefit of Emergency Contraception Available without a
    Prescription
Better Tolerated and More Effective Emergency
    Contraception
Bisphosphonate Reduces Risk of Breast Cancer
    Recurrence and Mortality
Spermicide (Nonoxynol 9) Does Not Reduce
    Transmission of STDs
Calcium Supplements Ameliorate PMS and May Provide
    Other Benefits

Fosamax Prevents Bone Loss in Postmenopausal Women. The approval of alendronate (*Fosamax*) was a welcome addition to the choices available for the prevention of osteoporosis and bone fractures—a common and frightening condition in postmenopausal women. *Fosamax* is an orally effective bisphosphonate. This class of drugs inhibits bone resorption and increases bone mineral density. Another bisphosphonate, etidronate, is widely used in Europe for postmenopausal osteoporosis. Before *Fosamax,* a woman's choice was limited to estrogen, which has discomfiting side effects and is feared because of the risk of breast cancer, and calcitonin, a hormone available as an injection or nasal spray. Calcitonin is both expensive and inconvenient to use. Now, the selective estrogen modulator raloxifene (*Evista*) joins alendronate as an oral drug for the prevention of osteoporosis.

Fosamax reduces the incidence of vertebral and other fractures in postmenopausal women with osteoporosis. How does *Fosamax* compare with estrogen in preventing bone loss in this at-risk population? Seeking an answer, investigators compared the effects of *Fosamax* with placebo in nearly 1,200 postmenopausal women under the age of 60. Another 435 women were assigned to either *Fosamax* or a combination of estrogen (*Premarin*) and progestin, medroxyprogesterone (*Provera*). When given with an estrogen, a progestin decreases the risk of endometrial changes that could lead to cancer. All patients were followed for two years.

The women who received placebo lost bone mineral density (BMD) at all measured sites. *Fosamax* 5 mg daily increased BMD by 3.5% at the lumbar spine and 1.9% at the hip, but only slowed the loss at the forearm. The estrogen-progestin combination prevented bone loss at all sites and was more effective than *Fosamax*. Although estrogen outperforms *Fosamax* in preventing the loss of BMD, there is no certainty that the same applies in preventing bone fractures.

There are reports of esophageal ulceration and upper gastrointestinal symptoms in people taking *Fosamax;* these problems were not encountered in this study. Some receiving the estrogen-progestin combination complained of withdrawal bleeding and breast tenderness. Until there is more information, estrogen taken with a progestin remains the first-line drug to prevent or treat osteoporosis in postmenopausal women. It is more effective than *Fosamax* in preventing bone loss and may have favorable effects on cardiovascular outcomes and cognitive function in the elderly. *Fosamax* is an effective alternative for women who do not tolerate estrogen therapy or who refuse to use it. Whether *Evista,* with its promise of a reduced risk of breast cancer, will overtake *Premarin* in the osteoporosis market remains to be seen.

Estrogen/Bisphosphonate Combination for Osteoporosis. Hormone replacement therapy (HRT) remains the most effective agent to prevent and treat postmenopausal osteoporosis, but alendronate, a bisphosphonate, and raloxifene, a selective estrogen receptor modulator, are important alternatives. Some physicians also favor HRT because they believe that estrogen protects against coronary artery disease and may delay the onset and/or mitigate the symptoms of Alzheimer disease. Etidronate, another bisphosphonate, has been show to reduce bone loss by inhibiting osteoclastic activity and decreasing bone turnover. Continuous treatment with etidronate, however, may need to be limited in duration because of demineralization effects that may increase the risk of fracture. Cyclical etidronate is used for osteoporosis therapy outside of the US.

Some women may benefit from combination therapy with estrogen and a bisphosphonate. To this end, investigators randomized 72 postmenopausal women with established osteoporosis into one of four treatment groups, including a placebo group, and monitored their progress over four years. The HRT group received cyclical estrogen and progesterone, the etidronate group received intermittent cyclic etidronate, and the combined therapy group received both HRT and etidronate. All patients also received calcium and vitamin D. BMD was measured in the lumbar spine and hip before treatment and at two and four years during treatment [*Am J Med* 1998;104: 219–26].

Women who received combination therapy had a 10.4% increase in BMD in the lumbar spine and a 7.0% increase in the hip. Corresponding figures for the etidronate group were 7.3% and 0.9%, and for the HRT group, 7.0% and 4.8%, respectively. The group treated with only calcium and vitamin D lost 2.5% and 4.4% of BMD in the lumbar spine and hip, respectively. Height loss, an indicator of new vertebral fractures, was significantly less in all three active treatment groups, in comparison with the control group. The combination group, however, did not have a significant loss of height, in comparison with the HRT and the etidronate groups. Despite the relatively small number of participants, the trial convincingly suggests that combination therapy is superior to either HRT or etidronate alone.

Fluoride Decreases Vertebral Fracture Rates. Although fluoride salts are effective to increase bone mass, none is approved for osteoporosis because there is conflicting evidence concerning their effect on osteoporotic fractures. Discrepant results have been seen in studies evaluating the quality of newly synthesized bone; discrepancies may be related to differences in fluoride dose, formulation, regimen, duration of continuous therapy, and patient population.

Although fluoride appears to work primarily by increasing bone mineral content without necessarily restoring disrupted bone tissue integrity, it may be useful for patients with mild to moderate osteoporosis in whom the microarchitecture is not excessively damaged. To test this hypothesis, investigators compared the effects of low-dose fluoride (sodium monofluorophosphate) plus calcium with the effects of calcium alone over four years in 200 postmenopausal women with moderately low BMD of the spine. Measured endpoints were vertebral fractures and BMD of the hip and spine.

The combination of fluoride and calcium markedly reduced the rate of new vertebral fractures compared with calcium alone (2.4% vs. 10%), and increased BMD of the spine more so than calcium alone. Both treatments increased BMD of the hip nearly equally. Sodium monofluorophosphate used in conjunction with a calcium supplement may be a useful alternative for the treatment of early osteoporosis in postmenopausal women.

Parathyroid Hormone Prevents Bone Loss in Women Treated for Endometriosis. There is evidence that short-term intermittent administration of parathyroid hormone (PTH) prevents bone loss from the spine of women with endometriosis who are estrogen deficient because of treatment with gonadotropin-releasing hormone (GnRH). A recent report describes efforts to determine whether more prolonged administration of PTH can prevent estrogen deficiency bone loss from the spine as well as from other sites in young women with endometriosis receiving intranasal nafarelin (*Synarel*), an analog of GnRH [*JAMA* 1998;280:1067–73].

The investigators enrolled 43 women between 21 and 45 years old with symptomatic endometriosis. Over a period of 12 months, the participants received twice-daily doses of nafarelin alone or nafarelin plus a single subcutaneous injection of human PTH. After 12 months, BMDs in the spine, femoral neck, trochanter, and radial shaft were 4% to 5% lower than at baseline in the women receiving only nafarelin. In contrast, the addition of PTH increased BMDs throughout the body, despite severe estrogen deficiency. Whether PTH prevents bone loss in women entering the natural menopause remains to be determined.

Aspirin Does Not Prevent Preeclampsia. Preeclampsia, defined as hypertension and proteinuria after 20 weeks' gestation, is a common, sometimes life-threatening complication of pregnancy. In principle, aspirin seems a reasonable choice for therapy because the disease is thought to result in part from an imbalance between vasodilating and vasoconstricting prostaglandins. Aspirin selectively inhibits prostaglandins and may result in a more favorable balance. Early, single-center trials in women at increased risk reported that low-dose aspirin reduces the incidence of preeclampsia and significantly improves outcomes in the newborn. These findings prompted widespread prophylactic use of aspirin. Subsequently, however, large multicenter trials found no beneficial effects of aspirin. These later studies are difficult to interpret because, although they were designed to enroll women at increased risk, preeclampsia occurred in less than 10% of the women in the placebo arms of the trials.

In light of the confusion, researchers initiated a well-controlled trial comparing low-dose aspirin, 60 mg daily, and placebo in about 2,500 pregnant women. The investigators were careful to enroll only women with well-defined risk factors. The enrollees included women with pregestational insulin-treated diabetes mellitus, chronic hypertension, and multifetal gestations, as well as women who had had preeclampsia during a previous pregnancy. Between gestation weeks 13 and 26, the participants received either aspirin 60 mg or placebo daily.

The investigators report that the incidence of preeclampsia was similar in the aspirin group and in the placebo group (18% vs. 20%). The incidences in the aspirin and placebo groups for each of the four high-risk categories were also similar. Furthermore, aspirin had no effect on the incidence of perinatal death, preterm birth, or infants small for gestational age [*N Engl J Med* 1998;338:701–05]. The investigators conclude that aspirin should not be given to prevent preeclampsia. A commentary on the report, however, suggests that the door is not permanently closed to the possibility that low-dose aspirin may prevent the disease in certain high-risk women [*N Engl J Med* 1998;338:756–57].

Isosorbide Mononitrate for Cervical Ripening before Abortion. Cervical ripening before first-trimester surgical termination of pregnancy facilitates the procedure and reduces perioperative morbidity. In the US, a natural product called laminaria is favored for this purpose, while in the UK, physicians prefer a prostaglandin such as gemeprost. Prostaglandins, however, are not ideal because they may cause abdominal pain, nausea, vomiting, and diarrhea.

Nitric oxide is a primary mediator of cervical ripening in animals, and sodium nitroprusside, a nitric oxide donor, results in effective ripening when applied locally to the cervix. A controlled trial in women in the first trimester of pregnancy showed that vaginally administered isosorbide-5-mononitrate and glyceryl trinitrate, other nitric oxide donors, induce effective ripening, compared with no treatment [*Br J Obstet Gynaecol* 1997;104:1054–57].

Postulating that nitric oxide donors can ripen the cervix with fewer side effects than prostaglandins, researchers randomly assigned 66 women, pregnant for the first time and scheduled for surgical termination of pregnancy, to receive isosorbide mononitrate or gemeprost before surgery [*Lancet* 1998;352:1093–96]. The primary outcome was the onset of new unwanted symptoms before termination of pregnancy.

The investigators found that more women remained symptom-free after isosorbide mononitrate than after gemeprost (64% vs. 14%). Gemeprost produced abdominal pain in 73% of women, compared with 3% receiving isosorbide mononitrate. Vaginal bleeding occurred in 32% of the women given gemeprost, while no bleeding was reported in women treated with isosorbide mononitrate. Headache occurred in more than a quarter of the group receiving the mononitrate, but was not a problem in women treated with the prostaglandin. Gemeprost was more effective in cervical ripening than 20 or 40 mg isosorbide mononitrate, but the nitric acid donor was sufficiently effective to be used as an alternative to gemeprost for this indication.

Benefit of Emergency Contraception Available without a Prescription. Family planning experts estimate that emergency postcoital contraception could prevent 1.7 million unwanted pregnancies and nearly one million abortions each year in the US. An increasing number of women are learning about this option but it remains underused because, with few exceptions, the method must be prescribed by a physician and taken within 72 hours of intercourse. Some fear that easier access to emergency contraception might encourage promiscuity and unsafe sexual relations, and discourage the use of more reliable contraception. With these considerations in mind, investigators in the UK have studied how women behave if emergency contraceptives are immediately available and the effect such availability has on the number of unintended pregnancies [*N Engl J Med* 1998;339:1–4].

They assigned more than 500 women to be given either a replaceable supply of hormonal emergency contraceptive pills to use at home (the treatment group) or to avail themselves of emergency contraception by calling or visiting a physician and having a prescription ordered and filled (the control group). The emergency contraceptive regimen consisted of four tablets, each containing 50 μg of ethinyl estradiol and 0.25 mg of levonorgestrel. The frequency of use of emergency contraception, the use of other contraceptives, and the incidence of unintended pregnancy were determined in both groups of women one year later.

The researchers found that 47% of women in the treatment group, compared with 27% of women in the control group, used emergency contraception at least once. There were no serious side effects. The women given the discretion to use emergency contraception as required were no more likely to use this method repeatedly than those required to seek a prescription. Their use of other methods of contraception was no different from that of the women in the control group. There were 18 unintended pregnancies in the treatment group and 25 in the control group. The authors conclude that making emergency contraception obtainable does no harm and may reduce the rate of unwanted pregnancies.

Another strategy to improve access to emergency contraception has been introduced in Washington State. There, women may obtain emergency contraception without a prescription at any time of the day or night, seven days a week, from certified pharmacists by calling a telephone number to determine the nearest location of a participating pharmacy. The program began in March and by June pharmacists had filled 2700 requests for emergency contraceptives [*Scrip*, August 14, 1998, p 18].

Better Tolerated and More Effective Emergency Contraception. Emergency contraception works by either inhibiting or delaying ovulation or preventing implantation of the fertilized ovum. It is not a form of abortion. Improvements in emergency contraception and its availability may lead to lower rates of induced abortion, a welcome proposition.

The most widely used approach to emergency contraception is the Yuzpe method. It is based on a modified regimen of combined oral contraceptive pills and involves taking 500 μg levonorgestrel and 100 μg ethinylestradiol. The first dose must be taken within 72 hours of unprotected sex and repeated after 12 hours. Although the regimen is safe, about half the women using it report nausea and about 20% vomit after treatment. A new study shows that 750 μg levonorgestrel alone is better tolerated and more effective as post-coital emergency contraception than the standard Yuzpe regimen [*Lancet* 1998;352:428–33].

To demonstrate the improvement, investigators enrolled nearly 2000 women at 21 centers worldwide to participate in a double-blind randomized comparison of the two regimens when started within 72 hours of unprotected intercourse. Pregnancy rate was 1.1% in the levonorgestrel group and 3.2% in the Yuzpe group. The proportion of pregnancies prevented was 85% in the levonorgestrel-only group and 57% in the Yuzpe group. Nausea (23.1% vs. 50.5%) and vomiting (5.6% vs. 18.8%) were significantly lower with the levonorgestrel regimen that with the Yuzpe regimen. The effectiveness of both treatments declined with increasing time after unprotected coitus. Among women receiving levonorgestrel alone, the pregnancy rate was 0.4% when medication was taken within 24 hours of coitus and 2.7% when taken 49 to 72 hours of coitus. The corresponding rates for the Yuzpe regimen were 2.0% and 4.7%. Neither regimen substantially delayed the onset of next menses. This is an important finding because such delays can worry women who are already concerned about the possibility of an unintended pregnancy.

A privately held US company, The Women's Capital Corporation (WCC), is planning to submit a new drug application to the FDA for emergency contraception using levonorgestrel only. The organization was established in 1997 with the aim of bringing emergency contraception to US and Canadian women. WCC is closely tied to the program in Washington State that permits pharmacists to provide emergency contraception with no prescription necessary [*Scrip*, August 14, 1998, p 18].

Bisphosphonate Reduces Risk of Breast Cancer Recurrence and Mortality.

Bone is the most common site of metastases in breast cancer, and bone metastases are the cause of substantial morbidity and complications [*N Engl J Med* 1998;449:974–84]. A recent report shows that clodronate (*Ostac*), a new bisphosphonate that is not yet available in the US, provides significant benefit to women with breast cancer [*N Engl J Med* 1998;339:357–63].

Bisphosphonates inhibit the loss of bone caused by excess osteoclast activity. Alendronate (*Fosamax*) is approved for the prevention and treatment of osteoporosis, and etidronate (*Didronel*) is used outside the US for the same purpose. Pamidronate (*Aredia*) has FDA approval for use in patients with metastatic cancers that involve bone. Clinical trials have demonstrated the anti-osteolytic effects of bisphosphonates in patients with breast cancer and metastatic bone disease. Clodronate has been shown to reduce the number of new skeletal metastases in patients with breast cancer who have advanced disease without preexisting bony metastases.

In the new study, investigators evaluated the effect of treatment with oral clodronate in 302 patients with primary breast cancer and tumor cells in the bone marrow—a risk factor for the development of distant metastases and disease recurrence. After surgery, patients were randomly assigned to receive either oral clodronate for two years or standard follow-up, in addition to customary hormone therapy or chemotherapy. Three years after surgery, only 21 of 157 patients in the clodronate group developed distant metastases, compared with 42 of 145 in the standard therapy group. Only six patients treated with clodronate died, compared with 22 in the control group.

Some experts say that bisphosphonates are effective against breast cancer because they slow the growth of new tumors in the bone by turning off growth factors, rather than by attacking cancer cells directly. This mechanism, however, does not explain why clodronate decreases both bone and visceral metastases, the most interesting finding of the study. Bisphosphonates do not appear to have cytotoxic effects, but they may induce apoptosis.

Spermicide (Nonoxynol 9) Does Not Reduce Transmission of STDs.

Nonoxynol 9 is a nonionic surface-active agent used as a spermicide for the past 40 years. It inactivates many sexually transmitted pathogens *in vitro* by disrupting membranes. Evidence from *in vitro* studies and animal models shows that nonoxynol 9 can inactivate HIV, but clinical studies have had conflicting results.

To resolve this important issue, researchers enrolled 1292 HIV-negative female sex workers in the Cameroon in a double-blind placebo controlled study in which the women were randomly assigned to use either a film containing nonoxynol 9 or a placebo film. The film was inserted into the vagina before intercourse. The film—5 cm by 5 cm and paper thin—dissolves in two to five minutes. The women were also given condoms and urged to have sex partners use them. At monthly follow-up visits, the investigators looked for genital lesions and tested for gonorrhea, chlamydia, and HIV infection.

Rates of HIV infection were 6.7 cases per 100 women-years in the nonoxynol 9 group and 6.6 in the placebo group. The rates of gonorrhea were 33.3 and 31.1 in the nonoxynol 9 and placebo groups, respectively, and the corresponding rates of chlamydia infection were 20.6 and 22.2. Nonoxynol 9 appeared to increase the rate of genital lesions, compared with placebo. The authors caution that although the spermicide product tested did not show evidence of protection against sexually transmitted diseases (STDs), the disappointing results should not be overly generalized. Other formulations of nonoxynol 9, as well as other microbicidal agents with different mechanisms of action, need testing. They conclude that, ". . . barrier methods controlled by women are urgently needed . . ." [*N Engl J Med* 1998;339:504–10].

Calcium Supplements Ameliorate PMS and May Provide Other Benefits. Women who experience the discomfort of premenstrual syndrome (PMS) may find relief by taking supplemental calcium, according to a new report in the *American Journal of Obstetrics and Gynecology* [1998;179:444–52]. For the study, investigators randomly assigned about 500 women with mild to moderate PMS to take either two 300 mg tablets of a chewable calcium supplement (*Tums E-X*) or placebo twice daily. Over the next three months, the participants maintained a diary to track the severity of 17 physical and emotional symptoms within four categories—mood swings, water retention, food cravings, and pain. The research found that within two to three months calcium carbonate was effective in all four categories of symptoms, as well as in 15 of the 17 individual symptoms. Women receiving calcium experienced a 50% reduction in pain, while the women assigned to placebo reported a modest increase in pain. Twice as many women on calcium said they felt less moody and depressed than did women not receiving calcium. The researchers raise the provocative idea that PMS might be a sign of chronic calcium deficiency and a predictor of osteoporosis in the future. The *Prescriber's Letter* [September 1998, p 53] observes: "It's hard to get young women to increase calcium intake to prevent osteoporosis 30 years down the road. Getting them to take calcium to improve PMS is much easier."

According to a report in *The New York Times* [October 13, 1998, pp D1,D9], ". . . calcium is fast emerging as the nutrient of the decade." The importance of calcium in the formation and maintenance of bone and teeth is long recognized, but other benefits may also accrue. The ongoing remodeling of bones continually releases calcium into the system, where it may play a key role in controlling blood pressure, reducing the risk of colon cancer, as well as ameliorating premenstrual syndrome. The focus on calcium is timely because the US population is becoming increasingly deficient in calcium and vitamin D—the agent that allows the body to absorb and utilize calcium. Calcium deficiency in children is a harbinger of osteoporosis in the future.

Among the recent findings is a reduction in blood pressure among women with mild hypertension after exposures to ultraviolet-B radiation, which stimulates the production of vitamin D [*JAMA* 1998;28:1704–09]. In another study, researchers found that women who were given calcium supplements during pregnancy had children whose blood pressure remained below average for at least the first seven years of life. Previous studies suggest that these children would have a lower risk of developing hypertension. Still another study reported that adding calcium to the diet lowered blood pressure in a group of female teenagers who normally consumed little calcium.

Investigators are now exploring the possibility that low intake of calcium-rich products may partly account for the high rates of hypertension among African-Americans. Some experts now believe that increased consumption of calcium-rich foods is more effective than a low-sodium diet to curb hypertension. A study called DASH (Dietary Approaches to Stop Hypertension) found that a diet rich in low-fat dairy products, fruits, and vegetables significantly lowered blood pressure in adults with high-normal pressure or mild hypertension, although participants lost no weight and continued to consume sodium as desired. The high-calcium diet used in DASH provided up to 1200 mg calcium per day. Nearly half of Americans consume less than 450 mg calcium a day.

Studies have linked high fat diets to colon cancer and shown that fatty acids and bile acids secreted in the digestive process stimulate abnormal cell proliferation in the colon. Calcium binds to these acids and renders them poorly water soluble and benign. Clinical studies suggest that calcium supplements or calcium-rich foods can inhibit cell proliferation in the colon, which may reduce the risk of cancer. The most recent study shows that increasing the daily intake of calcium by up to 1200 mg by means of a diet containing low-fat dairy foods in subjects at risk for colonic neoplasia reduces proliferative activity of colonic epithelial cells.

Men's Health

Proscar Effective for Men with Enlarged Prostate Glands. Benign prostatic hyperplasia (BPH) is common among older men and its symptoms are a significant distraction. BPH, if left untreated, can progress and present serious urological complications. Only recently have drugs been introduced to treat the condition medically. Finasteride (*Proscar*) is the first drug to receive approval for use in BPH. *Proscar* is an inhibitor of 5-alpha reductase, the enzyme required to convert testosterone to dihydrotestosterone (DHT). DHT stimulates the proliferation of prostatic tissue and leads to an enlarged prostate gland. Two large clinical trials show that *Proscar* is effective in men with BPH.

The introduction of *Proscar* was followed by the approval of several other agents with a different mechanism of action—terazosin (*Hytrin*), doxazosin (*Cardura*), and tamsulosin (*Flomax*). These agents are long-acting $alpha_1$-adrenergic antagonists, a class of drugs once often-prescribed to lower blood pressure. These drugs work by relaxing smooth muscle and reducing bladder-outlet obstruction. They too have been found to be safe and effective. Which of these two types of medication is better?

In 1996, in a head-to-head comparison, investigators reported that *Hytrin* is significantly more effective than *Proscar* at improving symptoms and increasing peak urinary-flow rate in men with BPH and that *Proscar* is no more effective than placebo. What is the explanation for the divergence of results from this study and the original placebo-controlled trials of *Proscar*? The answer lies in patient selection. The original studies enrolled men with enlarged prostates. In the comparison study, on the other hand, enlarged prostate was not one of the entrance requirements. Average prostatic volume among the men in the comparison study was significantly smaller than the average volume among those participating in the original studies.

To set the record straight, a new placebo-controlled trial shows that *Proscar* significantly decreases symptoms, improves urinary flow rates, and reduces prostate volume in men with BPH and an enlarged prostate gland [*N Engl J Med* 1998;338:557–63]. The average prostatic volume among men participating in the new trial was 55 ml, compared with an average volume of 37 ml for men in the comparison study reported in 1996. The new trial also shows, for the first time for any agent, that finasteride reduces the risk of acute urinary retention and the need for surgery.

The data now available indicate that physicians should consider prescribing *Proscar* only for symptomatic men with an enlarged prostate gland. In the absence of enlargement, symptomatic patients will do better on a long-acting alpha$_1$-adrenergic antagonist such as *Hytrin*. Alpha$_1$-adrenergic antagonists may be as effective as or even more effective than *Proscar* in reducing symptoms of urinary obstruction in men with enlarged prostates, but there is no current evidence that alpha blockers reduce acute complication of BPH or the need for surgery.

CHILDREN'S HEALTH

Growth Hormone for Short Normal Girls
Sertraline (*Zoloft*) in Children and
Adolescents with OCD

Growth Hormone for Short Normal Girls. Many pediatricians and pediatric endocrinologists prescribe human growth hormone off-label for short normal children, especially boys. There is, however, little information on long-term outcomes. Most studies in boys have shown no significant improvement over predicted or target (genetic potential) height. In light of the differences between boys and girls at the start and progression of puberty, investigators became interested in studying the effects of growth hormone in short normal girls [*Lancet* 1998;351:940–44].

The researchers identified 40 girls with a mean age of eight years and height two standard deviations or more below the mean for their age as potential candidates for a randomized controlled study. Completing the six-year study were seven girls who received an injection of growth hormone daily, six girls who were randomly assigned to no treatment, and 19 girls whose parents did not consent to randomization.

During the course of the study there was no difference in growth patterns between girls in the no-treatment control group and girls who refused to participate. Girls treated with growth hormone grew significantly more than did girls in the two untreated groups. At a mean age of about 16 years, girls in the growth hormone group were taller than the girls in the control and non-consent groups by 7.5 cm and 6.0 cm, respectively. Treatment did not compromise or affect any stage of puberty. While growth hormone was effective in young girls, the cost of treatment worked out to be $18,000 per cm of height gained.

Sertraline (Zoloft) in Children and Adolescents with OCD. Surveys estimate that 1 in 200 young people have obsessive-compulsive disorder (OCD). People with OCD attempt to ignore or suppress obsessive thoughts by carrying out compulsions—repetitive, purposeful behavior. Compulsions can be observable behavior (e.g., hand washing) or covert mental acts (e.g., counting). The clinical literature indicates that potent SSRIs are effective treatments for adults as well as for children and adolescents, although the evidence is less robust for young patients. Clomipramine (*Anafranil*) is quite effective but causes a wide range of adverse effects, including excessive sedation, weight gain, adverse cardiovascular complications, and increased risk of seizures.

Seeking a safer treatment strategy, investigators carried out a 12-week well-controlled trial of the SSRI sertraline (*Zoloft*) against placebo in 187 children 6 to 12 years old and 80 adolescents 13 to 17 years old with OCD. Comparison of scores on two-standard obsessive compulsive scales, a severity of illness scale (CGI-S), and an improvement scale (CGI-I) was used to evaluate outcomes.

Patients treated with sertraline showed significantly greater improvement than did placebo-treated patients according to three of the scales. Significant differences between treatments emerged at week three and persisted for the duration of the study. Based on CGI-I ratings, 42% of patients receiving sertraline and 26% of patients receiving placebo were very much or much improved. However, the incidence of side effects—insomnia, nausea, agitation, and tremor—was significantly greater in patients receiving sertraline. Thirteen percent of sertraline-treated patients compared with 3% of placebo-treated patients dropped out of the study because of adverse events. The authors conclude: "Sertraline appears to be a safe and effective short-term treatment for children and adolescents with OCD" [*JAMA* 1998; 280:1752–56].

Health in the Elderly

Lowering Blood Pressure Prevents Dementia in the Elderly. A report in 1997 suggested that indicators of atherosclerosis, such as hypertension, are associated with vascular dementia and Alzheimer's disease [*Lancet* 1997;349:151–54]. The hypothesis, however, that antihypertensive treatment would reduce the incidence of dementia, was not consistent with earlier findings from a large well-controlled trial—the SHEP trial—of systolic hypertension and its treatment in the elderly [*JAMA* 1991, 265:3255–64]. Now, researchers report the results of a vascular dementia project explicitly intended to determine whether antihypertensive drugs could reduce the incidence of dementia [*Lancet* 1998;352:1347–51]. The project is part of another large study—the Syst-Eur trial—of systolic hypertension in the elderly [*Lancet* 1997;350:757–64]. The project was stopped early because an interim analysis showed a significant benefit for the primary endpoint of stroke.

Eligible patients had no dementia, were at least 60 years old, and had a seated blood pressure of greater than 160 mm Hg systolic and less than 95 mm Hg diastolic. They were randomly assigned active treatment or placebo and followed for two years. Active treatment consisted of nitrendipine, up to 40 mg/day. Target systolic blood pressure reductions were 20 mm Hg and lower than 150 mm Hg. When patients on nitrendipine alone could not reach these goals, the calcium antagonist was combined with or replaced by enalapril, hydrochlorothiazide, or both.

Compared with placebo, active treatment reduced the incidence of dementia by 50% from 7.7 cases to 3.8 cases per 1000 patient years. Fifteen cases of dementia were seen in the placebo treatment group and seven in the active treatment group. The corresponding numbers for Alzheimer's disease were 13 and 5. The investigators calculated that 19 cases of dementia might be prevented if 1000 hypertensive patients with isolated systolic hypertension were treated with antihypertensive drugs for five years.

That antihypertensive treatment with a thiazide diuretic did not protect against cognitive impairment in the SHEP trial suggests that simply lowering blood pressure may not prevent dementia. There is the possibility that calcium antagonists confer neuroprotection. The authors of the report conclude: "The potential reduction by 50% of the incidence of dementias by antihypertensive drug treatment, initiated with the dihydropyridine nitrendipine, may have important public health implications in view of the increasing longevity of populations worldwide."

OTHER INDICATIONS

Therapy to Ameliorate Steroid-Induced Osteoporosis
Subcutaneous Compared with Intraveneous
Erythropoietin in Hemodialysis
Tacrolimus for Atopic Dermatitis

Therapy to Ameliorate Steroid-Induced Osteoporosis. Osteoporosis is the most debilitating complication of long-term glucocorticoid therapy. Bone loss leads to fractures in up to 50% of patients. Potential therapy includes the bisphosphonates pamidronate (*Aredia*) and etidronate (*Didronel*), which increase spinal bone mineral density. The most commonly used bisphosphonate in the US for the treatment of osteoporosis in postmenopausal women is alendronate (*Fosamax*).

A report in *The New England Journal of Medicine* [1998;339:292–99] presents the combined results of two similar, well-controlled 48-week studies of alendronate for the prevention and treatment of glucocorticoid-induced osteoporosis. Participants were 477 men and women ranging in age from 17 to 83 years, all of whom were receiving long-term glucocorticoid therapy. The primary endpoint was the difference in the mean percent change in lumbar spine bone density from baseline to week 48 among groups.

The mean bone density of the lumbar spine increased by 2.1% and 2.9%, respectively, in the groups that received 5 and 10 mg of alendronate each day, and decreased by 0.4% in the placebo group. The investigators observed a similar pattern of bone density changes in the femoral neck and trochanter. The rate of new vertebral fractures was lower in the alendronate group than in the placebo group (2.3% vs. 3.7%). When used as directed, alendronate is tolerated well and seems to offer a benefit to those who require long-term treatment with systemic steroids.

Some practitioners think that patients starting therapy with more than 7.5 mg prednisolone daily for at least six months should receive prophylactic therapy [*Lancet* 1998;352:1327–28]. A survey in the UK estimated that over 250,000 patients take continuous oral glucocorticoids, yet no more than 14% receive any therapy to prevent bone loss [*J Intern Med* 1998;244:271–92]. Studies have shown that alendronate [*Calcif Tissue Int* 1997;61:382–85] and cyclic etidronate [*N Engl J Med* 1997;337:382–77; *J Clin Endocrinol Metab* 1998;83:1128–33] are effective for primary prevention.

Another recent report concludes that treatment of corticosteroid-induced osteoporosis with a daily subcutaneous injection of parathyroid hormone is also safe and effective [*J Clin Invest* 1998;102:1627–33]. Bone mass in the lumbar spine of post-menopausal women who were on estrogen replacement therapy and had been taking an oral steroid for a least a year was significantly improved within three months of initiating treatment with parathyroid hormone. After one year of treatment, bone-mineral density was one third greater in women taking parathyroid hormone than in women assigned to placebo.

Subcutaneous Compared with Intraveneous Erythropoietin in Hemodialysis. There are approximately 200,000 patients with end-stage renal disease in the US who require dialysis therapy and nearly 70,000 new patients each year. About 90% of patients undergoing dialysis develop anemia as a consequence of erythropoietin deficiency. The introduction of human erythropoietin (epoetin) in 1989 substantially improved cardiovascular function and quality of life. However, epoetin is expensive and Medicare reimburses use only for patients with a hematocrit of 36% or less. Many physicians believe that this policy results in undertreatment. Consequently, strategies have been sought to improve the effectiveness of epoetin and reallocate savings. One recommendation from 1997 guidelines calls for administration of epoetin by subcutaneous rather intravenous injection. Although the bioavailability is lower, the apparent half-life of epoetin is longer after subcutaneous administration than after intravenous administration.

This recommendation is addressed in a recent article describing a study that compares the effectiveness of subcutaneous epoetin with that of intravenous epoetin [*N Engl J Med* 1998;339:579–83]. The investigators randomly allocated 208 patients who were receiving long-term hemodialysis and epoetin therapy to treatment with one or the other method of administration. For the 107 patients treated with subcutaneous epoetin, the average weekly dose was, on average, 32% less than that for the 101 patients treated with intravenous epoetin. Only one patient withdrew from the study because of pain at the subcutaneous injection site and 86% of the patients rated the pain associated with subcutaneous administration as ranging from absent to mild. The researchers estimate, based on the mean difference in the dose, that the average savings realized by giving epoetin subcutaneously would exceed $1100 per patient-year, enough to stretch available Medicare funds to treat less acute patients with epoetin.

An accompanying editorial, however, points out that 23% of patients who were switched from intravenous to subcutaneous administration needed more, rather than less, epoetin. Therefore, the switch, while sound strategy for some, must be individualized, ". . . to ensure that the most effective dose and route of administration are chosen" [*N Engl J Med* 1998;625–26].

Tacrolimus for Atopic Dermatitis. Atopic dermatitis is a chronic inflammatory skin disorder. It is characterized by extreme itching that leads to scratching and rubbing and in turn results in lesions. Topical corticosteroids are the most effective therapy, but may cause adverse local and systemic effects. The use of other immunosuppressants is of interest but studies with cyclosporine have been disappointing. Now, researchers have turned to tacrolimus, an agent finding increasing use to prevent transplant rejection [*J Allergy Clin Immunol* 1998;102:637–44].

The investigators randomly gave 180 seven to sixteen year-old patients with moderate-to-severe atopic dermatitis an ointment vehicle or the same vehicle with one of three doses of tacrolimus. The patients were asked to apply the preparation twice daily for three weeks. A clinical response of at least 75% was seen in 38% who were given the vehicle alone but in 69%, 67%, and 70% of patients given ointment with 0.03%, 0.1%, or 0.3% tacrolimus, respectively. Improvement was seen within one or two weeks after initiating therapy. Tacrolimus also decreased itching. Promisingly, no side effects were associated with the use of topical tacrolimus. If these findings are confirmed, topical tacrolimus would be the first new agent for atopic dermatitis since the introduction of topical steroids in the 1950s.

LATE BREAKING REPORTS

Cardiovascular Disease

β-Blockers: More Evidence of Benefit in Heart Failure. A third controlled clinical trial of a β-blocker in heart failure, the MERIT-HF study, was stopped early because of substantial benefit in the treatment group. The study enrolled nearly 4000 class II to class IV heart failure patients who received a long-acting formulation of metoprolol or a placebo. The trial was stopped after an average follow-up of one year when an interim analysis determined that metoprolol reduced mortality by 35% compared with placebo. Together with the results from the carvedilol (*Coreg*) and bisoprolol (*Zebeta*) trials, the new findings convince most experts that β-blockers have a net benefit for heart failure patients [*Scrip*, November 18, 1998, p 27].

Carvedilol (Coreg) Prevents Nitrate Tolerance in Heart Failure Patients. Patients treated with continuous nitrate therapy for 24 hours or less develop tolerance and lose anti-ischemic effects. Carvedilol combines α/β-blockade with antioxidant activity. It is the only β-blocker indicated for the treatment of chronic heart failure. To evaluate the effect of carvedilol on nitrate tolerance, investigators randomized 40 chronic heart failure patients to one of four treatment groups—carvedilol, metoprolol, doxazosin, or placebo. Vasodilatory response to sublingual nitroglycerin was unchanged in each treatment group on day 3 of the study compared with baseline. At that time, subjects continued assigned medication and also received transdermal nitroglycerin. Vasodilatory response to sublingual nitroglycerin 3 days after initiating continuous nitrate therapy decreased significantly compared with study day 3 and baseline for all treatment groups except the carvedilol group [*J Am Coll Cardiol* 1998;32:1194–1200]. In another study with the same protocol, the investigators again found that carvedilol attenuates nitrate tolerance development, whereas arotinolol, a pure β-blocker, does not [*Ibid*, pp 1201–06]. These studies suggest that carvedilol may prevent nitrate tolerance in chronic heart failure patients during continuous nitroglycerin therapy. β-blockers without antioxidant activity (i.e., metoprolol and arotinolol) seem to have no effect on nitrate tolerance development.

Aggressive Statin Therapy Benefits Diabetics. Yet another report from the CARE trial urges more aggressive management of risk-factors in diabetic patients who have had heart attacks [*Circulation* 1998;98:2513–19]. Compared with placebo, pravastatin reduced the relative risk of having another coronary event by 25% and the relative risk of needing coronary artery bypass or angioplasty by 32%. Benefit was not observed in glucose intolerant non-diabetic patients.

Gemfibrozil Benefits Patients with Coronary Heart Disease. Raising HDL-cholesterol and reducing triglycerides reduces coronary events according to VA-HIT trial investigators who presented their findings at the American

Heart Association in November 1998. A low HDL-cholesterol and a high triglyceride level characterizes about 25% of coronary heart disease (CHD) patients. The trial enrolled 2500 male CHD patients with HDL-cholesterol less than 40 mg/dl and LDL-cholesterol less than 140 mg/dl. The patients received the fibric acid derivative gemfibrozil or placebo. They were followed for five to seven years [*Scrip*, November 18, 1998, p 26]. Gemfibrozil increased HDL-cholesterol by 7.5% to 33 mg/dl and decreased triglycerides by 25% to 115 mg/dl. A healthy male adult usually has a HDL-cholesterol level of 45 mg/dl. Gemfibrozil reduced the primary combined endpoint of CHD death or MI by 22%. Treatment also reduced the incidence of stroke by 26% and decreased the number of transient ischemic attacks (TIAs).

Diltiazem May Be an Alternative to β-Blockers After a Heart Attack. A new study suggests that the heart rate-lowering calcium antagonist diltiazem may be an alternative to a β-blocker in the treatment of MI patients. According to INTERCEPT trial investigators, patients who received diltiazem within 36 to 96 hours of heart attack onset had a 33% reduction in the 36-day composite endpoint—CHD death, repeat MI, or refractory ischemia. The trend, however, was not statistically significant. Generally, calcium channel blockers are thought to be detrimental for MI patients, but this applies mainly if not exclusively to dihydropyridines (e.g., nifedipine). Unlike diltiazem, dihydropyridines do not lower heart rate [*Scrip*, November 18, 1998].

Abciximab (ReoPro)-Stent Combination Reduces Mortality After Angioplasty. The EPISTENT trial, described previously, compared the use of *ReoPro*, stents, or the combination in patients undergoing coronary angioplasty. One-year results show a significant reduction in mortality in patients given both a stent and *ReoPro*. Mortality rates were 1% in the combination group, 2.1% in the *ReoPro*-only group, and 2.4% in the stent-only group. EPISTENT is the first interventional cardiology trial to demonstrate a reduction in mortality. The investigators say that the reduction is particularly remarkable because the trial enrolled only 2400 patients who were not at especially high risk.

Simple Strategy May Reduce Mortality after Acute MI. A simple and inexpensive intravenous infusion of glucose, insulin, and potassium (GIK) could be an important adjuvant for the immediate treatment of acute MI patients. In a well-controlled trial of 407 patients, a combination of reperfusion therapy and GIK (given over 24 hours) reduced mortality from 15% to 5% compared with reperfusion therapy alone [*Circulation* 1998;98:2227–34]. Side-effects were infrequent and minor.

Gastrointestinal Disease

***Helicobacter pylori* and Nonulcer Dyspepsia.** Dyspepsia—upper abdominal pain and discomfort, bloating, fullness, early satiety, nausea, anorexia, heartburn, regurgitation, and belching—is experienced by 25% to 40% of Western populations. Management of the disorder is unsatisfactory. Recognition of the role of *Helicobacter pylori* in peptic ulcer has led to suggestions that the infection may also be the cause of dyspepsia in some patients with a nonulcer form of the condition. The end-of-year issue of *The New England Journal of Medicine* reports two well-controlled studies that examined eradication of *H pylori* and healing, but reached opposite conclusions regarding efficacy.

Both enrolled more than 300 patients with persistent dyspepsia and *H pylori* gastritis. Participants were randomly assigned to receive a course of the proton-pump inhibitor omeprazole and two antibiotics (to eradicate the organism) or omeprazole alone. Patients were reassessed one year later. In each study, *H pylori* was eradicated in at least 79% of the patients treated with omeprazole and antibiotics, but in few patients treated with omeprazole alone. In the first study, symptoms resolved in 21% of patients who were treated with omeprazole and antibiotics as compared with only 7% of patients treated with omeprazole alone. The authors conclude that treatment with omeprazole and antibiotics is more likely to resolve symptoms of dyspepsia than treatment with only a proton-pump inhibitor [*N Engl J Med* 1998; 339:1869–74].

In the second study, however, dyspepsia resolved in 27% of patients treated with omeprazole and antibiotics and in 20% who received only omeprazole. The authors conclude that *H pylori* infection does not have a major role in nonulcer dyspepsia [*N Engl J Med* 1998;339:1875–81]. The different outcomes may stem from differences in patient selection and in the symptom scales used to assess efficacy. The bottom line, however, is that for most patients with nonulcer dyspepsia and *H pylori* gastritis, eradicating the organism will not relieve symptoms. Antisecretory agents or drugs that promote motility may be effective in some patients [*Ibid*, pp 1929–30].

Pain Management

Anticonvulsant Gabapentin for the Treatment of Neuropathic Pain. Pain resulting from neuropathies is common but difficult to manage. Drugs currently prescribed for the treatment of painful neuropathies block pain transmission pathways and provide symptomatic relief. They include analgesics, tricyclic antidepressants (TCAs), antiarrhythmics, and local anesthetics. TCAs are standard therapy but they have serious side effects. In this light, two recent well-controlled 8-week studies on the treatment of painful diabetic neuropathy and postherpetic neuralgia with gabapentin (*Neurontin*) monotherapy are welcome. In one report, gabapentin-treated diabetic neuropathy patients' mean daily pain score at the end of the study was significantly lower than their mean baseline score, and significantly lower than placebo-treated patients' mean end-of-trial score [*JAMA* 1998;280:1831–36]. The other study showed a similar pattern of pain scores in postherpetic neuralgia patients treated with gabapentin or placebo following herpes zoster infection [*Ibid,* pp 1837–42]. Both studies demonstrate clinically important reductions in daily pain severity and improvement in secondary end points—sleep interference scores and quality of life measures. A commentary on the reports concludes that TCAs should remain first-line therapy for painful diabetic neuropathy and recommends gabapentin for those who do not tolerate the older agents. The authors seem persuaded, however, that gabapentin may be the drug of choice for postherpetic neuralgia [*Ibid,* pp 1863–64].

Women's Health

Alendronate Decreases Risk of Fracture in Fracture-Free Postmenopausal Women with Low Bone Density. The bisphosphonate alendronate (*Fosamax*) increases bone mineral density (BMD) and reduces the risk of vertebral fractures in women with osteoporosis. Three years of alendronate also reduces the risk of hip and wrist fractures by about 50% among women who have low BMD and vertebral fractures. The effectiveness of treatment, however, in the larger group of women who have low BMD but no vertebral fractures has not been investigated. A new study shows that four years of alendronate safely increases BMD and decreases the risk of first vertebral deformity [*JAMA* 1998;280:2077–82]. In the study, alendronate reduced clinical fractures in women with baseline osteoporosis at the femoral neck (>2.5 standard deviations below the normal young adult mean) but not among women with higher BMD. An editorial suggests that women most likely to benefit from alendronate prophylaxis are those with very low BMD scores, those who have had a fracture since turning 40 or a maternal history of hip fracture, as well as those starting corticosteroid therapy or needing prolonged immobilization. For women without these indications, other strategies that include a calcium intake of at least 1500 mg/day and a vitamin D intake of 600 to 1000 IU may be more appropriate [*Ibid*, pp 2119–20].

Other Indications

Treatment for Urge Incontinence. A research report in *JAMA* [1998; 280:1995–2000] shows that both behavioral treatment and drug therapy are more effective for urge incontinence in older women (55 to 92 years old) than placebo, and that a behavioral strategy is more effective than drug treatment. In the study, women with bladder dysfunction were randomized to four two-week sessions of biofeedback-assisted behavioral treatment, drug treatment with up to 5 mg oxybutynin daily, or placebo. The mean reduction of incontinence episodes was 81% in patients assigned to behavioral treatment, 68% in those receiving oxybutynin, and 39% among those randomized to placebo. Only 14% of people receiving behavior treatment sought to change to another treatment compared with 75% in each of the other groups.

3 Drug Evaluation
Other Studies and Reports

CARDIOVASCULAR DISEASE

Statins for the Prevention of Stroke
High-Dose Simvastatin Lowers Cholesterol and Triglycerides
Stopping Antihypertensive Medication May Pose Risks
β-Blockers—Not First-Line Therapy for Hypertension in the
  Elderly
Heparin Therapy for Treatment of Acute MI in the Elderly
Long-Term Benefit of a Thrombolytic Agent and Aspirin
  after MI
New Indication for Aprotinin in Bypass-Graft Surgery
Bleeding Risk Index May Improve Safety of Warfarin
Underuse of Warfarin in Patients with Atrial Fibrillation and
  Ischemic Stroke
β-Blockers in Chronic Heart Failure

Statins for the Prevention of Stroke. Pravastatin (*Pravachol*) and simvastatin (*Zocor*) are now available for the prevention of stroke. Approval was based on two recent meta-analyses. In an overview of 16 trials, which included about 29,000 patients who received an HMG-CoA reductase inhibitor or a placebo, the treatment group showed an average reduction in LDL-cholesterol of 30%. Patients assigned to a statin had a 29% reduction in stroke and a 22% reduction in total mortality [*JAMA* 1997;278:313–21]. The second overview investigated the incidence of stroke, death from coronary-heart disease, and overall mortality through the analysis of 28 randomized controlled trials of any cholesterol-lowering therapy that included more than 100,000 patients. The risk ratio for stroke was 0.76 with HMG-CoA reductase inhibitors but close to 1.0 with fibric acid derivatives, non-absorbable resins, and dietary interventions. Statins were also better than other lipid-lowering measures in reducing overall mortality [*Ann Intern Med* 1998;128:89–97]. The benefits of statins, compared with other interventions, are related, in part, to their greater effectiveness in lowering cholesterol. Two large individual trials with simvastatin [*Lancet* 1994;344:1383–89] and pravastatin [*N Engl J Med* 1996;335:1001–09] report that the overall reduction in fatal and nonfatal strokes was 30% and 31%, respectively. All patients with cardiovascular disease and elevated levels of cholesterol, unless otherwise ineligible, should receive statin therapy. Patients with average cholesterol levels may also benefit.

High-Dose Simvastatin Lowers Cholesterol and Triglycerides. Atorvastatin (*Lipitor*) profoundly decreases levels of low-density lipoprotein (LDL) cholesterol and is also effective in reducing triglyceride levels. Because *Lipitor* lowers LDL-cholesterol better than any other marketed drug, it has dominated new prescriptions for lipid-lowering drugs. On gaining FDA approval of a new high-dose preparation of simvastatin (*Zocor*), which contains twice the former maximum approved 40 mg dose, Merck will now offer an alternative to *Lipitor*. The *Prescriber's Letter* [1998;5:44] says that the new tablet reduces LDL-cholesterol by nearly 50% and reduces triglycerides by about 35%. These effects are approximately equivalent to those of 40 mg atorvastatin. The *Prescriber's Letter* cautions, however, that because high-dose *Zocor* also increases the risk of hepatotoxicity, liver function must be monitored closely. *Zocor*, like *Lipitor*, is now approved for patients with homozygous familial hypercholesterolemia, a condition characterized by very high cholesterol levels and coronary heart disease at a young age.

Stopping Antihypertensive Medication May Pose Risks. Patients who stop taking their medication for hypertension are at risk of hemorrhagic stroke. Analyzing 331 consecutive cases of documented intracerebral hemorrhage, investigators found that high blood pressure doubles the risk of bleeding into the brain (odds ratio OR, 2.45). The risk of hypertension-associated intracerebral hemorrhage was greater among those who stopped taking medication (OR, 5.0) compared with those who did not (OR, 2.0). Terminating medication presented an even greater risk in people younger than 55 years and in smokers. This is the first direct evidence for a link between stopping antihypertensive medication and the risk of stroke. The authors speculate that thinning of the arterial wall caused by antihypertensive agents might render the wall more vulnerable to injury when drug therapy is stopped and the arterial wall is exposed to elevated blood pressure. Since discontinuation of medication usually represents a failure to follow medical advice, the authors suggest that targeting these individuals and educating them on the importance of faithfully taking their medication may reduce the impact of hemorrhagic stroke [*Hypertension* 1998;31:1223–29].

β-Blockers—Not First-Line Therapy for Hypertension in the Elderly. The purpose of antihypertensive medication is to reduce the incidence of cardiovascular morbidity and mortality and overall mortality. Studies have shown the safety and effectiveness of diuretics in this regard, but the evidence supporting the use of β-blockers is less clear. The 1997 report of the Joint National Committee (JNC) no longer recommends β-blockers as first-line antihypertensive therapy for elderly patients. A systematic review of the literature found ten randomized trials involving more than 16,000 elderly patients that allowed a rigorous estimation of outcomes for patients treated with a β-blocker or a diuretic. Analysis of the reports found that two-thirds of the patients assigned to diuretics were well controlled, compared with less than one-third of the patients on β-blocker monotherapy. Diuretic therapy was superior to β-blockade in preventing stroke, fatal stroke, cardiovascular mortality, and all-cause mortality. β-blockers reduced the risk for stroke, but were ineffective in preventing coronary heart disease and mortality. The authors conclude that β-blockers should not be considered first-line therapy of uncomplicated hypertension in the elderly patient [*JAMA* 1998;279:1903–07]. A companion report examining why physicians do not routinely prescribe diuretics to manage hypertension concludes that diuretics should be used more frequently and that they would reduce the number of resistant hypertensive patients [*JAMA* 1998;279:1813–16].

Heparin Therapy for Treatment of Acute MI in the Elderly. While intravenous heparin is widely used in the treatment of acute myocardial infarction (MI), especially among patients who do not receive early treatment with a thrombolytic agent, its value is controversial. To shed some light on this issue, investigators conducted a cohort study using hospital records of Medicare beneficiaries [*J Am Coll Cardiol* 1998;31:973–79]. The researchers identified nearly 7000 patients 65 years of age or older with a diagnosis of acute MI but not receiving thrombolytic therapy. About half of these patients received early full-dose heparin. The adjusted 30-day mortality rate among those that did and did not receive intravenous heparin was about the same. While it is likely that heparin is not effective in this setting, we must take note that the nonrandom allocations of patients to the two groups did result in two different populations. Younger patients and patients with lower risk were more likely to receive heparin than not. While the investigators adjusted for differences in known risk factors, differences in unknown risk factors cannot be ruled out.

Long-Term Benefit of a Thrombolytic Agent and Aspirin after MI. The *British Medical Journal* [1998;316:1337–43] recently published a ten-year update of results from the second international study of infarct survival (ISIS-2), first reported in 1998. Trial investigators randomized patients who presented with a suspected MI to receive intravenous streptokinase, aspirin, both, or neither for one month. Assignment to streptokinase resulted in 29 fewer deaths per 1000 patients up to 35 days after treatment. This early benefit persisted so that there were 23 fewer deaths per 1000 patients treated with streptokinase after ten years. The early survival benefit in patients allocated to the combination of streptokinase and aspirin, 55 fewer deaths per 1000 at day 35, was still evident at ten years with 42 fewer deaths per 1000 patients. Thus, the early survival advantage provided by streptokinase and aspirin, when given during an evolving MI, is maintained for at least ten years. Other studies show that continuing aspirin treatment for some years after a heart attack can increase these benefits.

New Indication for Aprotinin in Bypass-Graft Surgery. Aprotinin (*Trasylol*), effective in reducing the number of blood transfusions required during surgery, is now approved for use in all patients who undergo coronary artery bypass graft surgery (CABG) [*The Pink Sheet* 1998;60(No38):6]. Until now, aprotinin was indicated only for high-risk CABG patients. The new indication doubles the population eligible to receive aprotinin to 400,000–500,000 patients. New labeling states that among primary CABG patients, 36% of patients given *Trasylol,* compared with 53.5% of patients on placebo, required donor blood. Because the drug will now be used in lower-risk patients, a warning of possible anaphylactic reactions to the drug, particularly on re-exposure, has been made more prominent in the revised labeling. The updated labeling also contains new information on mechanism of action. Aprotinin was previously thought to inhibit fibrinolysis and turnover of coagulation factors. Now, aprotinin is recognized as a broad-spectrum protease inhibitor that attenuates the systemic inflammatory response to CABG surgery.

Bleeding Risk Index May Improve Safety of Warfarin. Researchers have developed a simple algorithm called the Outpatient Bleeding Risk Index (OBRI) to minimize the risk of major bleeding in outpatients treated with warfarin. The index includes the four risk factors of age 65 or older, history of gastrointestinal bleeding, history of stroke, and at least one of four comorbid conditions. The conditions are a recent heart attack, a hematocrit of less than 30%, a serum creatinine of greater than 1.5 mg/dl, and diabetes mellitus. Those patients with three or all four risk factors are vulnerable and have a 23% chance of a major bleed when taking warfarin for three months; these patients have a 48% chance when anticoagulated for 12 months. Patients with one or two risk factors have an intermediary probability of bleeding and patients with no risk factors have a low probability of bleeding. A recent study prospectively evaluated the accuracy and utility of the index in 264 outpatients starting warfarin therapy [*Am J Med* 1998;105:91–99]. The cumulative incidence of major bleeding at 48 months was 3% in patients classified as low-risk according to the OBRI, 12% in patients classified as intermediary risk, and 53% in patients classified as high-risk. The index performed better than did physicians who used standard clinical criteria to estimate warfarin dosage. Of the 18 episodes of serious bleeding that occurred in high-risk patients, 17 could have been prevented by using the minimum effective dose of warfarin or deciding that the risk of major bleeding was too high to allow anticoagulation with warfarin.

Underuse of Warfarin in Patients with Atrial Fibrillation and Ischemic Stroke. Elderly patients with ischemic stroke and atrial fibrillation are at high risk of recurrent stroke. However, a recent survey shows that only 62% of patients ideally suited for secondary prevention therapy with an anticoagulant actually received a prescription for warfarin on hospital discharge [*Arch Intern Med* 1998;158:2093–100]. The authors conclude: "Anticoagulation of elderly stroke patients with atrial fibrillation, even among ideal candidates, is underused. The increased use of warfarin among these patients represents an excellent opportunity for reducing the risk of recurrent stroke in this high-risk population."

β-Blockers in Chronic Heart Failure. Researchers have reported findings from a meta-analysis of 18 double-blind placebo-controlled trials of β-blockers in patients with heart failure. From the combined database of 3023 patients, the investigators estimated that β-blockade increases ejection fraction by 29% and reduces the combined risk of death or hospitalization for heart failure by 37%. Although β-blockade reduced all-cause mortality by about one-third, the effect varied according to the type of β-blocker used in the study. The risk of dying was less for nonselective blockers than for β_1-selective drugs. Carvedilol (*Coreg*) is the only drug with β-blocker activity specifically approved in the US for the treatment of patients with chronic heart failure. A recent study with bisoprolol also provides convincing evidence of benefit [*Can J Cardiol* 1998;14:1045–53].

DIABETES

Type 1 Diabetes, Weight Gain, and Coronary Artery Disease
Caution Needed in Prescribing Acarbose (*Precose*)

Type 1 Diabetes, Weight Gain, and Coronary Artery Disease. Insulin therapy often results in weight gain, and intensive treatment of diabetics results in greater weight gain than conventional treatment. An understanding of the effect of weight gain resulting from intensive diabetes therapy on the risk factors for coronary artery disease (CAD) is important because CAD is a leading cause of mortality in adults with diabetes. Using updated data from the Diabetes Control and Complications Trial, which involved more than 1000 patients with type 1 diabetes and compared intensive treatment with conventional therapy, investigators determined the effects of weight gain on lipid levels and blood pressure [*JAMA* 1998;280:140–46]. The final lipid levels reflect improvements from intensive diabetes therapy offset by changes due to weight gain. Patients receiving intensive therapy and in the first quartile of weight gain had a significantly improved lipid profile compared with baseline, demonstrating the cardiovascular benefits of improved glycemic control. On the other hand, those in the fourth quartile had a significant deterioration of lipid levels and an increase in blood pressure. The deleterious changes included higher triglyceride levels, higher total and LDL-cholesterol levels, and lower HDL-cholesterol levels. The authors warn that despite improved glycemic control, these changes in lipid profile may contribute to an increased risk of heart disease in the subset of patients who gain an excessive amount of weight with intensive therapy.

Caution Needed in Prescribing Acarbose (Precose). Acarbose (*Precose*), a relatively new and novel agent that reduces the absorption of glucose from the gastrointestinal tract, has run into a higher incidence of liver toxicity than expected. Affected patients present with fatigue, abdominal pain, and jaundice. These reports prompted Bayer Corporation in February 1998 to change the labeling of *Precose* to reflect the greater risk. It now says that elevations of liver enzymes as high as three times the upper limit of normal were found in 3% of patients studied. The original label stated that transaminase levels during clinical trials were asymptomatic, reversible, more common in females, and not associated with other evidence of liver dysfunction. Acarbose is poorly absorbed after oral administration—less than 2% of the dose. However, the drug is metabolized in the gut and about one-third of formed metabolites are absorbed. An unusual metabolite may be responsible for the hepatotoxicity. According to the *Prescriber's Letter* [1998;5:51], patients who take acarbose should have liver function tests every three months during the first year of therapy and periodically thereafter.

GASTROINTESTINAL DISEASE

New Ten-Day Regimens for Eradicating *H pylori* and Peptic Ulcer

Proton Pump Inhibitors for Bleeding Peptic Ulcer

New Ten-Day Regimens for Eradicating* H pylori *and Peptic Ulcer. Until now, all of the approved drug combinations for the treatment of gastrointestinal ulcers by eradicating *H pylori* called for 14 days of dosing. The FDA has now approved two similar regimens for 10-day use. Each one contains a proton pump inhibitor, either omeprazole (*Prilosec*) or lansoprazole (*Prevacid*), as well as clarithromycin (*Biaxin*) and amoxicillin. Some physicians are even prescribing these regimens for seven days [*Prescriber's Letter* 1998; 5:45]. The shorter regimens cost less and may be better tolerated and improve compliance. Although the new course of treatment is not quite as effective as 14-day regimens, most patients will benefit.

Proton Pump Inhibitors for Bleeding Peptic Ulcer. The success of histamine-2 receptor blockers in the treatment of symptomatic, uncomplicated peptic ulcer led to their widespread use in patients hospitalized for bleeding ulcers. In 1985, a meta-analysis summarized the results of 27 randomized trials of cimetidine and ranitidine in nearly 1700 patients with bleeding gastric or duodenal ulcer. The investigators concluded that treatment with an H2-blocker appears to be "moderately promising." However, a subsequent, large randomized trial in 1000 patients comparing intravenous famotidine and placebo failed to support that conclusion. This outcome led some clinical scientists to believe that the reduction of gastric acidity afforded by H2-blockers was not enough to prevent rebleeding. Since then proton pump inhibitors have gained widespread use. These agents are more effective in lowering gastric acidity and might also be more effective in preventing rebleeding. Researchers seeking to update the evidence supporting the use of proton pump inhibitors for bleeding peptic ulcer identified and evaluated 8 well-controlled trials in eligible patients, all of which used omeprazole as the experimental treatment [*JAMA* 1998;280:877–78]. The authors conclude that while early treatment of a bleeding ulcer with a proton pump inhibitor may not confer a large benefit in terms of rebleeding, these agents should be used in patients whose bleeding ulcer has an overlying clot or a nonbleeding visible blood vessel.

INFECTIOUS DISEASE

British Guidelines for Anti-retroviral Treatment of HIV
  Infection
Anti-HIV Therapy Reduces Morbidity and Mortality
Treating STDs May Reduce Sexual Transmission of HIV
Eradicating HIV in the Central Nervous System
Managing Protease Inhibitor-Related Lipid Abnormalities
Hydroxyurea May Benefit Patients with HIV Infection
Directly Observed Therapy for Tuberculosis
Optimizing the Dose of Interferon for Hepatitis C
Restriction of Cephalosporin Use Reduces Resistant Klebsiella
  Infection
Influenza Vaccination Benefits Low-Risk Elderly
Concerted Effort to Eliminate Trachoma

British Guidelines for Anti-retroviral Treatment of HIV Infection. The British HIV Association recently issued a consensus statement on optimal treatment for HIV seropositive individuals. The British group continues to recommend delaying treatment until the benefits of therapy outweigh the potential morbidities associated with anti-HIV drugs and the patient is at risk of irreversible damage to the immune system. They also say that it is important to start treatment with regimens that reliably reduce individuals' plasma viral load to below detectable limits of current assays (200 to 500 copies per ml) and preferably to less than 50 copies per ml. Most clinicians believe that allowing a high level of viral replication to persist will lead to drug resistance. The Association favors starting treatment with two nucleoside reverse transcriptase inhibitors (RTIs) plus a non-nucleoside RTI (NNRTI) or a protease inhibitor. It also recommends the use of two protease inhibitors with or without an RTI. An initial combination of two RTIs is no longer considered a reasonable standard of care. The guidelines also suggest that initial therapy with two RTIs and an NNRTI is attractive because it allows the use of a protease inhibitor to be reserved for later. The group acknowledges that the definition of treatment failure following a period of successful therapy remains elusive [*Lancet* 1998;352:314–16].

Anti-HIV Therapy Reduces Morbidity and Mortality. The HIV Outpatient Study, ongoing since 1992, collects summaries of physician-patient interactions and data on the course of disease from more than 3500 HIV-infected ambulatory patients. A recent report concerns the use of this database to examine changes in morbidity and mortality that may have followed the introduction of combination therapy including a protease inhibitor [*N Engl J Med* 1998;338:853–60]. For purposes of their investigation, the researchers selected 1255 patients, seen from January 1994 through June 1997, who had at least one CD4+ count below 100 cells per cubic millimeter. Morality declined from 29.4 per 100 patient-years in 1995 to 8.8 per 100 patient-years in the second quarter of 1997. The incidence of any one of three major opportunistic infections—*Pneumocystis carinii* pneumonia, *Mycobacterium avium* complex disease, and cytomegalovirus retinitis—declined from 21.9 per 100 patient-years in 1994 to 3.7 per 100 patient-years by mid-1997. A failure-rate model of the data showed that increases in the intensity of antiretroviral therapy—none, monotherapy, combination therapy without a protease inhibitor, and combination therapy with a protease inhibitor—were associated with stepwise reductions in morbidity and mortality. The authors conclude: ". . . the routine use of increasingly intensive antiretroviral therapies has resulted directly in dramatic declines in morbidity and mortality among HIV-infected patients with advanced immune depletion." A more recently reported cohort study found that in the calendar year when potent antiretroviral therapy was introduced the time to development of AIDS and time to death were extended, and the rate of CD4 cell decline was arrested [*JAMA* 1998;280:1497–1503].

Treating STDs May Reduce Sexual Transmission of HIV. Observational studies link the risk of transmission of HIV to the presence of genital lesions. The most common infectious etiology of genital ulcers in North America and Europe is herpes simplex virus (HSV). To better understand the role of genital ulcers as a risk factor for transmission, investigators studied 12 HIV-infected men with a history of symptomatic HSV infection who, during an acute episode, underwent daily sampling of genital lesions for viral RNA [*JAMA* 1998;280:61–66]. They detected HIV RNA from swabs of the ulcer in 25 of 26 consecutively studied HSV episodes and on two-thirds of days in which genital lesions were noted. HIV RNA was present in 80% of swabs taken on days in which HSV was also isolated. However, HIV RNA in genital lesions was not associated with plasma HIV RNA levels. By day six, within two days of starting treatment with acyclovir, HSV could no longer be isolated from lesions. HIV RNA titer in genital lesions persisted at high levels until

HSV replication fell to low levels and then became undetectable. The authors conclude that genital herpes infection is likely to increase the efficiency of sexual transmission of HIV and that physicians must pay more attention to the treatment of genital ulcers.

Eradicating HIV in the Central Nervous System. Treatment of HIV-related neurological disease may depend on penetration of antiretroviral drugs into the central nervous system (CNS). In a recent study [*Lancet* 1998;351:1547–51], patients with HIV infection (viral load >10,000 copies/ml, CD4 cell counts >200/μl) who were free of neurological symptoms underwent lumbar puncture. HIV RNA was found in the cerebrospinal fluid (CSF) of all patients. They then were assigned to treatment with lamivudine (*Epivir*) plus zidovudine (*Retrovir*) or lamivudine plus stavudine (*Zerit*). After 12 weeks of therapy, a second lumbar puncture showed that both treatments reduced CSF HIV RNA levels to below detection in all patients. All three agents reached concentrations in the CSF greater than the 50% inhibitory concentration for wild-type HIV isolates. The authors conclude that both combinations were equally effective in decreasing HIV RNA in CSF. While zidovudine has been favored for the treatment of HIV infection in the CNS, other antiretroviral drugs might also be useful.

Managing Protease Inhibitor-Related Lipid Abnormalities. Troubling and potentially serious lipid abnormalities occur in patients receiving treatment with an HIV protease inhibitor. Elevated serum triglyceride and cholesterol levels may pose the risk of coronary atherosclerosis. A recent survey of 133 patients on protease inhibitors showed that people receiving ritonavir (*Norvir*) and saquinavir (*Inverase, Fortovase*) were almost twice as likely to have raised lipid concentrations compared with patients receiving nelfinavir (*Viracept*) or indinavir (*Crixivan*). These patients were then asked to participate in a lipid-lowering study. If they agreed, those with modest elevations in lipid levels were managed initially with a diet plus exercise program and patients with higher levels received gemfibrozil (*Lopid*) or atorvastatin (*Lipitor*). There were a large number of treatment failures among those assigned to diet/exercise and those assigned to gemfibrozil. The diet group failures were re-assigned to drug therapy and gemfibrozil failures added atorvastatin. Among patients receiving both drugs, mean cholesterol levels fell 30% and triglyceride levels fell 60% over six months. Atorvastatin also significantly lowered lipid levels but much less so than the combination. There are two issues, however, that need resolution before widely recommending the combination. One is a concern that administration of gemfibrozil with a statin may increase the risk of myopathy. The other is a concern of increased toxicity if atorvastatin is used with drugs, such as protease inhibitors, that inhibit drug metabolizing enzymes [*Lancet* 1998;352:1031–32].

Hydroxyurea May Benefit Patients with HIV Infection. Although most HIV production occurs in dividing, activated T lymphocytes, non-dividing, resting lymphocytes and macrophages are long-term reservoirs for the virus. One way to improve current anti-HIV therapy is to target simultaneously both reservoir cells and the virus, and to do so early in the course of the infection. A recently reported study evaluates this strategy [*Lancet* 1998;352:199–200]. Eleven individuals were treated within two months after onset of symptoms of primary HIV infection and before seroconversion with a novel combination therapy consisting of hydroxyurea (*Hydrea*), the RTI didanosine (*Videx*), and indinavir (*Crixivan*). Hydroxyurea blocks cellular activation needed for viral replication in CD4 T-lymphocytes, indinavir inhibits HIV replication in dividing cells, and hydroxyurea with didanosine is effective in non-dividing cells. Upon treatment, viral load fell from more than 500,000 copies per ml to undetectable levels, and remained so for up to 17 months. CD4 counts increased sharply by an average of 207. Examination of semen from six patients found no detectable HIV RNA. Lymph nodes from two of three patients studied were apparently free of HIV RNA. The investigators conclude: "These result show that treatment of acutely-infected individuals with potent antiviral drugs having different mechanisms of action and affecting multiple compartments results in a profound effect on the natural evolution of primary HIV-1 infection."

Directly Observed Therapy for Tuberculosis. The lengthy course of treatment needed to eradicate tuberculosis (TB) leads to poor compliance, particularly among the poor and homeless populations in which TB is a major problem. A patient's failure to complete treatment means that he or she continues to infect other people and may develop and transmit multidrug resistant organisms. To overcome this problem, public health officials conceived a strategy called directly observed therapy (DOT), wherein patients swallow each prescribed dose of medication under supervision. The introduction of DOT has been a success in the US and other developed nations. Some consider it the most significant advance in the treatment of TB in the past 25 years.

A recent report, called the Consensus Statement of the Public Health Tuberculosis Guidelines Panel, presented an evaluation of the evidence on the relative effectiveness of DOT in achieving treatment completion [*Chest* 1997;111:1151–53]. After reviewing the documentation, a panel of experts concluded that treatment completion rates for pulmonary tuberculosis are most likely to exceed 90% when treatment is based on a patient-centered approach using DOT. Less intensive interventions are unlikely to reach this level of treatment completion. They also suggest, although data are limited, that DOT appears to be cost-effective compared with self-administered therapy. We need keep in mind, however, that the development of policies has been based on observational studies in which DOT is a label for multifaceted programs that include improved laboratory services, investment in drug supply, punitive measures for recalcitrant patients, and rewards for compliance. An expert in the UK asks: "Is it direct observation of patients that results in better adherence, or other factors that accompany these initiatives? [*Lancet* 1998;352:1326–27]. Less than a total commitment to DOT, without supporting resources, is no better than self-supervised therapy [*Lancet* 1998; 352:1340–43].

Optimizing the Dose of Interferon for Hepatitis C. Chronic infection with hepatitis C virus (HCV) is a major worldwide health problem with a prevalence of up to 15% in some countries. As many as 30% of infected individuals develop cirrhosis and up to 3% may develop liver cancer. Treatment with interferon-α-2b (is successful in no more than 30% of cases, and some reports suggest an efficacy of only 10%. Higher daily doses of interferon-α-2b may be more effective than standard treatment for patients with hepatitis C according to a new study [*Science* 1998;282:103–07]. Researchers reported that in a group of 23 patients interferon doses of 10 and 15 million international units (IU) daily were significantly more effective than 5 million IU. Standard treatment is only 3 million units of interferon three times a week. Treatment with high doses of interferon resulted in a rapid dose-dependent decline in viral load at the start of therapy, followed by the death of infected liver cells. A mathematical model of viral load during interferon therapy suggests that patients should be treated aggressively at the outset to abolish production of the virus and to prevent drug-resistant mutations from developing. The investigators also suggest that monitoring of viral load can help guide therapy.

Restriction of Cephalosporin Use Reduces Resistant Klebsiella Infection. Since the development of penicillin-resistant *Staphylococcus aureus* more than

40 years ago, antibiotic resistance among nosocomial pathogens has been an evolving process. The use of antimicrobial agents encourages the development of resistance in bacterial strains and overuse invites disaster. Moreover, the genetic mechanisms used by bacteria to acquire antibiotic resistance not only promote the spread of resistance, but may also favor stability of resistance genes even in the absence of ongoing exposure to the antibiotic. Therefore, a recent report in *JAMA* [1998;280:1233–37] describing one institution's restriction of cephalosporin use that reduced the frequency of β-lactam resistance among *Klebsiella* species is good news. Facing an outbreak of multi-resistant *Klebsiella*, the hospital ordered an 80% reduction in cephalosporin use in 1996 compared with 1995. This was accompanied by a 44% reduction in the incidence of ceftazidime-resistant *Klebsiella* infection and colonization throughout the medical center. The unintended consequence of the restriction program was an increase in the use of imipenem and a concomitant increase in imipenem-resistant *Pseudomonas aeruginosa*. All but one imipenem-resistant *P aeruginosa* isolate, however, remained susceptible to other β-lactams, quinolones, or aminoglycosides.

Influenza Vaccination Benefits Low-Risk Elderly. Vaccination before each flu season provides a clear benefit for high-risk elderly individuals with chronic heart or lung disease. It is very likely to benefit intermediary-risk elderly citizens with diabetes, renal disease, stroke, or rheumatoid disease. Does vaccination benefit healthy elderly citizens? A cohort study with more than 20,000 elderly people shows that it does [*Arch Intern Med* 1998;158:1769–76]. For the cohort as a whole, vaccination rate was 60%. Vaccination over six seasons was associated with a reduction of 39% for pneumonia hospitalizations, 32% for hospitalizations for all respiratory conditions, and 21% for hospitalizations for congestive heart failure. Immunization also resulted in a 50% reduction in all-cause mortality. Within the risk subgroups, vaccination significantly reduced hospitalizations for pneumonia and influenza for high- and low-risk elderly citizens, and deaths from all causes for elderly citizens in each of the risk subgroups. An economic analysis suggests that vaccination is cost saving for each subgroup. The study confirms that healthy senior citizens as well as elderly individuals with underlying medical conditions are at risk for the complications of influenza and benefit from vaccination. "All individuals 65 years or older should be immunized with this vaccine."

Concerted Effort to Eliminate Trachoma. Trachoma is the leading cause of preventable blindness worldwide. The disease can be effectively treated by a single dose each year of the antibiotic azithromycin (*Zithromax*). It is caused by repeated infections with strains of chlamydia. Estimates are that six million people worldwide are blind because of trachoma. The barriers to getting the drug to the people who need it have, up until now, been insurmountable. The World Health Organization (WHO) recently developed a new strategy aimed at eliminating trachoma as a major cause of blindness by the year 2020. The strategy calls for purifying water supplies so people can wash and improve personal hygiene. More recently, Pfizer, azithromycin's maker, and a private foundation announced that they were starting a $66 million program to help carry out WHO's strategy in Ghana, Mali, Morocco, Tanzania, and Vietnam. Pfizer will donate enough *Zithromax* to treat three million people over the next two years [*The New York Times,* November 11, 1998, pp A1,A11].

Inflammatory Disease

Corticosteroids for the Treatment of Rheumatoid Arthritis
Cytotoxic Agents and Cyclosporine for Autoimmune Disease

Corticosteroids for the Treatment of Rheumatoid Arthritis. Despite 50 years of experience with potent anti-inflammatory corticosteroids, their role in the treatment of rheumatoid arthritis (RA) remains controversial. Initial hope that steroids might dramatically alter the course of the disease faded in the face of the serious adverse effects that accompany high-dose therapy. While low-dose steroids are safer, their effectiveness is uncertain. Investigators have recently reported the results of a meta-analysis of ten previously reported controlled trials [*BMJ* 1998;316:811–19]. Each trial evaluated whether short-term, oral, low-dose prednisolone (2.5 to 15 mg daily) is superior to placebo or a nonsteroidal anti-inflammatory agent (NSAID) for patients with RA. The investigators considered joint tenderness, pain, and grip strength. Prednisolone had a marked effect over placebo on all three measures. Prednisolone also had a greater effect than NSAIDs on joint tenderness and pain, but the difference in grip strength was not significant. The investigators recommend that patients with RA receive intermittent low-dose prednisolone, particularly if the disease cannot be controlled by other means. The results on effectiveness agree with the clinical impressions of most rheumatologists, but the authors' recommendations may not fully consider the serious side effects of corticosteroids, even at low doses, and the worry that tapering treatment may be difficult [*BMJ* 1998;316:789–90].

Cytotoxic Agents and Cyclosporine for Autoimmune Disease. Cancer chemotherapy with cytotoxic agents suppresses the immune system. As described in two reports from an NIH conference, this usually unwanted effect has been turned to advantage for the treatment on non-neoplastic disease in which autoimmune mechanisms are considered important to pathogenesis [*Ann Intern Med* 1998;128:1021–28; 129:49–58]. The first report concerns renal diseases and rheumatologic disorders—rheumatoid arthritis, systemic lupus erythematosus, and scleroderma. The second report concerns inflammatory bowel disease, systemic vasculitis, and therapeutic toxicity. The drugs reviewed are cyclophosphamide, chlorambucil, methotrexate, azathioprine, 6-mercaptopurine, and cyclosporine. The participants in the conference concluded that while these drugs are among the most useful and beneficial options in the treatment of autoimmune disease, they are probably not the ultimate therapeutic answer because they do not prevent relapse of disease in most cases and have side effects. Infection remains an important cause of illness and death because of the nonspecific actions of these agents. Drugs directed toward the disruption of more specific pathways of the immune response are under investigation and hold promise.

Mental Health

More Benefits of Current Generation of Antipsychotic Drugs
SSRI Antidepressants and Weight Gain

More Benefits of Current Generation of Antipsychotic Drugs. Reports at an international meeting demonstrate for the first time that the new atypical antipsychotic agents—risperidone, olanzapine, and clozapine—improve cognitive function in patients with schizophrenia. [*Scrip,* July 31, 1998, p 25; *JAMA* 1998;280:953–54]. This is an important advance over older drugs such as haloperidol. More than 85% of schizophrenics have impaired cognitive function, and of all their symptoms, cognitive function seems to correlate best with the potential for living independently and holding down a job. Conventional antipsychotic agents further depress cognitive function, an unwanted side effect. The atypicals already have the advantage of improving negative as well positive symptoms of schizophrenia and have a more favorable side-effect profile. These findings are commercially important to pharmaceutical companies who strive to differentiate their very expensive new drugs from older, far less expensive agents aimed at the same condition. Many experts at the meeting opined that the atypical antipsychotics should now be considered first-line treatment. In the US, atypicals now account for half of the antipsychotic market by volume.

SSRI Antidepressants and Weight Gain. Several reports suggest that short-term use of selective serotonin reuptake inhibitors (SSRIs) for the treatment of patients with clinical depression also results in loss of weight. If so, that "side effect" is a very welcome one. The weight gain frequently seen with tricyclic antidepressants is a deterrent to good compliance with prescribed therapy, particularly for women. Most experts agree that patients on SSRIs have less weight gain then those taking tricyclics. The weight loss seen with fluoxetine (*Prozac*) and other SSRIs usually occurs within 6 to 20 weeks after initiating therapy and averages two to four pounds. Trials evaluating fluoxetine as a diet drug confirm the early weight loss, but also report that most patients regain much or all of the lost weight after a year or more of therapy. Some patients on an SSRI actually gain weight [*Psychiatric Ann* 1998;28:89–97]. Weight gain is more pronounced for those under the age of 60 and for those treated for one year or more. A review of the literature suggests than in the long term, about one-third of patients lose weight, one-third gain weight (as much as 20 pounds), and one-third remain about the same. The *Prescriber's Letter* [September 1998, p 50] suggests that early weight loss may be related to an anorexic effect but prolonged use of SSRIs may reduce the sensitivity of serotonin receptors that regulate weight. Venlafaxine (*Effexor*), an antidepressant that acts on both serotonin and norepinephrine receptors, might be less likely to cause substantial weight gains.

OBESITY

Obesity Guidelines Caution on Drug Use. Obesity now affects nearly 100 million Americans. New guidelines, issued in June 1998, recommend that drugs to promote weight loss should be considered only after efforts to modify diet and increase physical exercise for at least six months. Patients who are not successful should initiate drug therapy with the lowest effective dose. An expert panel convened by the National Institutes of Health developed the guidance document [*Scrip*, June 24, 1998, p 23]. The panel defines the term overweight as a body mass index (BMI) of 25 to 29.9 and obesity as a BMI greater than 30. Appropriate patients for drug therapy are those with a BMI of 27 or above and obesity-related risk factors, and those with a BMI of 30 or above without additional risk factors. The expert panel recognizes that effective weight reduction is possible for most people only by prolonged drug therapy. The panel recommends that if there are no serious adverse effects, drug therapy can be continued in the weight maintenance phase of treatment, although safety and effectiveness beyond one year of treatment has not been established. The panel also says that physicians and their patients should aim to reduce weight initially by 10% from baseline over six months and that maintenance should be a priority after six months.

ONCOLOGY

Cyclosporine Improves Oral Therapy with *Taxol*
Arsenic Induces Complete Remission for a Form of Leukemia

Cyclosporine Improves Oral Therapy with Taxol. Intravenous paclitaxel (*Taxol*) causes unpredictable side effects mostly due to its injection vehicle—the commercial base Cremaphor EL. Oral administration is not an alternative because paclitaxel has a low bioavailability. Because of the drug's high affinity for the multidrug transporter P-glycoprotein, it is pumped out of intestinal cells and back into the lumen. The bioavailability of paclitaxel increases considerably in knockout mice lacking the transporter. Animal studies have identified several P-glycoprotein blockers and among them is cyclosporine. To determine if these findings also apply to humans and result in improved bioavailability of paclitaxel, investigators studied 14 patients with solid tumors. Five received oral paclitaxel (the intravenous formulation) alone and nine patients received oral paclitaxel with cyclosporine. Although there was considerable variability, cyclosporine increased the bioavailability of paclitaxel ninefold on average compared with the administration of paclitaxel alone. Following oral paclitaxel with cyclosporine, plasma concentrations were in the therapeutic range for four hours, comparable to levels achieved with an intravenous dose. The authors suggest that the idea of inhibiting P-glycoprotein may be applied to other drugs with poor bioavailability and high affinity for P-glycoprotein, such as HIV protease inhibitors [*Lancet* 1998;352:285].

Arsenic Induces Complete Remission for a Form of Leukemia. Acute promyelocytic leukemia (APL) is a variant of acute myeloid leukemia (AML), seen in 10 to 15% of cases. It is characterized by a specific cytogenetic abnormality. As a result of including a retinoid—all-trans-retinoic acid (*Vesanoid*)—into chemotherapy for APL, survival has more than doubled since 1990. Today, the risk of relapse in patients who achieve remission has decreased to about 20% compared with rates of 60% to 70% in the 1980s. Reports from China, dating back to 1992, say that arsenic trioxide may be another useful addition to chemotherapy for APL. More recently, a US study confirmed these reports [*N Engl J Med* 1998;339:1341–48]. The new study involved 12 patients with APL who had relapsed more than once after standard therapy. They were treated with daily doses of intravenous arsenic trioxide until leukemic cells were eliminated from the bone marrow. After treatment, 11 of the 12 patients had a complete remission that lasted from 12 to 30 days. Adverse effects were relatively mild. Arsenic induces terminal differentiation of some APL cells, followed by caspase activation and induction of apoptosis. Arsenic's striking effect and lack of specificity for APL proteins warrant further study of the drug as therapy for other neoplastic diseases [*Ibid,* pp 1389–91].

RESPIRATORY DISEASE

Competing Inhaled Corticosteroids Not Equipotent. A survey of computer records in New Zealand for 5930 patients who, over the course of one year, received nearly 17,000 prescriptions for inhaled beclomethasone or budesonide (*Pulmicort*), widely thought to be equipotent, showed that the daily prescribed dose was higher for patients on budesonide than for those taking beclomethasone (979 μg compared with 635 μg). The findings suggest that inhaled budesonide has about two-thirds of the potency of inhaled beclomethasone and may need to be given in higher doses [*Br Medical J* 1998;317:986–90]. Switching from one inhaled corticosteroid to the another may call for dosage adjustment.

Women's Health

Hormone Replacement Therapy Decreases Risk of Colorectal
  Cancer
Tamoxifen: Secondary Prevention of Breast Cancer
Chemotherapy for Early Breast Cancer Improves Survival
Estrogen Therapy: Effects on Cognitive Function and
  Dementia
Estrogen Replacement Therapy and Breast Cancer
Understanding and Treating Premenstrual Syndrome (PMS)
Oral Contraceptives and the Risk of Hereditary Ovarian Cancer
Does Acetaminophen Protect Against Ovarian Cancer?
Progestin-Only Oral Contraceptives May Increase the Risk of
  Type 2 Diabetes
Cancer Risk in Women Exposed to Diethylstilbestrol in Utero
Hormone Replacement Therapy Reduces Risk of Hip Fracture
Meeting Reports Hold Promise for the Treatment of
  Osteoporosis
Estrogen Replacement Therapy and Type 2 Diabetes
Birth Control Pill for Acne
Teenage Girls Favor Depot Contraceptive
Low-Dose OCs Do Not Increase the Risk of a Heart Attack
Sex Differences in Viral Load and Progression to AIDS
Erythromycin Poses Greater Risk of Arrhythmias for Women

Hormone Replacement Therapy Decreases Risk of Colorectal Cancer. Evidence suggests that postmenopausal hormone use may decrease the risk for colorectal cancer. Adding to the evidence is a recent report of a prospective cohort study [*Ann Intern Med* 1998;128:705–12]. The cohort consisted of about 59,000 postmenopausal women participating in the Nurses' Health Study. During the period of observation, 470 women developed colorectal cancer. Compared with the risk in women who had never used HRT, the risk for colorectal cancer was reduced by 35% in current users and by 30% in those who had stopped using HRT in the past five years. There was no evidence of benefit five years after stopping HRT. The historical view of cancer etiology gave rise to a sense that prevention efforts for middle-aged and elderly women were futile because the trigger had already been pulled.

This view has changed radically. Researchers have seen that excess risks for lymphoma related to immunosuppressive drugs and risks for endometrial cancer related to HRT appear shortly after initiation of treatment and decline rapidly after treatment. Scientists now believe that genetic changes that are required to initiate a tumor can take place late in the complex and prolonged process of carcinogenesis. The association between HRT and colorectal cancer, if real and causal, reinforces the idea that actions taken late, at a time close to when cancer might develop clinically, can indeed be preventive [*Ann Intern Med* 1998;128:771–72].

Tamoxifen: Secondary Prevention of Breast Cancer. A report from the Early Breast Cancer Trialists' Collaborative Group concerns a meta-analysis of 55 clinical trials involving 37,000 women. The trialists determined that tamoxifen, given to women with the most common type of breast cancer, estrogen receptor positive, for five years after surgery reduces the rates of recurrence by 42% and death by 22%. Tamoxifen prevents one in six recurrences of breast cancer and one in twelve deaths [*Lancet* 1998;351:1451–67]. Taken for five years, tamoxifen is more beneficial than if it is taken for one to two years. The drug benefits breast cancer patients of all ages, not only postmenopausal patients, and is effective whether the cancer is confined to the breast or has spread to lymph nodes. Among women who received chemotherapy and tamoxifen for five years, 61% had no disease recurrence after ten years, compared with 40% who received chemotherapy alone. Experts say that the key determinant of electing tamoxifen treatment should be whether the tumor is hormone sensitive. Hormone-sensitive breast cancers account for 75% of total breast cancers among women over 50 years old and 50% among women under 50.

Chemotherapy for Early Breast Cancer Improves Survival. A recent overview of data from randomized trials updates the benefits of chemotherapy with two or more cytotoxic agents after surgery for women with early breast cancer [*Lancet* 1998;352:930–42]. For recurrence of cancer, chemotherapy produces a 35% reduction among women younger than 50 years at randomization and a 20% reduction among women 50 to 69 years old. For mortality, the corresponding reductions are 27% and 11%, respectively. The proportional reductions in risk were similar for women with lymph node-positive and node-negative disease. The mortality reductions seen in women under 50 suggest that chemotherapy increases 10-year survival from 71% to 78% for those with node-negative disease, and from 42% to 53% in patients with node-positive disease. The review found no advantage in survival with the use of chemotherapy for more than three to six months. Anthracycline-containing regimens produced slightly greater reductions of recurrence and mortality than the combination of cyclophosphamide, methotrexate, and fluorouracil. The researchers conclude: "Some months of adjuvant polyche-motherapy . . . typically produces an absolute improvement of about 7–11% in 10-year survival for women aged under 50 at presentation with early breast cancer, and of about 2–3% for those aged 50–69. . . . Treatment decisions involve consideration not only of improvements in cancer recurrence and survival but also of adverse effects of treatment, and this report makes no recommendations as to who should or should not be treated."

Estrogen Therapy: Effects on Cognitive Function and Dementia. Loss of intellectual function (dementia) is a common and serious problem for elderly Americans. The number of people suffering Alzheimer's disease, the most prevalent cause of dementia, is approaching four million. Little is available to treat or prevent dementia. A growing number of observational studies suggest that estrogen taken by postmenopausal women may improve cognition, prevent the development of dementia, or improve the severity of dementia. In a recent report, researchers review biochemical and neurophysiological evidence to support the role of estrogen in cognition and describe the results of a meta-analysis of ten studies of postmenopausal estrogen use and risk of dementia [*JAMA* 1998;279:688–95]. They report that there are plausible biological mechanisms that might account for a beneficial effect of estrogen. Their meta-analysis suggests a statistically significant 29% reduction in risk. Nevertheless, the authors are reluctant to embrace the use of estrogen for dementia. They state that most reported studies have methodological problems and portray conflicting results. Moreover, the largest and soundest observational study of estrogen use on cognition in older women shows no benefit. The investigators conclude: "Given the known risks of estrogen therapy, we do not recommend estrogen for the prevention or treatment of Alzheimer's disease or other dementias until adequate trials have been completed."

Estrogen Replacement Therapy and Breast Cancer Evidence. In the absence of a randomized trial, there is uncertainty as to the significance of epidemiological studies associating the use of estrogen in postmenopausal women and the development of breast cancer. Seeking to determine the strength of that evidence, investigators carried out a meta-analysis of the extensive literature on the subject. They conclude that hormone replacement therapy (HRT) does increase the risk of breast cancer. Moreover, it seems that the longer a woman uses HRT, the greater the likelihood she has of developing breast cancer [*J Natl Cancer Inst* 1998;90:814–23]. Their analysis found that for each year of use, the risk of breast cancer increases by 2.3%. They estimate that for every 1000 women who begin HRT at age 50 and then take it for ten years, there are six additional cases of breast cancer; for fifteen years of use, there are twelve. The investigators believe that the relationship between HRT and breast cancer is causal, based on the following criteria: consistency, dose-response pattern, biologic plausibility, temporality, strength of association, and coherence. There are many, however, that are unlikely to be convinced that the issue is closed. The researchers conclude: "Strategies that do not cause breast cancer are urgently needed for the relief of menopausal symptoms and the long-term prevention of osteoporosis and heart disease."

The biology supporting the linkage between estrogen and the development of breast cancer is compelling. Estrogen powerfully stimulates cell proliferation and up until now has been seen as a promoter of cancer, but not as an initiator. Researchers have assigned the blame for initiating genetic damage to spontaneous mistakes in DNA replication and to damage triggered by external sources. New evidence, however, suggests a deeper involvement of estrogen and points to a new culprit for initiating carcinogenesis—estrogen metabolites [*Science* 1998;279:1631–33]. Cell culture studies show that estrogen metabolites can bind to DNA and trigger damage. Estradiol undergoes metabolic transformation to three primary metabolites, two of which, 4-HE and 16-alpha-HE, are problematic. Hamsters given 4-HE develop tumors within six months, whereas few of the animals given the natural hormone develop cancer. Other studies have shown that 4-HE is formed at susceptible sites. The enzyme that converts 17-β-estradiol to 4-HE is more abundant in the breast than in tissues not prone to estrogen-linked cancers. The enzyme is also present in the uterus and ovaries. Commenting on the link between estrogen and carcinogenesis, a leading researcher noted: "The evidence is building, but the burden of proof still lies in developing more direct evidence."

Understanding and Treating Premenstrual Syndrome. Recent studies show that psychoactive drugs such as alprazolam and SSRIs—fluoxetine (*Prozac*) and sertraline (*Zoloft*)—are effective for treating PMS. For years, however, physicians believed that women suffering PMS had a progesterone deficiency and prescribed progesterone suppositories as replacement therapy. This idea, however, has not withstood the test of time. Investigators have now reported that women with PMS have lower serum concentrations of the progesterone metabolite allopregnanolone during the luteal phase of the menstrual cycle than do symptom-free women [*Obstet Gynecol* 1997;90:709–14]. This observation suggests that women with PMS differ from symptom-free women in the metabolism of progesterone. Allopregnanolone is a psychoactive metabolite. It enhances gamma-aminobutyric acid A (GABA-A) receptor function and has anxiolytic effects. A deficiency in allopregnanolone might predispose to anxiety. Furthermore, women with PMS may preferentially metabolize progesterone to pregnenolone rather than allopregnanolone. Pregnenolone may antagonize GABA-A receptors and promote anxiety. Also worth noting, GABA agonists such as allopregnanolone may upregulate serotonin receptors and thereby ameliorate depression. Although the findings to date leave many questions unanswered, a refined hypothesis regarding the pathogenesis of PMS is emerging [*Lancet* 1998;351:465–66].

Oral Contraceptives and the Risk of Hereditary Ovarian Cancer. One in ten cases of ovarian cancer is hereditary. The majority of women at risk of the hereditary form of the cancer carry mutations in the BRCA1 or BRCA2 gene. There is evidence that oral contraceptives protect against ovarian cancer in the general population, but it is not known whether they protect against the hereditary form of the disease. To address this question, investigators enrolled 207 women with hereditary ovarian cancers and 161 of their sisters as controls in a case-control study. All the women with cancer carried pathogenic mutation in either BRCA1 (179 women) or BRCA2 (28 women). Study participants provided information concerning lifetime histories of oral contraceptive use. The researchers found that any past use of oral contraceptives reduced the risk of ovarian cancer by 50%, on average. Risk decreased with increasing duration of use. Use for six years or longer decreased the risk by 60%. The use of oral contraceptives protected both carriers of the BRCA1 mutation and the BRCA2 mutation [*N Engl J Med* 1998;339:424–28]. Some physicians are prescribing oral contraceptives for women at high risk for ovarian cancer and, as a result of this report, more are likely to do so. While cautioning against the potential bias that arises in case-control studies, an editorial on the findings concludes that the study provides the best available data on the subject, and that the results and conclusions are biologically plausible [*N Engl J Med* 1998;339:460–71].

Does Acetaminophen Protect Against Ovarian Cancer? Evidence that aspirin and other nonsteroidal anti-inflammatory agents reduce the risk for colorectal cancer encouraged investigators to undertake a case-control study to examine the association of over-the-counter analgesics with the incidence of ovarian cancer. Cases were 523 American women who had epithelial ovarian cancer. They were matched with 523 controls drawn from the general population. The investigators reported no significant association between the use of aspirin or ibuprofen and ovarian cancer, whereas the use acetaminophen at least once a week for at least six months significantly reduced risk by nearly 50% [*Lancet* 1998;351:104–07]. Similar findings are seen in a more recent report that examined the association between the use of acetaminophen and death rates from ovarian cancer in a prospective cohort of American women enrolled in a cancer prevention study [*Lancet* 1998;352:1354–56]. At the end of twelve years of follow-up, 1573 ovarian cancer deaths were observed among 616,189 women who were free of cancer at study entry. More than 12,000 women reported using acetaminophen in the month before enrollment and 5731 reported daily use. Women using acetaminophen every day had a 45% lower death rate from ovarian cancer than those who reported no use. The benefit, however, failed to reach statistical significance. A potential biological mechanism for a protective effect against ovarian cancer is the antigonadotropic effect of acetaminophen.

Progestin-Only Oral Contraceptives May Increase the Risk of Type 2 Diabetes. Progestin-only and low-dose estrogen-progestin combination oral contraceptives have little effect on glucose tolerance in the general population. However, women with recent gestational diabetes are at increased risk of developing type 2 diabetes and may be more susceptible to the effects of oral contraceptives. Ironically, these women require effective contraception because if they conceive after developing type 2 diabetes, their newborns are at increased risk of major congenital malformations. Researchers have reported recently the results of a cohort study of Latina women with recent gestational diabetes. At their first postpartum visit, 443 women selected a nonhormonal form of contraception, 383 chose a low-dose estrogen-progestin combination product, and 78 women, who wished to breast feed, chose a progestin-only oral contraceptive and then switched to a combination product after weaning.

The average annual incidence rates of type 2 diabetes over a 7.5-year period were about 9%, 10%, and 26%, respectively. After adjustment for potential confounding factors, the use of a progestin-only oral contraceptive nearly triples the risk of developing diabetes compared with the use of a combination product. Physicians should probably be cautious when prescribing progestin-only oral contraceptives for Latina women with recent gestational diabetes [*JAMA* 1998;280:533–38].

Cancer Risk in Women Exposed to Diethylstilbestrol in Utero. In the 1950s and 60s several million pregnant women were exposed to diethylstilbestrol (DES) in the US and Europe for the prevention of spontaneous abortion and premature delivery. As many as three million American women living today may have been exposed. Its use was stopped in 1971 following reports of a strong association between DES use in pregnancy and the occurrence of vaginal and cervical clear cell adenocarcinoma (CCA) in exposed female offspring. Not knowing the effects of DES exposure in utero on the development of cancers other than CCA, investigators have identified and queried a cohort of 4536 DES-exposed daughters and compared them with an age-matched cohort of 1544 unexposed daughters [*JAMA* 1998;280:630–34]. The researchers found that up until now, DES-exposed daughters have not experienced an increased risk for all cancers or individual cancer sites, except CCA of the vagina and cervix. Despite the encouraging results, the investigators point out that the exposed daughters included in the study were on average only 38 years old, and conclude that continued surveillance is warranted to see if any increases in cancer risk occur during the menopausal years.

Hormone Replacement Therapy Reduces Risk of Hip Fracture. A population-based case-control study covering six counties in Sweden, identified 1327 women 50 to 81 years old with hip fracture and 3262 randomly selected healthy controls. Current and past users of hormone replacement therapy (HRT) had odds ratios of 0.35 and 0.77, respectively, for hip fracture, compared with women who had never used HRT. For every year of replacement therapy, the overall risk decreased by 4% for HRT regimens without a progestin and 11% for regimens including a progestin. After five years without HRT, the protective effect on hip fracture was substantially diminished. For women currently using HRT, initiation of therapy nine or more years after the menopause gave equally strong protection against hip fracture as an early start of therapy. Estrogen treatment with skin patches gave similar risk estimates as oral regimens. The investigators conclude: "Recent use of HRT is required for optimum fracture protection, but therapy can be started several years after the menopause. The protective effect increases with duration of use, and an estrogen-sparing effect is achieved when progestins are included in the regimen" [*BMJ* 1998;316:1858–63]. Following the report, the National Osteoporosis Foundation released the "Physician's Guide to Prevention and Treatment of Osteoporosis." The report concludes that HRT represents the greatest benefit relative to cost as a pharmacologic treatment of osteoporosis [*The Pink Sheet* 1998;60(No46):21]. According to the guide, all postmenopausal women should be counseled to consider HRT and offered guidance in weighing its risks and benefits. Patients should also be counseled on risk factor reduction, which includes the use of calcium, vitamin D, and exercise. The guidance recommends alendronate (*Fosamax*) for patients who are unwilling to take HRT. The document more tepidly endorses calcitonin nasal spray (*Miacalcin*) and raloxifene (*Evista*) as other potential alternatives to HRT.

Meeting Reports Hold Promise for Treatment of Osteoporosis. Several reports at the European Congress on Osteoporosis in Berlin confirmed and extended existing evidence of the effectiveness of products marketed for the prevention and treatment of osteoporosis [*The Wall Street Journal,* September 15, 1998, p B4]. Merck scientists reported that alendronate (*Fosamax*) further increases bone density in older women with the disease who are receiving conjugated estrogens (*Premarin*). In the study, 428 women received *Fosamax, Premarin,* and a progestin, or *Premarin* and progestin alone, for one year. Combination treatment increased bone mass in the spine by 3.6% compared with an increase of only 1% in women receiving hormone therapy alone.

Another report presented data showing that women using raloxifene (*Evista*), Lilly's selective estrogen receptor modulator, were only half as likely to have their first spinal fracture after two years compared with women taking placebo. Women who had had a spinal fracture and used *Evista* were 38% less likely to have another. A third presentation reported that calcitonin-salmon (*Miacalcin*) nasal spray decreases new spinal fracture by 36% over a five-year period compared with placebo. *Miacalcin* is approved to treat osteoporosis in postmenopausal women who refuse or cannot tolerate estrogen replacement therapy.

Estrogen Replacement Therapy and Type 2 Diabetes. Presentations at the summer meeting of the American Diabetes Association suggest that replacement therapy may prevent or ameliorate type 2 diabetes in postmenopausal women [*Prescriber's Letter,* September 1998, p 51]. A survey of 14,601 women over the age of 50 with type 2 diabetes found that age-adjusted mean glycosylated hemoglobin levels were significantly lower in women using estrogen replacement therapy (ERT) than in nonusers. Among white and African-American women, patients using ERT could control elevated glucose levels with diet alone; nonusers of ERT required antidiabetic drugs or insulin. Women using ERT, however, were younger and better educated than their counterparts. Another presentation reported that among 418 postmenopausal women, those who had never used ERT were nearly five times more likely to develop type 2 diabetes than nonusers. A third report stated that among 128 postmenopausal Japanese-American women, those who used ERT had considerably lower levels of proinsulin than did nonusers. Elevated levels of proinsulin occur when this precursor is not efficiently converted to insulin by pancreatic beta cells. They reflect poor functioning of the beta cells, a hallmark of type 2 diabetes.

Birth Control Pill for Acne. *OrthoTriCyclen,* an oral contraceptive containing norgestimate and ethinyl estradiol, is the only birth control pill to have an indication for the treatment of acne in young women 15 years of age or older. According to the label, the combination of norgestimate and ethinyl estradiol may increase sex hormone binding globulin and decrease free testosterone, resulting in a decrease in the severity of facial acne in women with this condition. It is likely that other estrogen-containing oral contraceptives will also be effective. Ortho-McNeil, however, is the only company with permission, granted in January 1997, to promote the skin-clearing ability of its product. From 1996 to 1998, market share of *TriCyclen* increased 137%. Because of the additional indication, *TriCyclen* is the sales leader in the $1.6 billion per year oral contraceptive market [*The Wall Street Journal,* September 28, 1998, pp B1, B6]. Some health professionals complain that many young women are being distracted from making the wisest birth control choices because of their obsession with clear skin. They are worried that ads are coaxing teens to use birth control pills rather than condoms, which can prevent sexually transmitted diseases.

Teenage Girls Favor Depot Contraceptive. According to *The Wall Street Journal* [October 14, 1998, pp A1,A14] teenage girls are turning to *Depo-Provera* to prevent unwanted pregnancies because they have a difficult time remembering to take an oral contraceptive each day. The use of this long-acting medroxyprogesterone preparation, which reliably prevents pregnancy for three months after a single injection, may be a driving force behind a recent substantial decline in teen pregnancies, particularly in blacks. Although Pharmacia & Upjohn did not market the product until 1993, by 1995 it accounted for 19% of contraceptive use among black teens between 15 and 19 years old. The use of oral contraceptives and male condoms accounted for 32% and 38%, respectively, of contraceptive use in this population. More recent surveys find that the use of the depot injection in public health clinics is up sharply from 1995. Limiting more widespread use of *Depo-Provera* is the high cost of the product compared with most other forms of contraception.

Low-Dose OCs Do Not Increase the Risk of a Heart Attack. A case-control study of women in California and Washington state who ranged in age from 18 to 44 years, shows that oral contraceptives (OCs) containing a low dose of estrogen do not increase the risk of MI [*Circulation* 1998;98:1058–63]. Cases were 271 women with an MI who had no prior history of ischemic heart disease or cerebrovascular disease. They were matched with 993 controls. Compared with those not using an OC, current users had an adjusted odds ratio for MI of 0.94 Compared with women who had never used an OC, current users had an adjusted odds ratio for MI of 0.56 and past users had an adjusted odds ratio of 0.54. Among any-time users of OCs, duration of use was unrelated to the risk of MI.

Sex Differences in Viral Load and Progression to AIDS. Studies of white homosexual men and male African-American injection-drug users with HIV infection show that the number of HIV RNA copies (viral load) and CD4 T-lymphocyte counts are strong predictors for progression to AIDS. Clinical guidelines for initiation of treatment of HIV infection were developed based on these studies. There is little information, however, whether and to what extent, current treatment guidelines are applicable to women. To generate more information, researchers designed a study to analyze the relation between gender and viral load, and their joint impact in predicting disease progression [*Lancet* 1998;352:1510–14]. They found that women infected with HIV are at a more advanced stage of infection and at higher risk of developing AIDS than men with identical levels of virus in plasma.

The investigators examined 812 specimens from 650 injection-drug users at a clinic in Baltimore. Women had a lower median viral load than men. The association persisted even after adjustment for CD4 cell count, race, and drug use. Women with the same viral load as men had a 60% greater chance of progressing to AIDS; women with half the viral load of men had a similar time to progression to AIDS as men. Although the biological mechanism for this difference is not clear, the findings suggest that current recommendations for HIV viral load thresholds at which antiretroviral therapy is initiated should be revised downward for women. Other researchers, however, say that changing treatment guidelines now would be premature. The study has also fanned the flames that are rising from the debate over the best time for people with HIV infection to begin taking antiretroviral medication [*The New York Times,* November 6, 1998, p A18].

Erythromycin Poses Greater Risk of Arrhythmias for Women. The widely used macrolide antibiotic erythromycin is one of many drugs that prolong the QT interval on the ECG and pose a risk of severe or even fatal arrhythmias. In the general population, men have a shorter QT interval than women and may be less sensitive to proarrhythmic effects. To evaluate the potential influence of gender on the cardiac adverse effects of erythromycin, investigators searched FDA's MedWatch Spontaneous Reporting System for such events. They estimated usage of erythromycin from the National Disease and Therapeutic Index (NDTI), a proprietary database that contains information about the patterns and treatment of disease encountered in office-based medical practice in the US. NDTI shows no gender imbalance in the prescription pattern for intravenous erythromycin. The investigators found a total of 346 cardiac arrhythmia reports in the FDA database. Fifty-eight percent were women, 32% men, and 10% unspecified. Among the cases were 49 episodes of life threatening ventricular arrhythmias and deaths directly related to intravenous erythromycin: 67% were women and 33% were men. A laboratory study included in the report found that perfusion with erythromycin causes significantly greater QT-prolongation in female rabbit hearts than in male hearts. The authors hypothesize that an increased sensitivity to erythromycin in women could facilitate, especially at low heart rates, the induction of ventricular arrhythmias [*JAMA* 1998;280:1774–76].

Men's Health

Treatment of Sexual Deviation in Men
Aging Men Lose Testosterone
Aging Men Also Lose Estrogen and Develop Osteoporosis

Treatment of Sexual Deviation in Men. Deviant sexual behavior (paraphilia) in men is a serious problem. At least 100,000 children are sexually molested by men in the US each year and the number may be as high as 500,000. There is considerable interest in chemical castration but several strategies have had only partial success. Selective suppression of pituitary-gonadal function may abolish the deviant sexual fantasies, urges, and behavior of men with paraphilia by reducing serum testosterone to very low levels. Researchers have reported the results of treating men with severe paraphilia with monthly injections of triptorelin, a long-acting agonist analogue of gonadotropin-releasing hormone, and psychotherapy [*N Engl J Med* 1998;338:416–22]. Before treatment the average number of deviant sexual fantasies experienced by the men participating in the study was 48 per week and the average number of incidents of abnormal sexual behavior was 5 per month. Three to ten months of treatment abolished all deviant fantasies and abnormal behavior. Effects persisted for at least one year. The men's mean serum testosterone concentration fell from 545 ng/dl before treatment to 23 ng/dl during treatment. Main side effects were erectile failure, hot flashes, and a decrease in bone mineral density. Up until now the FDA has approved no agent for the treatment of paraphilia, despite its seriousness. Perhaps the findings with triptorelin will encourage the pharmaceutical industry and the regulatory agency to work at solving this problem.

Aging Men Lose Testosterone. *The Wall Street Journal* (February 2, 1998) reported that male aging is "a red hot field" and the subject of a world congress attracting researchers to discuss, among many facets of aging, what happens to testosterone and what men can do about it. Unlike women, whose menstrual cycle stops at about age 50, resulting in abrupt hormonal changes, men experience a gradual change in hormone levels over many years. According to the National Institutes of Health, testosterone subsides about 1% to 2% per year from age 30. By age 75 to 80, about 50% of men have subnormal levels of testosterone. Should elderly men, like postmenopausal women, receive hormone replacement therapy? Some researchers say that testosterone can improve lean muscle mass and bone strength in deficient elderly men. The decision to prescribe, however, is complicated because testosterone stimulates the growth of prostate cancer, which may be present in an as yet undetectable form. Testosterone may also increase the risk of stroke. The *Journal* reports that despite concerns about safety, ". . . men are embracing testosterone more readily than women accept estrogen." Replacement is available in the form of skin patches, scrotal patches, implants, and self-administered injections. The author of a book entitled *Male Menopause* warns: "In the business of youth elixirs, benefits are always trumpeted loudly and risks, if they are mentioned at all, are always whispered softly."

Aging Men Also Lose Estrogen and Develop Osteoporosis. New studies, presented at a meeting of the American Society for Bone and Mineral Research, suggest that osteoporosis is more prevalent in men than previously thought and that the main cause of the bone loss is an age-related decrease in estrogen [*The New York Times*, December 8, 1998, p D6]. Two studies presented at the meeting, one from the US and the other from Germany, indicate that estrogen plays a more central role than does testosterone in the development of osteoporosis in men. One investigator is sufficiently emboldened by the preliminary findings that she plans to study the use of estrogen supplements to treat men with osteoporosis. The National Osteoporosis Foundation estimates that of the 10 million Americans who have osteoporosis, more than 1.5 million are men. About one-half of women and 1 in 8 men over 50 years old will have an osteoporosis-related fracture.

CHILDREN'S HEALTH

Growth Hormone Therapy for Children
Survey Reveals Alarming Overuse of Antibiotics in Children
Antidepressants Pose Low Risk to Fetus
Cesarean Delivery May Reduce Risk of Vertical Transmission
   of HIV
Risk Factors for Perinatal Transmission of HIV in Women
   Receiving AZT
Abbreviated AZT Regimens Reduce Risk of Perinatal HIV
   Transmission
Attempted Abortion with Misoprostol Increases the Risk of
   Birth Defect
Pamidronate for Osteogenesis Imperfecta

Growth Hormone Therapy for Children. Evidence support the use of human growth hormone (GH) in children with classical GH deficiency, with renal insufficiency, and in children with short stature due to Turner's syndrome, a disorder that occurs in female children with only one X chromosome. Although GH is also prescribed for short children who do not have a defined medical disorder, there is little information to support this use. Investigators interested in comparing health coverage policies of insurers with the treatment recommended by physicians for short children developed a survey to acquire pertinent information [*JAMA* 1998;279:663–68]. Physician recommendations and insurance coverage decisions differed widely. Overall, treatment decisions by physicians resulted in recommendations for GH therapy in 78% of children with primary deficiency, Turner's syndrome, or renal failure. Insurers denied coverage to 28% of those recommendations. More than half of the recommendations for children with Turner's Syndrome were rejected. Physicians surveyed indicated they would recommend GH for about 10% of children with idiopathic short stature, but insurers would not cover GH for the vast majority of these children. Considerations that are influencing insurers include the somewhat elective use of GH therapy—it is rarely needed for life-threatening situations—and medication costs of about $14,000 per year.

Survey Reveals Alarming Overuse of Antibiotics in Children. Researchers wishing to evaluate antibiotic-prescribing practices for children with colds, upper respiratory tract infections (URIs), or bronchitis, went to the information contained in the Medical Care Survey conducted in 1992 [*JAMA* 1998;279:875–77]. Participating office-based physicians reported a total of 531 pediatric visits that included a principal diagnosis of cold, URI, or bronchitis. They prescribed antibiotics to 44% of patients with common colds, 46% with URIs, and 75% with bronchitis. Prescribing rates for pediatricians were about 50% lower than for other physicians. Extrapolating these figures to the entire population of office-based physicians in the US suggests that in 1992 more than 10 million prescriptions were written for children diagnosed as having conditions that typically do not benefit from antibiotics. Concern about patient/parent satisfaction and retention is a key factor promoting overprescribing as is a physician's lack of experience with medical conditions in children. When time management is a problem, writing a prescription for an antibiotic is perceived as more efficient than explaining why an antibiotic is not needed [*JAMA* 1998;279:881–82]. These practices contribute directly to the calamitous increase in the rate of resistance to antibacterial agents.

Antidepressants Pose Low Risk to Fetus. Many women of childbearing age suffer depression and are using an antidepressant agent, usually a SSRI such as fluoxetine (*Prozac*). Because more than half of all pregnancies are unplanned, the safety of these agents for the exposed fetus is a concern. Studies of fetal exposure to *Prozac* in the first trimester or during the entire pregnancy show no evidence of major malformation or behavioral teratology. There is no human data, however, on the reproductive safety of newly approved SSRIs. To assess fetal safety of these agents, investigators working with nine Teratology Information Service centers identified a cohort of 267 depressed women who reported taking an SSRI—fluvoxamine (*Luvox*), paroxetine (*Paxil*), or sertraline (*Zoloft*)—during the first trimester of pregnancy. The same number of controls was randomly selected from pregnant women counseled at the same center who reported exposure to a benign substance. The investigators found no association between exposure to SSRIs and either increased risk for major malformations or higher rates of miscarriage, stillbirth, or prematurity. Mean birth weight among offspring of SSRI users was about the same as the birth weight of nonusers.

Cesarean Delivery May Reduce Risk of Vertical Transmission of HIV. Investigators in France have reported the results of a prospective cohort study of 2834 children born to mothers with HIV infection [*JAMA* 1998;280:55–

60]. No zidovudine (*Retrovir*) was used in 1917 pregnancies. Emergency cesarean deliveries were performed in 10.9% of the mothers; 8.3% opted for elective cesareans, performed before labor or membrane rupture. Among mothers who did not receive zidovudine prophylaxis, 17.2% transmitted the virus to their child. Mode of delivery was not related to transmission. In mothers who did receive zidovudine, overall transmission was 6.4%, and elective cesarean delivery was associated with a lower transmission rate than emergent cesarean or vaginal delivery (0.8%, 11.4%, and 6.6%, respectively). The role of elective cesarean to prevent vertical transmission in clinical practice remains to be determined. If a planned cesarean with zidovudine prophylaxis decreases the risk of transmission from 6% to 1%, 20 surgical procedures would be necessary to prevent one case of transmission. This benefit, however, is offset by the risk of maternal morbidity and mortality, which is greater with cesarean delivery than with vaginal delivery.

Risk Factors for Perinatal Transmission of HIV in Women Receiving AZT.

The protection offered by zidovudine (AZT, *Retrovir*) against the vertical transmission of HIV from a pregnant mother to her offspring is not absolute. Researchers from the Centers for Disease Control and Prevention recently reported the results of a prospective cohort study of 1533 children born to HIV-infected women in the US. The objective was to determine risk factors for transmission among women receiving antiviral therapy including zidovudine. The overall risk of transmission was 18%. Membrane rupture more than four hours before delivery doubled the risk. A gestational age of less than 37 weeks, a maternal CD4+ count of less than 500, and a birth weight less than 2500 g increased the risk of transmission by 70% to 80%. For all infants exposed to zidovudine before and after delivery, the transmission rate was 13%, but decreased to 9% with term delivery, and 7% when membrane rupture occurred less than four hours before delivery. The investigators conclude that while zidovudine is effective in reducing transmission, further reductions may be possible by lowering the incidence of potentially modifiable risk factors [*AIDS* 1998;12:301–08].

Abbreviated AZT Regimens Reduce Risk of Perinatal HIV Transmission. A

three-part regimen of zidovudine given ante partum, intra partum, and to the newborn reduces the rate of perinatal transmission of HIV from 25% to 8%. Some women, however, do not seek medical care until shortly before delivery and the *ad hoc* administration of abbreviated regimens of zidovudine is common. How well do these more limited strategies protect against transmission? Data from the New York State Department of Health's pediatric diagnostic testing service that covered the period from August 1, 1995 to January 31, 1997 are reassuring [*N Engl J Med* 1998;339:1409–14]. HIV status of 939 exposed infants indicates that the rate of perinatal transmission of the virus depends on when treatment begins. When treatment was begun in the perinatal period, the rate of HIV transmission was 6.1%; when begun intra partum, the rate was 10.0%; and when begun within the first 48 hours of life, the rate was 9.3%. However, when zidovudine was begun on day three of life or later, the rate was 18.4%. In the absence of zidovudine prophylaxis, the rate of HIV transmission was 26.6%. These findings generally confirm the results from a perinatal HIV transmission trial in Thailand [*MMWR* 1998;47:151–54]. The findings add weight to the argument that HIV infection can be prevented after exposure [*N Engl J Med* 1998;339: 1467–68].

Attempted Abortion with Misoprostol Increases the Risk of Birth Defect. Mifepristone combined with a prostaglandin is available in France and a few other countries to terminate an early pregnancy. The drug is also approved, but not marketed, in the US. When it does become available, mifepristone will be used with misoprostol. Misoprostol, a synthetic prostaglandin, stimulates uterine contractions. It has been used to terminate pregnancies in some countries that prohibit elective abortions. There have been reports of birth defects, notably Mobius Syndrome—congenital facial paralysis, with or without limb defects—in infants whose mothers took misoprostol in an unsuccessful attempt at abortion. More recently, a study based in Brazil compared the frequency of misoprostol use during the first trimester of pregnancy between mothers of infants born with Mobius syndrome and mothers of infants with neural-tube defects [N *Engl J Med* 1998;338:1881–85]. The investigators identified 96 infants with Mobius syndrome and matched them with 96 infants with neural-tube defects. Among the mothers of the infants with Mobius syndrome, 49% had used misoprostol, compared with 3% of the mothers of the infants with neural-tube defects. Infants, carried to term, of mothers who fail to terminate a pregnancy by using misoprostol are at considerable risk of a serious birth defect.

Pamidronate for Osteogenesis Imperfecta. Osteogenesis imperfecta— brittle-bone disease—is an inherited connective-tissue disorder characterized in its severe form by frequent fractures, short stature, deformity, loss of mobility, and chronic bone pain. At this time, there is no effective treatment for this devastating disorder. However, there is interest in using a bisphosphonate, and some evidence to support the idea. Bisphosphonates are potent inhibitors of bone resorption, a hallmark of osteogenesis imperfecta. A recent report concerns an uncontrolled observational study of 30 children, who ranged in age from 3 to 16 years, with severe osteogenesis imperfecta. Each child received intravenous pamidronate (*Aredia*) at four- to six-month intervals for 1.3 to 5.0 years. The treatment resulted in sustained reductions in serum alkaline phosphatase levels and in the urinary excretion of calcium and collagen. The children had a mean annualized increase in bone mineral density of 42%. On average, the number of fractures decreased by 1.7 per year. Mobility and ambulation improved in 16 children and remained unchanged in the others. All the children reported substantial relief of chronic pain and fatigue. The findings indicate that pamidronate should be considered for the treatment of this difficult disease [*N Engl J Med* 1998;339:947–52].

Health in the Elderly

Vitamin D Deficiency in the Sick and Elderly
No Advantage of SSRIs Over TCAs in Risk of Falls and
  Hip Fracture
Inhaled Steroids and Cataracts in the Elderly

Vitamin D Deficiency in the Sick and Elderly. Hypovitaminosis D is common in the elderly and house-bound and is an important risk factor for osteoporosis. Dietary supplementation with vitamin D and calcium reduces bone loss and nonvertebral fractures. Persons with chronic liver and renal diseases and those receiving certain drugs (e.g., phenytoin, carbamazepine, and rifampin) are also at risk of vitamin D deficiency. A recent survey of 290 consecutive adult patients on a medical ward revealed that 57% of the patients were deficient in vitamin D, including 22% who were severely deficient [*N Engl J Med* 1998;338:777–83]. Deficient levels of vitamin D were also found in 37% of those who reported consuming the newly defined adequate intake of 400 international units (IUs) of vitamin D per day for people 51 to 70 years of age and 600 IUs per day for people over 70. Until recently, the recommended daily allowance of vitamin D for all people was only 200 IUs per day [*N Engl J Med* 1998;338:828–29]. The investigators identified two important risk factors for hypovitaminosis D: insufficient dietary intake of the vitamin and inadequate exposure to sunlight to stimulate production of vitamin D in the skin. Because of the morbidity associated with vitamin D deficiency, the researchers recommend that the amount of vitamin D in the diet, in supplemental multivitamins, and in calcium supplements be increased to achieve a total intake of 800 IUs per day for all adults.

No Advantage of SSRIs Over TCAs in Risk of Falls and Hip Fracture. Medications, particularly antidepressants, increase the risk of falls and hip fracture in older people. Prognosis after hip fracture is poor. This presents a dilemma because many older people benefit from treatment with an antidepressant. The prevailing view is that fluoxetine (*Prozac*) and other second generation antidepressants (SSRIs) have a more favorable safety profile than amitriptyline and other first generation agents (TCAs). Does the difference in side-effect profile lead to a lower risk of hip fracture with SSRIs than with TCAs? To answer this question, investigators reviewed administrative health care data from Canada and identified 8239 cases who were 66 years or older and treated in hospital between 1994 and 1995 for hip fracture. Compared with matched control subjects who had no exposure, the use of an antidepressant from either class significantly increased the risk of hip fracture and there was no significant difference between them. Current use of either type of antidepressant was associated with a higher risk of hip fracture than former use and the risk was higher for new current users than continuous current users. The study suggests that SSRIs do not offer an advantage over TCAs with respect to hip fracture [*Lancet* 1998;351:1303–07]. Another study demonstrates little difference in rates of falls between nursing home residents treated with TCAs and those treated with SSRIs [*N Engl J Med* 1998;339: 875–82].

Inhaled Steroids and Cataracts in the Elderly. Oral corticosteroids are a known risk factor for the development of cataracts. This adverse outcome may also occur in older people who regularly use inhaled steroids for asthma or other respiratory diseases. The effectiveness of inhaled steroids for the treatment of asthma has considerably increased their use over extended periods of time. Using the Quebec health insurance database, researchers have recently completed a case-control study that involved 3677 elderly patients who developed cataracts that required extraction and 21,868 controls who did not have a diagnosis of cataract. After excluding patients who used oral steroids and adjusting for a host of potential confounding factors, the investigators found that the use of inhaled steroids for more than three years was associated with a threefold increase in the risk of undergoing cataract extraction. This level of increased risk was observed after only two years for patients who used relatively large daily doses of beclomethasone or budesonide. Low to medium doses of inhaled steroid posed less of a risk, decreasing the possibility of developing cataracts by about 60% compared with high doses [*JAMA* 1998;280:539–43].

OTHER STUDIES AND REPORTS

Nasal Corticosteroids or Nonsedating Antihistamines for
  Allergic Rhinitis
Liver Disease Selectively Decreases Activity of Drug-
  Metabolizing Enzymes
Secretin Improves Behavior in Children with Autism

Nasal Corticosteroids or Nonsedating Antihistamines for Allergic Rhinitis.
Allergic rhinitis is prevalent and takes a heavy toll in terms of cost of medication, work productivity, and quality of life. The lifetime prevalence in the US
population exceeds 20%. Nonsedating antihistamines (e.g., *Claritin, Allegra*)
are the most common and most expensive therapy. Nasal corticosteroids are
a less expensive alternative, but are not as widely promoted as nonsedating
antihistamines. Investigators have recently reviewed 13 randomized, blinded
studies reported in the biomedical literature that compared intranasal steroids
with nonsedating antihistamines for the management of allergic rhinitis [*Am
J Managed Care* 1998;4:89–96]. The evidence tables derived from the data
show that in all studies in which total nasal symptoms and nasal obstruction
were recorded, the nasal steroid was superior to the nonsedating antihistamine. Indeed, for nasal blockage, the nonsedating antihistamine was no more
effective than placebo. For all other nasal symptoms, the steroid was statistically superior in most reports and equal or numerically better in the rest of
the reports. Linking these findings with data from cost-analysis and quality-
of-life studies strongly suggests that nasal steroids should be first-line therapy
for adult patients with allergic rhinitis. The authors conclude: "Like asthma,
allergic rhinitis is an inflammatory disease and should be managed with anti-
inflammatory medication."

***Liver Disease Selectively Decreases Activity of Drug-Metabolizing En-
zymes.*** The drug-metabolizing enzymes in the liver play a central role in the
elimination of a countless number of organic molecules. Patients with liver
disease may have an impaired ability to eliminate potent drugs, which may
lead to accumulation and toxicity. It remains unclear, however, how the
activities of specific drug-metabolizing enzymes are influenced. Consequently
there is no way to predict if or how much the dose of a drug need be lowered
in a patient with liver disease to avoid adverse effects. To address this question,

investigators determined the activities of two isozymes of cytochrome P450—2C19 and 2D6—in a group of patients with mild or moderate liver disease and a group of healthy control subjects. They found that the elimination of S-mephenytoin, a marker for the activity of 2C19, was decreased by 79% in patients with liver disease compared with the clearance of S-mephenytoin in healthy subjects. The change was related to the severity of the disease. Liver disease had no effect on the clearance of debrisoquin, a marker for the activity of 2D6. The authors conclude that the recommendations to change the dose of a drug for patients with liver disease should be based on knowledge of the particular enzyme involved in the metabolism of the drug [*Clin Pharmacol Ther* 1998;54:8–17].

Secretin Improves Behavior in Children with Autism. Autism is a pervasive developmental disorder with a prevalence of about 15 per 10,000. Approximately 400,000 Americans, predominantly males, are affected by the disorder. Media interest in autism dates back to a popular film *Rainman*. Since there is no known treatment, a case report describing three young boys with autism who seemed to benefit from treatment with secretin, though published in an obscure medical journal, provoked considerable attention. A large proportion of patients with autistic spectrum disorder has gastrointestinal symptoms. Three autistic children presented with chronic diarrhea. They underwent upper gastrointestinal endoscopy and received intravenous secretin to stimulate pancreaticobiliary secretory response for the purpose of examining the fluid. Within five weeks of the secretin infusion, the physicians observed a significant improvement of gastrointestinal symptoms as well as a dramatic improvement in the children's behavior—improved eye contact, alertness, and an increase in the use of expressive language [*J Assoc Acad Minority Physicians* 1998;9:9–15]. These preliminary observations suggest a role for secretin in the treatment of both gastrointestinal and behavioral/developmental symptoms in young autistic children.

ADVERSE DRUG EFFECTS

Acetaminophen is a Risk Factor for Excessive Warfarin
  Anticoagulation
Regular Use of Aspirin May Increase the Risk of Stroke
Ticlopidine May Result in TTP after Stenting
Grapefruit Juice, Statins, and Adverse Effects
Drug for CMV Retinitis May Lead to Renal Failure
Benzodiazepines and Other CNS Drugs Impair Driving Skills
Over-the-Counter NSAIDs May Cause Liver Damage in
  Patients with Hepatitis C
Side Effects of Alendronate (Fosamax)
Safety of Long-Term Use of Nicotine Replacement Products
  Questioned
Risk for Intracranial Bleed after TPA for Acute MI

Acetaminophen is a Risk Factor for Excessive Warfarin Anticoagulation.
Warfarin is effective in preventing thromboembolism but increases the risk
of bleeding. Major hemorrhage in those patients receiving warfarin is strongly
associated with the intensity of anticoagulation. The international normalized
ratio (INR), measured *ex vivo,* is an index of anticoagulation. Investigators,
seeking to identify causes of excessive anticoagulation, followed outpatients
taking warfarin therapy with a target INR of 2.0 to 3.0, the usual therapeutic
range [*JAMA* 1998;279:657–662]. Case patients (93) were those reaching
a measured INR of 6.0 during the course of therapy; controls (196) were
randomly selected from patients having INRs between 1.7 and 3.3. The
researchers found that the commonly used nonprescription analgesic acetaminophen was independently associated with an INR greater than 6.0. Risk
increased with the dose of acetaminophen. For the highest-dose category (28
tablets of *Tylenol* 325 mg per week or more), the odds of having an INR
greater than 6.0 increased tenfold above those taking no acetaminophen.
This is a troubling report. Aspirin and other NSAIDs increase bleeding time
and should not be used with warfarin. Acetaminophen is the only nonprescription alternative. The authors believe that acetaminophen remains a valuable
therapy for patients taking warfarin but urge that those who also require
sustained high doses of acetaminophen need close monitoring of their
INR levels.

Regular Use of Aspirin May Increase the Risk of Stroke. There is considerable evidence that regular use of aspirin by high-risk patients decreases the chance of having a fatal or ischemic stroke. On the other hand, controlled trials consistently show small increases in stroke associated with the use of aspirin by *low-risk* people [*Stroke* 1998;29:885–86]. To explore this paradox, a research team analyzed the relationship between the regular use of aspirin and ischemic and hemorrhagic stroke among more than 5,000 elderly people (at least 65 years old) [*Stroke* 1998;29:887–94]. Twenty-two percent of the patients used aspirin frequently, on more than ten days of a defined two-week period, whereas 17% used aspirin less frequently. The rest did not use aspirin. The investigators followed the cohort for an average of 4.2 years. They found, after adjustment for other risk factors, that frequent use of aspirin by women, but not by men, was associated with a significantly increased rate of ischemic stroke compared with nonusers (relative risk, 1.8); women who used aspirin less frequently had a relative risk of 1.6. As expected, both men and women who used aspirin had a fourfold increase in the risk of hemorrhagic stroke whether they were infrequent or frequent users. The authors stress that a conclusion that aspirin increases the risk of ischemic stroke in elderly women is premature. The question of aspirin for primary prevention of stroke can be settled only by randomized clinical trials.

Ticlopidine May Result in TTP after Stenting. Ticlopidine (*Ticlid*), a recently introduced antiplatelet agent, has been associated with thrombotic thrombocytopenic purpura (TTP), a serious and sometimes life-threatening condition characterized by a massive loss of platelets [*Ann Intern Med* 1998;128:541–44]. *Ticlid* is often used with aspirin following coronary revascularization and stent placement to prevent restenosis. A recent study assessed the frequency of TTP with ticlopidine and cardiac stents in a single large metropolitan area in the US over an 18-month period [*Lancet* 1998;352:1036–37]. The investigators estimated a frequency of about one in 1600 treated patients. The estimate is similar to that offered by Roche Laboratories for the incidence of TTP in stroke patients given ticlopidine. The investigators speculate that ticlopidine or a metabolite could induce an autoantibody that inactivates the protease required to cleave von Willebrand factor. Persistent high levels of von Willebrand factor may lead to platelet adhesion, aggregation, and the formation of platelet thrombi typical of TTP. Cardiologists who wish to use ticlopidine after stenting should consider a two-week rather than a four-week course of treatment. Recently approved clopidogrel (*Plavix*) may be an alternative to *Ticlid*.

Grapefruit Juice, Statins, and Adverse Effects. *The Prescriber's Letter* [1998;5 (No 7):38] reports that grapefruit juice can increase blood levels of the HMG Co-A reductase inhibitors lovastatin (*Mevacor*) and simvastatin (*Zocor*). Grapefruit juice inhibits cytochrome P450 enzymes in the small intestine and allows more unmetabolized drug to reach the systemic circulation. Both lovastatin and simvastatin are widely prescribed for patients with elevated levels of cholesterol. The use of grapefruit juice by patients receiving high doses of these drugs may result in serious toxicity—myopathy and rhabdomyolysis. The effect of grapefruit juice on drug-metabolizing enzymes is prolonged. Patients receiving statins should entirely avoid it. Differences in metabolic pathways suggest that grapefruit juice is not likely to affect pravastatin or fluvastatin. Whether or not grapefruit juice inhibits the metabolism of the newest statins, atorvastatin (*Lipitor*) and cerivastatin (*Baycol*), is not yet evident. Grapefruit juice also inhibits the metabolism and increases the toxicity of many other drugs including felodipine (*Plendil*) and other dihydropyridine calcium antagonists, cyclosporine (*Neoral*), and cisapride (*Propulsid*).

Drug for CMV Retinitis May Lead to Renal Failure. Cidofovir (*Vistide*), a nucleotide analogue, is one of three antiviral drugs used for the treatment of cytomegalovirus (CMV) retinitis, an opportunistic infection seen in patients with advanced HIV disease. Ganciclovir (*Cytovene*) and foscarnet (*Foscavir*) are the other agents [*N Engl J Med* 1997;337:105–14]. Initial labeling of cidofovir included a boxed warning stating that renal impairment is the drug's major toxicity. Cidofovir is contraindicated for patients with elevated serum creatinine and for patients receiving other nephrotoxic agents, including NSAIDs. Co-administered probenecid decreases the risk of nephrotoxicity [*Med Letter* 1997;39:15–16]. In August 1998, *Vistide's* manufacturer, Gilead Sciences, sent a letter to health care professionals reiterating the warning of reports of renal failure, adding that toxicity is seen sometimes after only a few doses of cidofovir. The letter also alerted them to recent reports of uveitis and iritis, both listed in the labeling as rare adverse events, and the previously unreported side effect of hearing loss [*Scrip*, August 26, 1998, p 15].

Benzodiazepines and Other CNS Drugs Impair Driving Skills. Drugs acting on the central nervous system (CNS) can have adverse effects that impair driving performance. In the elderly, investigators have associated benzodiazepines and tricyclic antidepressants with increased risks of driving accidents causing injury. Many suggest a causal link between the use of psychotropic drugs and driving accidents, but the data supporting that premise are scant. To study the possible link, researchers worked with local police to examine the records of more than 400,000 individuals [*Lancet* 1998;352:1331–36]. They determined that 19,386 were involved in a traffic accident during the study period. Of those, 1731 were using a psychoactive drug. The use of an antidepressant on the day of the accident was not a significant risk factor. The use of benzodiazepines, on the other hand, increased risk by 60%. Risk increased with dose and was highest in drivers younger than 30 years of age. The use of benzodiazepines for anxiety increased risk more than twofold, whereas their use as hypnotics, with one exception, had a modest non-significant effect on risk. The exception was the short-acting hypnotic zopiclone, which increased the risk of a traffic accident fourfold. Zopiclone is a cyclopyrrolone rather than a benzodiazepine, but its acts on the same receptors as benzodiazepines. The drug seems to have residual effects that impair driving performance. The authors conclude: "Users of anxiolytic benzodiazepines and zopiclone should be advised not to drive."

Over-the-Counter NSAIDs May Cause Liver Damage in Patients with Hepatitis C. According to a case report describing three patients with chronic hepatitis C infection, even low doses of over-the-counter (OTC) ibuprofen can cause liver damage [*Am J Gastroenterol* 1998;1563–65]. Ibuprofen use led to a marked rise in hepatic transaminases. In all cases liver enzyme levels fell when ibuprofen was discontinued. A re-challenge in one patient again led to elevated transaminases. If a patient requires a nonprescription analgesic, acetaminophen is likely to be a better choice than an NSAID.

Side Effects of Alendronate (Fosamax). The marketing of alendronate (*Fosamax*) and raloxifene (*Evista*) has intensified competition among a spectrum of agents indicated for the treatment of osteoporosis. Merck's *Fosamax* is popular because it is free of the side effects posed by estrogen replacement, but can cause gastrointestinal (GI) problems if not taken correctly. Novartis, the manufacturer of intranasal calcitonin (*Miacalcin*), a competitor to *Fosamax*, provided funds to investigators at Kaiser Permanente to gauge the extent of the problem created by the misuse of *Fosamax*. Their telephone survey of 812 women taking the drug found that 56% did not follow specific dosage recommendations to minimize the possibility of esophageal erosion [*Am J Managed Care* 1998;4:1377–82]. The label directs that *Fosamax* be given with water, on an empty stomach, in an upright position. The investigators also report that one-third of patients using *Fosamax* complained of new upper GI symptoms. They warn that elderly alendronate users, or those concurrently taking NSAIDs, should be monitored carefully because of their high risk of having an "acid-related upper GI disorder." Merck argues that these conclusions are not justified as the study had no control group. Moreover, the survey was started before Merck intensified its education campaign about dosing instructions for *Fosamax*. Since the initiation of this campaign, surveys have shown that more than 90% of patients on the drug are aware of these instructions [*Scrip*, October 23, 1998, p 18].

Safety of Long-Term Use of Nicotine Replacement Products Questioned. Nicotine replacement products, developed to help people to stop smoking, now include chewing gum, skin patches, a nasal spray, and a product called an inhaler that has the form of a cigarette. There is broad agreement that replacement nicotine is safer than smoking and worth a modicum of risk if it helps people to quit. Some experts, however, are becoming concerned because a growing number of smokers are using nicotine products not just for the three to six months recommended by manufacturers, but for years. They are especially worried about inhalers. Recent studies suggest that nicotine can damage cells that line blood vessels and the airways in the lungs. These tissues are maintained by stimulation of acetylcholine receptors of tegumental cells. Nicotine displaces acetylcholine, binds to the receptor, and desensitizes it [*The New York Times*, November 17, 1998, pp D1,D8].

Risk for Intracranial Bleed after TPA for Acute MI. The efficacy of thrombolytic therapy to reduce mortality from acute MI is somewhat compromised by bleeding complications, including intracranial hemorrhage. To determine the frequency of and the risk factors for intracranial bleeding after alteplase (TPA, *Activase*) administration, researchers examined data in a large national registry of patients who have had acute MI. The registry includes 71,000 patients who had had a heart attack during the period from June 1994 to September 1996 and received alteplase as the initial reperfusion strategy. The database revealed that 673 of those patients (0.95%) were reported to have had intracranial hemorrhage during hospitalization; 625 patients (0.88%) had the bleed confirmed by computed tomography or magnetic resonance imaging. Among those with a confirmed event, 53% died during hospitalization and 25%, who survived to hospital discharge, had residual neurologic deficit. Significant risk factors were older age, female sex, black ethnicity, blood pressure of 140/100 mm Hg or higher, history of stroke, alteplase dose more than 1.5 mg/kg, and low body weight. The authors conclude that intracranial hemorrhage is a rare but serious complication of alteplase therapy, and that careful selection of dose may reduce the risk. They suggest that other therapies, such as coronary angioplasty, may be preferable in patients with acute MI who have a history of stroke [*Ann Intern Med* 1998;129:597–602].

PHARMACOECONOMICS

Introduction. Pharmaceutical manufacturers, drug purchasers, the government, and academia have embraced, to a greater or lesser degree, the idea that economic evaluation of pharmaceuticals is an integral part of health care evaluation. There is much disagreement, however, as to the techniques for evaluating pharmaceutical products. A primary issue is whether economic evaluations should be based on well-controlled clinical trials or decision models. The FDA clearly favors the use of data from controlled trials, but this information is not always available. A recent review article [*Pharmaceutical News* 1998;5:7–10] describes other important issues facing those who attempt economic evaluations.

Preventing AIDS-Related Opportunistic Infections: Economic Implications. AIDS is a complex illness with treatment options directed at both the virus itself and the complications associated with profound immunosuppression. Evidence shows that the occurrence of *Pneumocystis carinii* pneumonia (PCP), *Mycobacterium avium* complex (MAC) infection, cytomegalovirus (CMV) disease, and other opportunistic infections can be reduced with drug therapy. The annual cost of prophylactic medication ranges from $60 for prevention of PCP with trimethoprim-sulfamethoxazole (TMP-SM) to more than $15,000 for the treatment of CMV disease with ganciclovir. While prophylaxis is expensive, its effectiveness may minimize overall health care costs by reducing other medical costs. Whether this is the case was the subject of a cost-effectiveness study [*JAMA* 1998;279:130–36].

Using a simulation model, researchers found that for patients with CD4 cell counts of 200/μl or less prophylaxis for PCP and toxoplasmosis with TMP-SM increased quality-adjusted life expectancy at an incremental cost of $16,000 per quality-of-life-year (QUALY) saved. The incremental cost for preventing MAC with azithromycin in patients with CD4 counts of 50/μl or less is $35,000 per QALY saved, but the cost for preventing CMV infection with oral ganciclovir is more than $300,000 per QALY saved. With costs of QALY saved of less than $50,000, TMP-SP for PCP and azithromycin for MAC are relatively cost effective; scarce resources should be directed toward these therapies.

Cost-Effectiveness of STD Treatment to Prevent HIV Infection in Africa. Studies show that the sexual transmission of HIV is increased when other sexually transmitted diseases (STDs) are present [*Lancet* 1995;346:530–36]. The World Health Organization and other international bodies advocate improved management of STDs as an effective and potentially cost-effective strategy to control the spread of HIV infection. The first comprehensive effort to assess the cost-effectiveness of this strategy has recently been reported, using data from several communities in Tanzania [*Lancet* 1998:350:1805–99]. The investigators followed a cohort of 12,537 patients for two years and treated 11,632 cases of STDs. The incidence of HIV during the study period was 1.16% in those communities that treated STDs and 1.86% in those communities that did not have a STD intervention unit. Intervention decreased the occurrence of infection by 40%. The data indicate that the program prevented about 250 HIV infections each year. Program costs were only 39 cents per patient served. The incremental annual cost of the intervention was about $55,000, equivalent to $218 per HIV infection averted and $10 per life year saved. This is remarkably low and compares favorably with childhood immunizations. From a societal perspective, the cost of averting one case of HIV infection is likely to be less than the cost of treatment.

Cost-Effectiveness of Drugs to Treat Schizophrenia. Janssen's *Risperdal* (risperidone) is in a pitched battle with Lilly's *Zyprexa* (olanzapine) to dominate the considerable market for anti-psychotic drugs. A new study suggests that *Risperdal* is more cost effective than *Zyprexa,* while another shows that *Zyprexa* is more cost effective than traditional therapy with haloperidol [*Scrip,* July 22, 1998, p 26]. A Canadian study, based on 60 patients with schizophrenia, shows that treating patients with *Risperdal* costs only about one-third of what it costs to treat them with *Zyprexa*, based on the costs of the two products in Canada. The study, funded by Janssen, also found *Risperdal* to be more effective than *Zyprexa*. *Risperdal* realized cost saving by reducing the duration and rate of hospitalization. Lilly says that this small short-term study does not provide a realistic comparison of the cost-effectiveness of the two products because it does not take into account the impact on total health care costs. A study from the United Kingdom reported at about the same time as the Canadian study, shows that *Zyprexa* is more cost effective than haloperidol in the treatment of schizophrenia when the costs of medical services and hospital care are taken into account. *Zyprexa* generated cost savings by reducing relapse rates, alleviating symptoms, and reducing the need to switch to alternative medication. These results will find their way into promotional material for the competing products.

Cost-Effectiveness of Smoking-Cessation Services. The cost effectiveness of smoking cessation interventions as compared with other medical services is documented. Nevertheless, broad adoption of coverage for smoking-cessation services has not occurred. Results of a small number of studies of the effects of out-of-pocket costs on the use of nicotine gum suggest that offering it at a reduced cost or at no cost increases the amount of gum that is used and the rate of smoking cessation. No studies have examined the effects of cost-sharing health insurance plans for combined coverage of behavioral modification and nicotine-replacement therapy.

Now, investigators from a large managed care organization, Group Health Cooperative of Puget Sound, report the results of a study comparing the use and cost-effectiveness of alternative forms of insurance coverage with those of a standard form of coverage for smoking-cessation services. The services include a behavioral program and nicotine-replacement therapy [*N Engl J Med* 1998;339:673–79].

The standard plan offered 50% coverage of the behavioral program and full coverage of nicotine-replacement therapy. The reduced coverage plan offered 50% coverage of both the behavioral program and nicotine-replacement therapy. The full coverage plan required no co-pay for either therapy.

Estimated annual rates of use of smoking-cessation services ranged from 2.4% (among smokers with reduced coverage) to 10% (among those with full coverage). For those who used the services, smoking cessation rates were 38% in the standard coverage group, 31% in the reduced coverage group, and 28% in the full coverage group. While offering the services at no charge increases the number of people taking advantage of the benefit, the additional people seem to be less committed to stop smoking than are those paying half the costs of nicotine-replacement therapy. Nevertheless, the additional number of people who decided to try the services was sufficiently large so that full-coverage had the greatest success. With full coverage, an estimated 2.8% of smokers stopped smoking per year, as compared with 1.3% with standard coverage, and 0.7% with reduced coverage.

Factoring in the costs of the benefit the authors estimate that, "This increase in the annual rate of cessation among smokers with full coverage can be achieved at a cost of $328 per benefit user, which is clearly a bargain as compared with the average annual cost of medical treatment for hypertension ($5291) or heart disease ($6941)." Extending the analysis suggests that the fully covered smoking-cessation program cost $883 per year of life saved, compared with $11,300 for the treatment of moderate hypertension and more than $65,000 for the treatment of elevated cholesterol levels.

The researchers conclude that policy decisions regarding coverage for smoking must also take into account the social benefits of smoking cessation— reduced exposure to secondhand smoke and associated illnesses, decreased access to tobacco in the home leading to a reduction in the rate of smoking among teenagers, and decreased rates of morbidity and mortality of offspring of women who quit smoking before pregnancy.

The Cost of Gastroesophageal Reflux Disease. Heartburn, the primary symptom of gastroesophageal reflux disease (GERD), occurs in 40% of Americans at least once a month. In one survey, 10% of respondents reported taking prescription medication for heartburn or acid regurgitation or having GERD symptoms at least twice a week. In light of these estimates, it comes as no surprise that the cost of diagnosing and treating GERD is high. To determine economic impact in a more comprehensive manner, researchers developed a decision analytic model to calculate clinical and direct economic outcomes for patients with GERD treated for two years with antacids, H_2-receptor antagonists, prokinetic agents, or proton pump inhibitors [*Am J Managed Care* 1998;4:1450–60].

Data in the literature show that maximizing the percentage of patients who would be symptom-free at the end of two years is best achieved in patients with either mild GERD or moderate to severe disease by treatment with proton pump inhibitors. Patients with mild GERD, who were treated with the least costly therapy of antacids or no drugs had the highest total cost per case ($2040) because of low efficacy. On the other hand, the drug class with the highest acquisition costs, proton pump inhibitors, had the lowest cost per case ($938). The authors note: "The reduced need for diagnostic testing and hospitalization associated with products with higher efficacy are likely key reasons for proton pump inhibitors having the lowest cost per case." Proton pump inhibitors also give best value in patients with moderate to severe GERD.

Cyclosporine (Neoral) Faces Competition. In the next few years, an unusually large number of important and costly drugs will lose patent protection and face competition from lower-priced alternatives. This could reduce drug costs, unless pharmaceutical companies can persuade physicians to prescribe line extensions and "new and improved" products.

The first blockbuster drug to face price competition is Novartis' *Neoral* (modified cyclosporine), expected to have worldwide sales of $1.3 billion in 1998 [*The New York Times,* November 13, 1998]. Sales may not approach that level in 1999. FDA has approved a product called *Sangcya,* which is therapeutically equivalent to *Neoral.* Sangstat said that it would price *Sangcya* about 20% below *Neoral.* The new product will cost $4800 to $5500 per patient per year, saving about $1200 a year for each transplant patient. FDA's designation of therapeutic equivalence means that patients would not need a new prescription to switch from *Neoral* to *Sangcya.*

Although therapeutically equivalent and bioequivalent, *Sangcya* differs from *Neoral* in that it is a liquid formulation with an unusually helpful dispensing device, rather than a capsule. A liquid form of *Neoral* is available for children but is not as easy to use as *Sangcya.* Some analysts say that the transplant community will not take the entry of a new form of cyclosporine lightly. Physicians will want experience before switching patients to the new product. Moreover, companies including Novartis are developing new immunosuppressant agents for organ transplantation that may prove more effective than cyclosporine.

America's Soaring Drug Costs. "America has a new drug problem," starts the first of a series of articles in *The Wall Journal* titled Hard to Swallow: *America's Soaring Drug Costs.* A revolution in pharmaceutical research, a billion-dollar advertising blitz, and Americans' voracious appetite for the newest and most heavily promoted drugs have come together to drive spending for pharmaceuticals to record levels [*The Wall Street Journal,* November 16, 1998, ppA1,A10].

Community pharmacies are expected to ring up more than $100 billion in sales of prescription drugs in 1998, up 85% from five years ago. Drug sales in the US are increasing at an annual rate more than four times the rate of increase in health care spending overall. Profits for US drug companies are expected to grow by at least 16% per year for the next four years. The trend is ominous for those trying to control health care costs and for the uninsured. For health insurance providers, drug outlays now represent 25% or more of total health care expenditures. The financial relief expected from the approval of generic versions of blockbuster drugs has not materialized because of the skillful marketing ability of the pharmaceutical industry. The industry has consistently succeeded in persuading physicians to write prescriptions for new, "improved," and much more expensive drug therapies. The problem will worsen as our population ages because older people use more drugs than young adults do.

While prices of some drugs have increased sharply in recent years, higher prices of marketed products contributes only 3.2 percentage points to the 16.6% increase in drug spending in 1998. The most important factor is the pricing of new pharmaceuticals, which Americans, prompted by direct-to-consumer promotions, are increasingly demanding to preserve their health and, in some cases, their youth. Sales of safe and effective drugs that racked up millions of dollars of profit fall sharply when patent protection is lost and their continued use is no longer promoted.

Drug companies say that pharmaceuticals are the most cost-effective portion of the health care system. Drug therapy alleviates pain and suffering, extends life, and improves quality of life. There is justification for this argument, but the US is virtually alone in forgoing price controls and allowing the market to set prices. In too many cases, the price in the US is what the market will bear. Drugs that can prevent hospital visits are priced high because of the purported savings and "value" they offer. Industry observers warn drug companies that it is only a matter of time until spiraling drug costs raise the ire of the public and politicians.

A related story in the same issue of the *Journal* examined large and expensive clinical trials that go beyond the studies required by the FDA to gain marketing approval [*The Wall Street Journal*, November 16, 1998, A10]. The reporter suggests that such trials needlessly increase the price of a prescription drug. He chides Bristol-Meyers Squibb for launching large outcomes trials with pravastatin (*Pravachol*) after the drug had received FDA approval for use in patients with elevated cholesterol levels. He accuses the company of mounting these trials merely to improve marketing position in a competitive therapeutic area. This accusation may be true but it does not detract from the importance of the additional clinical trials. These studies were essential to demonstrate that lipid lowering with a statin reduces overall mortality and benefits a wide range of people, not only those with coronary artery disease and elevated serum cholesterol.

The second article in the series concerns the crushing burden of prescription drug prices on the elderly [*The Wall Street Journal*, November 17, 1998, ppA1,A15]. The principal health insurance for the elderly is Medicare. But Medicare has a glaring deficiency. With few exceptions, it does not cover the cost of drugs—"the single largest health-care expenditure for the elderly." About 19 million elderly people in the US have little or no coverage for prescription drugs. Nor do an estimated 43 million younger Americans who lack any health insurance. Those age 65 or older constitute only 12% of the population but consume almost 35% of all prescription drugs. One in five elderly people takes at least five prescription drugs each day.

About half of Medicare-eligible patients get some drug assistance because they are also covered under employer-sponsored insurance plans for retirees, are members of managed care organizations, or are poor enough to qualify for Medicaid programs, which do provide coverage for pharmaceuticals. The other half goes it alone. These people incur debt, implore physicians for free samples, cross the borders to Canada and Mexico where drug prices are lower, and forego basic necessities. Others do not fill prescriptions for costly drugs or skip doses to stretch their supply. Ironically, the uninsured pay higher prices for prescription drugs because community pharmacies cannot get the steep discounts offered to government agencies and managed care organizations.

Expanding Medicare to pay for drugs would cost an additional $20 billion a year. Congress has resisted such action because of intense opposition from the drug industry. The industry fears that Medicare coverage of drugs for the elderly would open the way for price controls.

The third article explains why generic drugs often cannot compete against brand name products [*The Wall Street Journal*, November 18, 1998, ppA1,A14]. In a few words, lower prices are usually not enough to overcome the demand for the new and improved. As generic copies of popular brand-name medications are planned in anticipation of the loss of marketing exclusivity, the brand-name companies are developing new generations of even more expensive products. More directly, pharmaceutical companies use every legal tactic available to delay the marketing of generic products. When legal strategies are exhausted, some companies pay generic manufacturers millions of dollars to keep their products off the market.

The last article in the series explores the conflict experienced by an individual who is both the chief executive of a small community hospital and the victim of cystic fibrosis. As an administrator, one of his greatest worries is how to keep demand for new pharmaceuticals from busting his budget. As a patient, he realizes, sometimes dramatically, the importance of the two newest drugs for cystic fibrosis—one costing $1000 per month and the other $2000 per month—that keep him functioning. He very much wants to see his eight-year old son and his five-year old daughter graduate from college. At current prices, that will take about $200,000 in drug costs alone [*The Wall Street Journal,* November 19, 1998, ppA1,A8].

FTC Challenges Major Generic Drug Manufacturer's Prices. Generic products reduce the cost of drug therapy and are especially attractive to consumers on fixed incomes. This year, however, prices of many popular generic drugs have risen dramatically. Mylan, one of the most important generic manufacturers in the world, has been particularly aggressive in its pricing. So aggressive that that the staff of the Federal Trade Commission (FTC) has recommended filing a civil suit accusing Mylan of anti-competitive practices after it raised the price of several generic products including the anti-anxiety drug lorazepam [*The New York Times,* December 5, 1998, pp A1,B14]. Mylan has tripled lorazepam's price to more than a dollar per tablet and plans a new round of price increases on 20 of its products. The FTC inquiry has focused on whether Mylan sought to illegally corner the market on crucial raw materials supplied by an Italian bulk manufacturer. Mylan has an exclusive arrangement with the company. Mylan representatives scoffed at the accusation and said that the price increases of their products this year were needed to reverse sharp losses on 41 of the 97 drugs it sold. Despite the company's contention, some consumer groups and pharmacy associations have said the increases are inexplicable.

LATE BREAKING REPORTS

Cardiovascular Disease

New Guidelines to Prevent Stroke in Atrial Fibrillation Patients. The American College of Chest Physicians has published updated guidelines to prevent stroke in patients with atrial fibrillation [*Chest* 1998;114:39S–40S]. Patients at high risk for stroke are those older than 70 years as well as those with hypertension, poor left ventricular function, or a prior stroke, transient ischemic attack, or systemic embolism. Patients at low risk are those younger than 65 years with no additional cardiovascular risk factors. The expert panel strongly recommends warfarin for all high-risk patients. Warfarin's safety profile is greatly improved if the international normalized ratio (INR) is maintained at no higher than 3.0. At the other end of the spectrum, the efficacy of warfarin drops sharply when the INR falls below 2.0. The updated guidelines recommend a target INR of 2.5 (range 2.5 to 3.5) for most indications. Aspirin is also efficacious, but not as effective as warfarin. Aspirin therapy is useful for those patients who cannot take warfarin or are at low risk for stroke.

Inadequate Management of Elevated Blood Pressure. Treatment for hypertension protects against cardiovascular disease and stroke. Despite the availability of effective medication and increasing awareness of the hazards of even small elevations in blood pressure, hypertension is poorly controlled in large numbers of people. This is the conclusion of a two-year Veterans' Affairs study of 800 hypertensive men (mean age 65.5 years; mean duration of hypertension 12.6 years). Mean blood pressure at the first visit was 146.2/ 84.3 mm Hg. Despite two years of regular medical-clinical visits that included blood pressure measurements, patients' systolic blood pressure was virtually unchanged, and diastolic blood pressure decreased by less than 2 mm Hg. The percentage of patients with a blood pressure of $\geq160/90$ mm Hg decreased only modestly during this period, from 46% to 39%. The authors urge physicians to examine, " . . . their approach to individual patients and identify situations in which more aggressive management of hypertension may be appropriate." They added: "Inadequate control of blood pressure can no longer be ascribed solely to the lack of access to medical care and noncompliance with therapy; physicians themselves must accept some responsibility for the problem" [*New Engl J Med,* 1998;339:1957–63].

Choice of Lipid-Lowering Drugs. *The Medical Letter* [1998;40:117–22] closed the year with a review of lipid-lowering agents. The editors conclude: "HMG-CoA reductase inhibitors ("statins") are the drugs of first choice for treatment of most patients with hypercholesterolemia. A beneficial effect on cardiovascular disease is documented best with pravastatin, simvastatin and lovastatin. For patients with low LDL-cholesterol, but also low HDL, with or without elevated triglycerides, gemfibrozil appears to have beneficial effects on the incidence of coronary events."

Infectious Disease

Semen: Yet Another Reservoir for HIV. Researchers report that replication-competent viruses can be recovered from seminal cells in some HIV-infected men who are receiving aggressive antiretroviral therapy and who have undetectable levels of viral RNA in plasma. This finding suggests that sexual transmission of HIV is possible, if not probable, despite the use of seemingly effective therapy [*N Engl J Med* 1998;339:1803–09].

Other Studies and Reports

Surgical Glue for Closing Wounds. *The Wall Street Journal* [December 28, 1998, p B1] alerted its readers to the availability of a liquid adhesive that may eventually replace sutures in up to 40% of their uses. This is important for both parents and pediatric practitioners because even the thought of needle and thread terrifies many children. In the summer of 1998, the FDA approved *Dermabond,* which contains cyanoacrylate and sets in about 50 seconds. A return visit to a physician is not necessary because the material sloughs off in 5 to 10 days. A similar product has been available to veterinarians to close surgical and other wounds in various creatures. The price of *Dermabond* is about the same as a suture kit but the adhesive saves time and eliminates the need for sedation or analgesia. A report in *JAMA* [1997;277:1527–30] says there is no cosmetic difference between wounds closed with stitches and those closed with surgical glue. The adhesive does not work well on elbows and knees because the degree of motion is likely to cause the adhesive to peel too soon. Also, it cannot be used in the mouth, groin, or other moist areas.

Adverse Drug Effects

Trovafloxacin and Liver Toxicity. The December 1998 issue of the *Prescriber's Letter* alerts readers to new precautions about hepatotoxicity with the quinolone antibacterial agent trovafloxacin (*Trovan*). The potential for hepatic dysfunction in patients taking trovafloxacin for more than 21 days is recognized. Now, there are reports of liver toxicity and pancreatitis in patients who take shorter courses of the drug. Some experts suspect that this might be the result of a sensitivity reaction. There is reason for concern. *Trovan* is used frequently because it has a broader spectrum than the other quinolones. Careful monitoring of therapy is called for.

New Warning for Anti-Cancer Monoclonal Antibody. European authorities have asked Roche to change the labeling of rituximab (*Rituxan, MabThera*), one of very few options to treat follicular or low-grade non-Hodgkin's lymphoma. The new labeling will reflect reports of severe life-threatening and fatal reactions, and emphasize that *MabThera* should not be used outside its approved indication [*Scrip*, December 4, 1998, p 17]. About half of patients experience adverse events; cytokine release syndrome, characterized by dyspnea, fever, and chills, accounts for about 10% of the cases. Observers say that the FDA is likely to ask Roche to issue a "Dear Doctor" letter in the US.

Aspirin and Risk of Hemorrhage Stroke. Aspirin is widely used for the prevention of cardiovascular disease. While it is relatively safe, it is not entirely free of risk. Adverse effects on the gastrointestinal tract are widely recognized and several studies have suggested that aspirin increases the risk of hemorrhagic stroke. To quantify the relationship between aspirin use and hemorrhagic stroke risk, investigators undertook a meta-analysis of 16 randomized controlled trials that enrolled more than 55,000 participants who received either aspirin or placebo for at least one month [*JAMA* 1998;280:1930–35]. Most of the studies selected patients with ischemic heart disease or ischemic stroke. Aspirin use was associated with an acute MI risk reduction of 137 events per 10,000 persons and an ischemic stroke risk reduction of 39 events per 10,000. However, use was also associated with an absolute risk increase in hemorrhagic stroke of 12 events per 10,000 persons. The analysis indicates that in the study population aspirin therapy reduces the risk of MI and ischemic stroke more than it increases the risk of hemorrhagic stroke. However, a net benefit may not accrue for patients with low risk of acute MI or ischemic stroke [*Ibid*, p 1949].

Pharmacoeconomics

Steep Markups on Generic Drugs. Generic drugs are priced significantly lower than the equivalent brand-name product. However, according to a report in *The Wall Street Journal* [December 31, 1998, pp B1,B3], patients pay many times more than the cost of the generic product to the pharmacy. The journal claims that drugstores are marking up the price of some generic drugs by more than 1000%. This practice delivers a double blow to uninsured patients; they pay for prescriptions out of pocket and often pay the highest prices. Using data from a market research firm, the journal cites several examples. An average prescription for the generic version of the antihypertensive drug *Captopen* (captopril) costs the uninsured patient about $25. This compares favorably with the average retail price of $66 for *Captopen*. However, the generic manufacturer's price for the drug is only $1.46. The gross profit for the pharmacy is greater when the generic rather than the brand-name version is dispensed. A pharmaceutical industry analyst suggests that this is the reason pharmacies promote generic prescribing. Pharmacies argue that to focus on generic drugs' high gross margins is misleading and unfair because it does not take into account the pharmacist's professional services, which are the same whether a generic or brand-name product is dispensed.

4 In the Pipeline

CARDIOVASCULAR DISEASE

Treatment of Ischemic Stroke. Intravenous alteplase (*Activase*) is the only therapy specifically indicated for the treatment of ischemic stroke. Its use, however, is limited because it requires a brain scan before treatment to rule out hemorrhagic stroke, and therapy must start no more than three hours after the onset of stroke. Safer, more effective, and more applicable treatment is needed. One strategy that has attracted interest is a combination of low-dose alteplase with a glycoprotein IIb/IIIa antiplatelet agent. Three of these agents are now available in the US for the treatment of unstable angina and to reduce complications after coronary angioplasty. This strategy is likely to be safer than full-dose alteplase and may be more effective. Although the idea is prime for clinical testing, most companies developing IIb/IIIa inhibitors are focusing on other indications.

Patients not eligible for alteplase usually receive anticoagulation therapy with unfractionated heparin, but its use remains controversial because it has not been shown to be effective or safe. Some evidence suggests that low molecular weight heparins or heparinoids may be more effective in people with stroke. A recent study, however, shows that favorable outcomes at three months after an acute ischemic stroke are about the same for patients receiving danaparoid, a heparinoid, and those receiving placebo [*JAMA* 1998; 279:1265–72]. Within ten days of initiation of treatment, however, serious intracranial bleeding occurred in 14 patients given danaparoid but in only 4 patients treated with placebo.

A potentially important treatment strategy for patients with an evolving ischemic stroke is the application of neuroprotective agents. Neuroprotective drugs may be effective in these patients because the cerebral ischemic region has varying levels of residual blood flow that results in a comparatively slow evolution of damage from ischemia to cell death. This residual circulation permits delivery of the drug to the therapeutic target [*JAMA* 1998; 279:1298–303].

A host of biochemical changes accompany a stroke. For example, ischemia causes glutamate release, which activates N-methyl-D-aspartate (NMDA) receptors and leads to the release of calcium. This results in the production of free radicals that cause necrosis of brain tissue. Several biotechnology companies are trying to develop agents that would prevent the further activation of NMDA receptors. Other neuroprotective compounds are directed to other points in the stroke cascade. Unfortunately, the experience to date with these kinds of agents has been disappointing. While many have been abandoned because of a lack of benefit and/or serious toxicity, a combination of alteplase and a neuroprotective agent is of interest.

Endothelin Antagonists for the Treatment of Cardiovascular Disease. Endothelin-1 is a potent vasopressor peptide derived from the endothelium that was discovered in 1988. Overexpression of the peptide is seen in a range of cardiovascular diseases, including hypertension and heart failure. Modulation of nitric oxide and endothelin levels may contribute to the protective effects of estrogen replacement therapy (ERT) on heart disease. Nitric oxide causes vasodilation, inhibits platelet aggregation, and has anti-atherogenic activity. Endothelin-1 opposes the effects of nitric oxide, causing vasoconstriction of the systemic and coronary vasculature, increasing monocyte adhesion, and activating macrophages. In turn, nitric oxide inhibits the production of endothelin-1 and modulates the number and affinity of endothelin receptors. Nitric oxide synthase is functionally coupled to an endothelin receptor. Imbalances between nitric oxide and endothelin-1 occur in patients with elevated levels of cholesterol, atherosclerosis, and congestive heart failure.

A recent report examines the hypothesis that ERT increases the ratio of plasma nitric oxide products and circulating enodthelin-1 [_Ann Intern Med_ 1998;128:285–88]. Investigators treated postmenopausal women with estrogen for six months and measured levels of total oxidized products of nitric oxide and endothelin-1 before and after treatment. Estrogen replacement increased baseline nitric oxide by 26% and decreased baseline plasma endothelin-1 levels by 24%. Treatment increased the mean baseline ratio of nitric oxide to endothelin-1 from 2.0 to 3.2. The investigators concluded that increasing the ratio of nitric oxide to endothelin-1 might be one mechanism by which ERT provides cardiovascular benefit.

Two types of endothelin receptors have been described: A and B. Both types are found on vascular smooth muscle cells and mediate vasoconstriction.

Only the B receptor has been identified on endothelial cells. Activation of this B receptor mediates vasodilation. The B receptor may also be involved in the elimination of endothelin. Bosentan, under development by Roche Laboratories, is an orally active mixed A- and B-receptor antagonist that lowers blood pressure in animals. This suggests that the overall effect of antagonism of mixed endothelin receptors is vasodilation. Most endothelial antagonists in development act only on the A receptor.

In a recent study, investigators randomized 293 patients with mild-to-moderate hypertension to receive four weeks of therapy with one of four oral doses of bosentan, placebo, or enalapril (*Vasotec*), an angiotensin-converting enzyme inhibitor [*N Engl J Med* 1998;338:784–90]. Daily doses of 500 mg or more of bosentan lowered blood pressure about as effectively as enalapril, with no significant change in heart rate. Bosentan did not activate the sympathetic nervous system or the renin-angiotensin system. The blood pressure-lowering effect of bosentan suggests that endothelin may contribute to essential hypertension.

Preliminary results in the development of bosentan were encouraging, but during a phase III trial for heart failure, toxicity problems arose [*Scrip*, September 11, 1998, p 19]. The REACH-1 trial was stopped prematurely because of signs of liver toxicity. Because no overt liver damage was observed, Roche believes that it still may be possible to develop a lower, safe, and effective dose of the drug.

The place of endothelin-receptor antagonists in the treatment of hypertension is controversial, but they may have an important role in the treatment of hypertensive blacks, because blacks have higher endothelin concentrations than whites. Organ recipients tend to be unresponsive to conventional antihypertensive agents and may also benefit from this new class of drugs [*Pharmacother* 1998;18:706–19]. Other potentially important cardiovascular indications for endothelin antagonists are still emerging. They include heart failure, stroke, subarachnoid hemorrhage, and renal failure. All are likely to be the subject of clinical trials within the next few years. New molecules with increasing selectivity for A and B endothelin receptors also continue to be developed and may prove valuable [*TiPS* 1998;19 (No1):5–7].

Will Oral Glycoprotein IIb/IIIa Inhibitors Replace Aspirin? The development of abciximab (*ReoPro*), a monoclonal antibody directed against the gp IIb/IIIa receptor on the surface of blood platelets, and other inhibitors of the IIb/IIIa receptor is an important breakthrough for the treatment of cardiovascular disease. Currently available inhibitors are expensive and must be given by continuous intravenous infusion. There is a compelling rationale for developing oral agents, which could prevent recurrent thrombus formation and extend the benefits of intravenous therapy to the chronic phase of coronary syndromes. Patients who have survived an episode of unstable angina or myocardial infarction may have persistent activation of the hemostatic system for several months after the acute event. In theory, oral IIb/IIIa inhibitors could share the same broad clinical indications as aspirin, at least in high-risk patients.

Genentech, Monsanto, and Boehringer Ingelheim have led the field and have effective oral IIb/IIIa blockers entering phase III trials. These agents seem more effective than aspirin but also more risky. Phase II studies have shown high rates of "nuisance bleeding" from the gums, nose, and shaving nicks. One reviewer observes that the usefulness of oral agents will be the measure of their efficacy at tolerated doses. A lower dose of an oral agent combined with aspirin may be a sensible strategy.

A recent report in *Circulation* [1998;97:340–49] describes a randomized phase II trial—TIMI-12—of an oral agent called sibrafiban in patients following an acute coronary syndrome. The authors conclude that sibrafiban achieves effective long-term platelet inhibition with a clear dose-response relationship, but at the expense of a relatively high incidence of minor bleeding. A commentary accompanying this report observed: "Although some degree of optimism should prevail about future potential efficacy for chronic oral gp IIb/IIIa inhibitors, the major challenge to be pursued at this time is safety" [*Circulation* 1998;97:312–314].

Novel Mechanism to Lower Cholesterol. Several drug companies are developing small molecules that inhibit a human microsomal triglyceride transfer protein (MTP), which plays an important role in modulating lipid levels [*The Wall Street Journal*, October 23, 1998, pp B1,B4]. The hope is that these agents will lower cholesterol even more effectively than HMG-CoA reductase inhibitors (statins) and eventually replace them.

The new strategy has emerged from studies in people with a genetic defect—abetalipoproteinemia—who do not produce apolipoprotein B-containing lipoproteins (chylomicrons, very low-density lipoproteins, and low-density lipoproteins), which promote coronary artery atherosclerosis. People affected have very low levels of cholesterol and little heart disease. By 1992, researchers had cloned the gene and found that it expresses MTP.

When they deactivated the gene in certain cholesterol-synthesizing cells, the cells were unable to secrete proteolipids. Pharmaceutical scientists quickly recognized that inhibitors of MTP might prevent the assembly and secretion of atherogenic lipoproteins.

Abetalipoproteinemia is an extreme example of MTP inhibition and would not be the intended goal of drug therapy. Hypobetalipoproteinemia, a related genetic disorder, is caused by mutations in apolipoprotein B. Heterozygotes with this disease have about half the usual levels of apolipoprotein B-containing lipoproteins and have a prolonged life span.

In a paper published recently in *Science* [1998;282:751–54], a research team at the Bristol-Meyers Squibb Pharmaceutical Research Institute reports that an experimental MTP inhibitor (compound 9) significantly reduced cholesterol levels in rabbits genetically altered to produce very high levels of cholesterol. These creatures manifest many of the characteristics of coronary heart disease. The results suggest that compound 9, or derivatives thereof, has potential applications for the therapeutic lowering of atherogenic lipoprotein levels in humans.

GASTROINTESTINAL DISEASE

Isomer of Cisapride (*Propulsid*) Could Be Safer and Expand
  Indications
Single Isomer Version of Omeprazole Better than Omeprazole

Isomer of Cisapride (Propulsid) Could Be Safer and Expand Indications.
Janssen's commercial prospects with cisapride (*Propulsid*), a unique agent
to promote gastrointestinal motility and mitigate reflux disease, have been
hobbled by the addition of label warnings of potential drug interactions
with dire consequences [*The Pink Sheet* 1998;60(No30):12]. To maintain
its franchise, Janssen is helping Sepracor develop the single-isomer version
of cisapride, norcisapride. The companies say that norcisapride has a different
receptor binding profile than cisapride and offers the opportunity for novel
indications. Sepracor will evaluate norcisapride for bulimia, emesis, and irritable bowel syndrome, as well for cisapride's current indication for gastroesophageal reflux disease. Preclinical studies suggest that norcisapride has a more
favorable drug interaction profile than cisapride. Sepracor successfully developed fexofenadine (*Allegra*), which is a single isomer active metabolite of
terfenadine (*Seldane*) with little potential for drug interactions.

Single Isomer Version of Omeprazole Better than Omeprazole. According
to a report in *Scrip* [October 14, 1998, p 24], phase II/III trials of a second
generation proton pump inhibitor, perprazole, demonstrate that it has greater
efficacy than omeprazole. Perprazole, a single isomer version of omeprazole,
is under development for the treatment of reflux esophagitis, symptomatic
gastroesophageal reflux disease (GERD) and, in conjunction with antimicrobial agents, for the eradication of *Helicobacter pylori*. The studies indicate
that perprazole is absorbed faster than omeprazole, provides more rapid relief,
and elicits a more predictable response from one patient to another.

Infectious Disease

New Pharmaceuticals May Mean Safer Sex for Women
New Combination of Antiviral Drugs May Simplify HIV
  Therapy
New Protease Inhibitor Offers Less Frequent Dosing
The Next Wave of Anti-HIV Agents
Treatment of Kaposi's Sarcoma
New Drugs for the Treatment of Colds and Flu
Oxazolidinone Antimicrobials for Multidrug-Resistant
  Infections

New Pharmaceuticals May Mean Safer Sex for Women. The only way for a woman to avoid the risk of sexually transmitted diseases (STDs) or HIV infection is to use a condom during sexual intercourse. The lack of options is a dilemma for women who wish to conceive without risking infection and for those who do not wish to become pregnant or risk disease, but whose partner resists the use of a condom. Existing products containing the spermicide nonoxynol-9 (N-9) are being tested against STDs and HIV but some studies have linked the drug to vaginal and vulval irritation.

Fortunately, according to reports presented at the May 1998 meeting of the American Society of Microbiology, new bactericidal and virucidal intravaginal products could offer women safe and effective prevention. A recent commentary in *The Lancet* (1998;351:964) summarized these reports. Generating interest at the meeting were presentations on PRO 2000, a naphthalene sulfonate polymer that is effective against HIV, genital herpes, and perhaps *Chlamydia trachomatis*. Also promising is an invisible condom. This intravaginal liquid is thermoreversible; it is liquid at room temperature, but quickly sets to a transparent, odorless gel at body temperature. Developers believe that the gel will adhere strongly to the vaginal mucosa and stay in place during sexual intercourse. The gel alone is a physical barrier to pathogens but it can also contain microbicides. Another gel in development contains chlorhexidine and small, nonirritating amounts of N-9.

Also on the horizon are protegrins. These peptides have antimicrobial activity against bacteria, fungi, and some viruses. Other investigators have developed a vaginal suppository containing desiccated *Lactobacillus crispatus*. The bacterium produces hydrogen peroxide and makes the vagina more acidic and thus more resistant to infection. This product may be particularly useful for women who douche frequently. The commentary concludes: "So the idea that we can put something in the vagina to prevent or cure infection is within the realm of medical science today" [*Ibid.*].

New Combination of Antiviral Drugs May Simplify HIV Therapy. Researchers at the 12th World AIDS Conference in Geneva described a seemingly effective and easy-to-use drug therapy for the treatment of HIV infection. The regimen is based on a new, investigational non-nucleoside reverse transcriptase inhibitor (NNRTI) called efavirenz (*Sustiva*). The scientists claim that the new therapy—*Sustiva* plus *Combivir* (zidovudine and lamivudine)—will reduce the number of doses of antiviral agents from 10 or more per day to 3 per day [*The Wall Street Journal*, June 30, 1998]. *Combivir* would be taken in the morning and at night while *Sustiva* need be taken only at night. The researchers also say that the new combination is as effective as current therapy consisting of a protease inhibitor and *Combivir* or two other RTIs.

A controlled clinical trial with 450 patients showed that 62% of the patients in the *Sustiva* combination therapy group had plasma HIV RNA levels below 50 copies per ml compared with 48% of those in the indinavir (*Crixivan*) triple therapy group after 24 weeks of treatment. At that time, 24 patients from the indinavir group had withdrawn from the study because of adverse effects, compared with ten from the efavirenz group [*Scrip*, July 3, 1998, p 16]. Eliminating the need for a protease inhibitor is a welcome possibility because these agents have been found in some patients to cause troubling long-term side effects, including a lipodystrophy syndrome.

There is the possibility that the new combination may serve as alternative therapy for people who have drug-resistant infection. *Sustiva* plus *Combivir* may also reduce the development of drug resistance. Because the new regimen is easier to use, patients may be more compliant; poor compliance is viewed as an important factor in the development of resistance. However, some participants at the conference urged caution. One observer said, "I think we are seeing a lot of hype over *Sustiva*," adding that the new combination is not without serious side effects. A small number of patients taking *Sustiva*, less than 1%, report a psychosis-like reaction.

Yet another simplified strategy for the treatment of HIV infection was presented at the conference. The second approach is based on the new RTI abacavir (*Ziagen*). The new agent shows remarkable suppression of the virus when combined with *Combivir*, comparable in efficacy to triple therapy containing a protease inhibitor. The combination of *Ziagen* and *Combivir* can be dosed as two tablets twice daily, with no food restrictions. Although abacavir provokes a hypersensitivity reaction in about 3% of patients and produces a high incidence of vomiting, clinical investigators say that the symptoms are manageable. Another issue is that prior exposure to nucleoside therapy can reduce the response to abacavir. Glaxo Wellcome has submitted an application for approval of *Ziagen* for the treatment of HIV infection in adults and children.

New Protease Inhibitor Offers Less Frequent Dosing. Data from the first phase III trial of Vertex's amprenavir, called a second-generation HIV protease inhibitor, was presented at an infectious disease conference in September [*Scrip,* October 9, 1998, p 23]. The findings confirm the effectiveness of a twice-daily dosing regimen of amprenavir to reduce viral load when given with lamivudine and zidovudine. Currently marketed protease inhibitors require dosing three times a day, so a twice-daily regimen offers an advantage over existing products. Glaxo, Vertex's development partner, has filed a new drug application with the FDA and hopes that amprenavir will be available in mid-1999. A pediatric formulation of the drug has been developed and is included in the NDA submission.

An intention-to-treat analysis of the data showed that 59% of never-treated patients receiving combination therapy with amprenavir achieved a viral load of fewer than 400 copies at 16 weeks. Only 17% of those receiving the two reverse transcriptase inhibitors alone achieved that target. There was no significant difference in the incidence of side effects between the two groups but nausea and other gastrointestinal symptoms were more intense in the group receiving amprenavir. The trial will continue for an additional 32 weeks.

The Next Wave of Anti-HIV Agents. Current antiretroviral therapy for the treatment of HIV infection decreases viral load in plasma to undetectable levels, delays the progression of the disease, and strikingly reduces mortality. Nevertheless, the serious limitations of these agents are well known. The next generation of anti-HIV agents is likely to come from research on chemokines and chemokine receptors. Chemokines control the attraction of leukocytes to tissues, which is essential for inflammation and the host response to infection. Chemokines induce cell migration by binding to specific cell-surface chemokine receptors on target cells [*N Engl J Med* 1998;338:36–45].

Pathogenic organisms bind to receptors on leukocytes to gain access to the cytoplasm and nucleus of cells. Chemokine receptors serve as co-receptors for two human pathogens—plasmodium and HIV. In 1996, investigators discovered two chemokine co-receptors on the surface of T-lymphocyte immune cells that the virus uses, together with its primary receptor (CD4), to dock onto and penetrate its target cells. The co-receptor CXCR4 appears to be used by highly virulent viruses from patients in the later stages of the disease. Another, CCR5, seems to dominate in early stages of HIV infection. These findings galvanized the search for ways to stop HIV entry.

Today more than a dozen co-receptors for HIV have been identified. Earlier hopes of developing drugs to block viral attachment are subdued. Scientists are divided over whether co-receptors other than CCR5 and CXCR4 play anything more than a minor role. A clear majority thinks that CCR5 is central. People with genetic mutations that cause production of defective CCR5 molecules are resistant to infection with HIV. Considerable interest remains in developing a CCR5 antagonist. People with CCR5 mutations are not only resistant to infection with HIV but seem to have normal immune systems, implying that blocking the receptor would not have serious side effects. There is some evidence to suggest that blocking CXCR4 may be more consequential [*Science* 1998;280:825-26].

Novel strategies to prevent the expression of chemokine receptors and make cells resistant to infection with HIV are reviewed in a recent issue of *Nature Medicine* [1998;4:563-68]. One approach is to inhibit the interaction of HIV with its co-receptor by administering a monoclonal antibody to the chemokine receptor. Nonprotein, small molecule inhibitors are also of great interest.

Another potential key target for antiviral therapy is an HIV protein called gp120, which studs the surface of the virus's outer coat. By linking up with receptors on the surface of T-lymphocytes, HIV's primary target, gp120 allows the virus to enter the cells and reproduce. Efforts to destroy the virus by attacking gp120 have been unsuccessful. In June 1998, investigators using X-ray crystallography determined, for the first time, the atomic structure of gp120 bound to CD4 and a stabilizing antibody [*Nature* 1998;393:648–59, 705–11; *Science* 1998;280:1949–53]. The work helps us understand why antibodies raised against HIV fail to destroy the virus, and suggests therapeutic strategies to prevent the virus from binding and entering T-cells [*Science* 1998;280:1833–34].

According to a report in *The Scientist* [1998;12 (No14):1,7]: "The glycoprotein gp120 binds to the CD4 receptor on the T-cell, causing the viral molecule to contort in a way that enables it to bind to the nearby chemokine receptor, too. This dual binding of HIV to two co-receptors triggers fusion of the viral and T-cell membranes. Infection begins." Because the second binding protein on the virus is hidden until the last moment, it is largely unseen by the immune system. Another reason for the virus's invisibility is that it is surrounded by sugars that are the same kind that are cloaked on human proteins. The immune system recognizes the virus as "self" and does not mount a response. The pictures also show a cavity that forms as gp120 and CD4 link. The cleft may be a therapeutic target for future drugs.

Treatment of Kaposi's Sarcoma. Once a medical curiosity, Kaposi's sarcoma (KS) is now more common and more virulent as a result of immunosuppressive drug therapy in transplant patients and HIV infection. In patients with AIDS, KS imposes life-threatening complications. In 1995, a research group reported that crude, urine-derived preparations of the human pregnancy hormone chorionic gonadotrophin (hCG) inhibit the growth of KS cell lines and cause regression of KS lesions in mice. Ever since, the race has been on to discover the mechanism of this effect and determine whether hCG might be effective in the clinic.

A recent study shows that a factor present in clinical preparations of hCG, but not part of the native hCG protein, is responsible for the anti-KS activity associated with hCG. This component, called hCG associated factor (HAF) not only inhibits KS cell growth but also blocks the replication of HIV and the expression of HIV transgenes in mice. The researchers ascribe these properties to a pro-hematopoietic effect [*Nature Med* 1998;4:428–34].

Clinical preparations of hCG, injected locally or systemically, ameliorate clinical manifestations in about half of patients with AIDS-related KS. Some patients also have a decline in their HIV plasma levels and an increase in CD4 counts. HAF holds promise for treating KS and researchers are working to purify enough to identify the key factor or factors. One hurdle in reaching this goal is that the only known source is first trimester human urine.

New Drugs for the Treatment of Colds and Flu. Early reports of work presented at the Interscience Conference on Antimicrobial Agents and Chemotherapy in September promised that highly effective pharmaceuticals are in the offing for the treatment of influenza. The viral infection affects about 40 million Americans each year [*The Wall Street Journal,* September 25, 1998, A3, A11]. The new agents, Gilead Sciences's GS4104, and Glaxo's zanamivir (*Relenza*), can significantly reduce the length and severity of a typical flu attack caused by major strains of the influenza virus.

Also described at the conference were two prophylactic trials in nearly 1000 healthy adults. The investigators report that 1.2% of patients given GS4104 once daily for six weeks developed influenza during January and February 1998, compared with 4.8% of patients receiving placebo [*The Pink Sheet* 1998;60(No40):14]. A similar benefit was seen in a prophylaxis trial with zanamivir. Zanamivir is administered by means of an oral inhaler and GS4104 by mouth. Experts attending the conference described both drugs as highly effective and well tolerated. Roche plans to submit a new drug application for GS4104 in 1999. Glaxo hopes to file a NDA for zanamivir by the end of 1998 so that it may market *Relenza Diskhaler* for the 1999–2000 flu season.

Both drugs disable neuraminidase, a viral enzyme required to make new viral particles from an infected cell. They work against A and B strains of influenza, the most common types of flu in the US. Studies show that the new agents reduce the usual six to eight day duration of the illness by about two days. The vaccine developed each year against the currently circulating strains of the virus can prevent influenza. Most Americans, however, do not get vaccinated.

At a parallel meeting, this one of the American Society for Microbiology, researchers reported on the new drug AG7088 that may be effective for the treatment of the common cold [*The New York Times*, September 29, 1998, p B15]. Agouron has studied the structure of rhinovirus and identified an enzyme called 3C protease, which splits viral precursor polyproteins that are essential for the proliferation of new viral particles. AG7088 inactivates the enzyme. Because the 3C protease is broadly similar in 46 out of 100 strains of human rhinovirus examined so far, AG7088 and related drugs may have broad efficacy.

Agouron started clinical trials of a nasal formulation of AG7088 in late 1998, focusing on patients with underlying pulmonary disease such as asthma, COPD, bronchitis, and cystic fibrosis. The company is likely to first seek approval in these areas.

Oxazolidinone Antimicrobials for Multidrug-Resistant Infections. Pharmacia & Upjohn is developing a novel group of antimicrobial agents called oxazolidinones [*Scrip*, October 7, 1998, p 26]. These agents are potential candidates for the treatment of infections caused by multidrug-resistant gram-positive microorganisms. Linezolid, now in phase III trials, is the lead compound. Oxazolidinones work by inhibiting bacterial messenger RNA translation, thereby blocking protein synthesis at an earlier stage than other antimicrobial agents. This novel mechanism of action may avoid the development of cross-resistance between linezolid and other antimicrobial agents. In the ongoing trials, investigators are studying the effects of linezolid in patients with serious staphylococcal, streptococcal, and enterococcal infections, including those caused by strains resistant to other antimicrobial agents. The product is being developed in both oral and intravenous forms.

MENTAL HEALTH

New Indications for SSRI Antidepressants
New Antidepressants Will Challenge Market Leaders
New Way to Treat Schizophrenia

New Indications for SSRI Antidepressants. Drug companies marketing selective serotonin reuptake inhibitors (SSRIs) have been diligent in expanding the indications for their products. These efforts continue. Lilly is preparing to seek approval for its antidepressant, fluoxetine (*Prozac*), to treat premenstrual syndrome (PMS) as well as its severe form called premenstrual dysphoric disorder (PMDD) [*Scrip*, July 24, 1998, p 19]. One expert estimates that as many as 20% of premenopausal women could benefit from treatment. A recent clinical trial in women with PMDD shows that fluoxetine provides more than 75% improvement from base line in mood symptoms in 75% of women treated over the 14-day period between ovulation to onset of menstruation. A shorter course of treatment may also be effective.

Fluoxetine provides prompt relief of the symptoms of PMS. However, when the drug is used to treat patients with depression, the time lag before resolution of symptoms is usually three to six weeks. This suggests that the two disorders have a different pathology and therefore, different symptoms. Irritability is much more important in PMS than in depression.

SmithKline Beecham has applied for a new indication for paroxetine (*Paxil*) for the treatment of social anxiety disorder, which has previously been called social phobia [*Scrip*, July 24, 1998, p 22]. *Paxil* is already approved for panic attack and obsessive-compulsive disorder, in addition to its primary indication for the treatment of depression. Embarrassment and a tendency to discount achievements and emphasize failure are hallmarks of the disorder. Antidepressants that work by inhibiting monoamine oxidase are also effective in treating social anxiety disorder, but side effects and the need for dietary restrictions relegates them to second-line status.

New Antidepressants Will Challenge Market Leaders. The World Health Organization estimates that there are 340 million people with depression. It is said to affect 1% of the US population. Dominating the antidepressant market in the US are SSRIs which have a better safety profile than do older agents—tricyclic antidepressants and monoamine oxidase inhibitors. A challenge may come from new drugs, however, that have novel mechanisms of action, are more effective, and have an even better safety profile.

One of the most promising agents is Pharmacia & Upjohn's *Edronax* (reboxetine) described by some as a breakthrough product [*Scrip* July 29, 1998, p 24]. Reboxetine is the first of a new class of agents that selectively inhibit norepinephrine re-uptake (NaRIs). Preliminary clinical studies suggest that reboxetine is more effective than SSRIs, even in patients with moderate depression. A better response is also claimed by Wyeth-Ayerst for venlafaxine (*Effexor*). Venlafaxine is the first drug to combine both norepinephrine and serotonin re-uptake inhibition (SNaRI). This product was launched in 1994 but its use has been limited by side effects, particularly nausea. The recent development of a once-daily slow-release formulation of venlafaxine has minimized side effects. Some experts say that *Effexor* is a drug to turn to when a patient is not responding to other agents. Another SNaRI, with few side effects is milnacipran. Mirtazapine is a norepinephrine and specific serotonin antidepressant (NaSSA). It too promises to have fewer adverse effects than SSRIs.

Depression and anxiety often occur together in the same patient, but regulatory bodies insist that efficacy be demonstrated for each condition separately. Wyeth-Ayerst seeks to have *Effexor* recognized as the first-line drug for depressed patients with anxiety, and to be a major product in both the anxiety and depression markets. The company has applied to the FDA for the additional indication of generalized anxiety disorder (GAD) [*Scrip*, August 26, 1998]. This disorder embraces a range of different anxiety states and includes elements of panic disorder and social phobia. Buspirone (*Buspar*) is usually selected for long term treatment of GAD. According to Wyeth-Ayerst, an eight-week trial shows that sustained-release venlafaxine (*Effexor XR*) has significant advantages compared with buspirone.

Another effort to develop a safer and more effective antidepressant centers on a chemical discovered in 1931 called substance P. Substance P is a neuropeptide found in the brain and peripheral neurons and is one of several dozen neurotransmitters that relay signals between brain cells. The role it plays in the central nervous system is not entirely clear. Merck, convinced that substance P regulates mood, has developed a substance P receptor blocker they are calling MK-869. A study in 210 patients with moderate to severe major depressive disorder shows that MK-869 is significantly more effective than placebo and at least as effective as paroxetine (*Paxil*), but with significantly fewer side effects [*Science* 1998:281:1640–45]. In the trial, 3% of the patients taking MK-869 reported sexual side effects, compared with 26% of those who received *Paxil.*

The Wall Street Journal [August 13, 1998, pp B1, B4] suggests that MK-869 could be a boon to the 20% of people with depression who are not helped by currently available antidepressant agents and to the thousands of patients who experience side effects and eventually stop taking conventional antidepressants. Merck cautioned that at least two more years of clinical testing is needed before the drug's promise is confirmed. The company believes that substance P receptor blockers may also be effective for other mental disorders, including anxiety and schizophrenia [*The Wall Street Journal,* September 11, 1998].

Novartis is also developing a substance P antagonist, while Lilly is working on a drug, duloxetine, that increases brain levels of norepinephrine and serotonin. SmithKline Beecham seeks success with an agent that increases brain levels of serotonin. Pfizer is also said to be developing a novel antidepressant, but information is scant [*The New York Times,* October 11, 1998, pp Bu1, Bu2].

New Way to Treat Schizophrenia. Schizophrenia afflicts about 1% of the population of the US. Current therapy—haloperidol, phenothiazines, and other agents—work by blocking the action of the neurotransmitter dopamine. These agents reduce the level of paranoia and the frequency of hallucinations, but offer little help for other symptoms characteristic of schizophrenia—poor attention span, jumbled thoughts, and difficulty interacting with other people. Furthermore, patients taking these agents, collectively called neuroleptics, often suffer troubling side effects including uncontrollable tremors. Clinical experts say there is an urgent need for anti-schizophrenic agents that are not primarily dopaminergic.

Research groups are studying drugs that lower brain levels of glutamate, another important neurotransmitter [*Science* 1998;281:1264–65]. Interest in these agents stems from the observation that phencyclidine, known as angel dust in street parlance, induces schizophrenia-like symptoms in healthy people. This effect is attributed to its ability to block N-methyl-D-aspartate (NMDA) receptors in the brain, through which glutamate exerts its effects. Experiments in rats show that phencyclidine induces symptoms thought to parallel psychotic symptoms in humans. As expected, phencyclidine raises dopamine concentrations in rat brain. Unexpected, however, is that phencyclidine also causes a surge in the levels of glutamate in the brain, suggesting that abnormally high glutamate activity might underlie the reaction of rats to phencyclidine.

Further study led to the identification of a drug called LY354740 that is under development at Lilly for other psychiatric disorders including anxiety. The experimental agent stimulates a subgroup of glutamate receptors that act as regulators of glutamate levels. As a result of this selectivity, LY354740 dampens the output of glutamate when its levels get too high, but does not interfere with normal levels. Experiments in rats show that LY354740 blocks the increase in glutamate levels in the brain and the "psychotic effects" ordinarily seen after administration of phencyclidine. There is also evidence that LY354740 reduces a phencyclidine-induced cognitive deficit not helped by the administration of conventional neuroleptics.

NEUROLOGICAL DISEASE

Anti-Cancer Drug Benefits Patients with Multiple Sclerosis. A presentation at a meeting of the European Committee for Treatment and Research in Multiple Sclerosis reported that mitoxantrone (*Novantrone*) provides significant benefit to patients with multiple sclerosis (MS), a progressive disease that leads to paralysis and early death [*Scrip,* September 16, 1998, p 23]. *Novantrone* is marketed in the US and other countries for the treatment of prostate cancer and acute non-lymphocytic leukemia. The basis of the report is a preliminary analysis of a phase III trial that compared two different doses of mitoxantrone, given intravenously every three months, against placebo.

According to the meeting report, the annual rate of disease progression was 21% for patients given the higher of the two doses of *Novantrone,* compared with 60% for patients on placebo. The median time to first relapse was 15 months for the placebo group and was not reached after 24 months for either of the *Novantrone* groups. The investigators reported no major toxicity. The most frequently reported side effects were neutropenia, infection, and loss of hair. A clinical investigator, who has worked with the drug, says that *Novantrone* compares favorably to the immunomodulators that are now available [*The Wall Street Journal,* September 10, 1998, p B6].

This is encouraging news because options for the treatment of MS are limited. Currently available are interferon beta-1a (*Avonex*) and interferon beta-1b (*Betaseron*). These agents affect the course of the disease only modestly and must be given by intravenous injection daily or weekly. Immunex will consult with the FDA to determine whether this single clinical trial is sufficient to file for a new indication for use in patients with MS.

Obesity

Orlistat (*Xenical*): Novel Drug for Weight Loss
Strategies and Potential Targets for the Treatment of Obesity

Orlistat (Xenical): Novel Drug for Weight Loss. Orlistat promotes weight loss by inhibiting lipases in the gastrointestinal tract, thereby reducing fat absorption. Evidence of efficacy is found in a controlled trial enrolling 683 subjects, mostly women, who had body mass indexes ranging from 28 to 47 kg/m^2 [*Lancet* 1998;352:167–73]. They were assigned to receive orlistat or placebo three times daily for 52 weeks. At the end of the year, 273 orlistat patients and 253 placebo patients either remained on assigned treatment or were reassigned for year two. Both groups were asked to maintain a low calorie diet.

At the end of the first year, participants receiving orlistat had an average weight loss of 10%, compared with a 6% average weight loss in those assigned to placebo. About 9% of the orlistat group compared with 2% of the placebo group lost 20% of initial body weight. On reassignment to orlistat, former placebo recipients lost weight, while those who stayed on placebo gained weight. On reassignment to placebo, former orlistat recipients gained twice as much weight as did orlistat patients who remained on the study drug. Total cholesterol, low-density lipoprotein cholesterol, and concentrations of glucose and insulin decreased more in the orlistat group than in the placebo group.

Gastrointestinal adverse events—changes in stool consistency, oily spotting, and increased defecation—were more common in the orlistat group than in the placebo group. Most complaints were made early in the course of treatment and faded by year two. Adverse reaction rates are likely to increase when orlistat is taken with a high-fat diet. Orlistat also has the potential to decrease the absorption of fat-soluble vitamins. During the study, patients on orlistat had lower concentrations of vitamins D and E and beta-carotene, but levels remained in the normal range.

In another study, investigators evaluated the role of orlistat in obese patients with type 2 diabetes [*Diabetes Care* 1998;21:1288–93]. Weight loss in patients with type 2 disease improves glycemic control and reduces cardiovascular disease risk factors. After one year of treatment, the researchers found that the orlistat group lost 6.2% of initial body weight, compared with a loss of 4.3% in the placebo group. Nearly half of the patients on orlistat lost 5% or more of initial body weight compared with 23% of those on placebo. Orlistat compared with placebo significantly improved glycemic control as reflected in decreases in glycosylated hemoglobin, fasting plasma glucose, and dosages of sulfonylurea medication. Orlistat also excelled in reducing total cholesterol, low-density lipoprotein cholesterol, and triglycerides.

In March 1998, a FDA advisory panel divided evenly on whether to recommend the approval of *Xenical*. The hurdle was whether orlistat increases the risk of breast cancer. Most observers are puzzled as to how a lipase inhibitor that is not absorbed and works primarily by blocking fat absorption in the gut could be linked to excess cases of breast cancer. The manufacturer, Roche, says that the relative risk of developing cancer, estimated as 3.6, compared with placebo, occurred by chance, and that studies in animals have not shown carcinogenicity [*Lancet* 1998;351:885]. Roche also argues that the weight loss resulting from treatment with orlistat might have allowed detection of existing cancers by changing breast architecture. The data, however, do not support that argument.

In May 1998, Roche received an approvable letter from the FDA, stating that final approval is subject to certain conditions including submission of follow-up safety data from ongoing clinical programs and agreement of final labeling. Roche estimated that the requirements would keep them from marketing *Xenical* in the US until the middle of 1999, two years later than the company had hoped [*The Pink Sheet* 1998;60 (No20):6].

In July, Roche announced that *Xenical* had been approved in Europe with clean labeling. There is no mention of breast cancer. The European Union label states that pooled data from five two-year studies demonstrated that 20% of patients lost 10% or more of their body weight while taking orlistat for one year, compared to 8% of patients receiving placebo. It warns, however, that *Xenical* should be discontinued after 12 weeks if patients have been unable to lose at least 5% of body weight. The European Public Assessment Report for orlistat stated that *Xenical* appears to have a positive effect on quality of life measures [*The Pink Sheet* 1998;60(No33):15].

Roche estimates that the maximum potential market for *Xenical* in the UK is 400,000 seriously overweight people. If prescribed for all eligible patients, *Xenical* would cost the health system $350 million a year, and it would rank among the most expensive medications covered by the health service. To counter concerns about the use of *Xenical* for cosmetic purposes, Roche's promotions will emphasize that the target audience is obese patients, who often have co-morbidities.

Strategies and Potential Targets for the Treatment of Obesity. Obesity is an increasingly prevalent and important health problem in much of the developed world, and especially in the US in both adults and children. Prevention and treatment are a challenge because of the complex etiology of obesity. The burgeoning research on the altered biochemical pathways caused by single gene mutatations in animal models of obesity has greatly increased the knowledge of these physiological mechanisms and led to intensified efforts to develop innovative anti-obesity drugs [*Science* 1998;280:1383–87].

The development of new drugs for obesity is paralleled by a growing interest in a new way to measure outcomes of treatment called "metabolic fitness." It is defined as the absence of biochemical risk factors associated with obesity. In this perspective, weight loss is viewed not as a goal but as a means to improve health. There is much evidence to support the association between weight loss and improvement in the profile of cardiovascular risk factors. The hope is that this new way to look at obesity treatment will shift the patient's focus from culturally imposed goals to the goal of better health.

There are several strategies to achieve weight loss. The only anti-obesity agent approved for use in the US, sibutramine (*Meridia*), is an appetite suppressant that reduces food intake by modulating concentrations of mono-amine neurotransmitters—serotonin and norepinephrine—in the brain.

The most publicized new target for treating obesity is the OB receptor. The recently isolated hormone leptin activates the OB receptor in the brain and reduces food intake, serum glucose and insulin levels, and increases metabolic rate, which leads to a reduction in fat mass and body weight. Leptin mediates its effects through a specific receptor called OB-R. Perhaps the next generation of anti-obesity agents may target the OB pathway. Bear in mind, however, that obese humans have elevated levels of serum leptin, suggesting that obesity is the result of a decreased sensitivity to leptin, not a deficiency of the hormone.

The most effective treatment for obesity is likely to be one that involves the use of a combination of drugs, each with a distinct mechanism of action, or a single drug with multiple activities. Drugs for obestiy treatment must have a favorable safety profile because they are taken continuously or intermittently throughout adult life. Innovative drugs will be most effective when they are used as adjuncts to, rather than substitutes for, lifestyle changes to improve metabolic fitness, health, and quality of life for obese individuals.

ONCOLOGY

Photodynamic Therapy for Cancer. Photodynamic therapy is based on the action of light on certain chemicals called photosensitizers. The FDA has so far approved only one photosensitizer, a porphyrin-like molecule called porfimer (*Photofrin*). Porfimer accumulates in tumors. When illuminated, it forms chemically reactive species that can kill cancer cells. In photodynamic therapy, the tissues meant to be destroyed are selectively illuminated and the damage confined only to those areas. In the US, *Photofrin* is approved only for the treatment of esophageal cancer, but it is used outside the US for the treatment of other cancers. A typical treatment consists of an intravenous dose of *Photofrin* 24 to 48 hours before the tumor is illuminated for 10 to 30 minutes, often using fiber optics. The one side effect of treatment with *Photofrin* is that the patient remains sensitive to light for 30 days and needs to wear protective clothes if venturing out into the sun.

Drug and chemical companies are developing compounds that improve on *Photofrin*. One way to improve current therapy is to increase light penetration. According to a report in *Chem & Engineering News* [November 2, 1990, pp 22–27], light penetrates deeper into tissues as its wavelength increases. *Photofrin* is activated at 630 nm. Consequently, its effect penetrates through only a few millimeters of tumor tissue. A photosensitizer excited at longer wavelengths will deliver its therapeutic effect deeper in the tumor. A second generation agent, called *Verteporfin,* is activated at 690 nm, builds up rapidly in target tissues, allowing light treatment to begin within five minutes of administration, and quickly clears from normal tissue. Other photosensitizers with similar characteristics are also being studied.

The photosensitizers used in photodynamic therapy have an affinity to lipoprotein, especially low-density lipoproteins (LDLs). Rapidly dividing cells have more LDL receptors than do quiescent cells. Porfimer and other photosensitizers under development for photodynamic therapy tend to concentrate in tissue with rapidly dividing cells and new blood vessels. It follows that photodynamic therapy could also be useful for non-cancer disease with characteristics similar to tumors, such as macular degeneration of the eye. This condition affects 10 million Americans, causes blurred vision, and eventually leads to blindness. Some experts think that photodynamic therapy is on the verge of becoming mainstream treatment for various diseases.

PAIN MANAGEMENT

New Nonopioid Analgesic
Enhancing the Effects of Morphine
New NSAIDs: An Array of Benefits without Stomach Damage

New Nonopioid Analgesic. Abbott is developing a novel nonopioid analgesic that is based on a natural compound isolated from the skin of a South American frog. The agent, epibatidine (ABT-594), is in early clinical trials. Studies in animal models of pain suggest that epibatidine may topple the centuries-old reign of morphine as the most effective analgesic [*Science* 1998;279:32–33]. The new agent appears to act through a nicotinic acetylcholine receptor and safely blocks both acute and chronic pain. Animal studies also show that in contrast to morphine, repeated administration of epibatidine does not appear to produce opioid-like withdrawal symptoms or physical dependence, nor does it cause respiratory depression or suppression of gastrointestinal activity.

Enhancing the Effects of Morphine. The *Prescriber's Letter* [1998;5 (No 4):23] reports that some physicians are prescribing dextromethorphan to enhance the analgesic effect of morphine and other opioids. Dextromethorphan seems to reduce sensitivity to pain by blocking N-methyl-D-aspartate (NMDA) receptors in the brain and spinal cord, thereby increasing and prolonging pain relief. A combination of 30 mg of morphine and 30 mg of dextromethorphan is said to be as effective as doubling the morphine dose. A product containing morphine and dextromethorphan, called *MorphiDex*, is under development.

New NSAIDs: An Array of Benefits without Stomach Damage. Aspirin and other nonsteroidal anti-inflammatory (NSAIDs) are effective for the treatment of pain and inflammation. But they can also erode the stomach lining, incur gastroduodenal ulcers, and damage the kidneys. The problem with marketed NSAIDs may be that they are not sufficiently selective. Their benefits probably derive from the ability to block COX-2, an isoform of cyclooxygenase that promotes inflammation, pain, and fever. Because the currently available NSAIDs were developed before knowledge of two forms of cyclooxygenase, these agents also inhibit COX-1, which is essential to maintain the integrity of stomach and kidney function.

The pharmaceutical industry is attempting to build a better aspirin by developing compounds that selectively inhibit COX-2. Monsanto/Searle and Merck are vying to be the first to market a specific COX-2 inhibitor. To improve its chances, Monsanto has invited Pfizer to co-develop their drug. According to Monsanto, a recent study comparing celecoxib (*Celebrex,* formerly called *Celebra*) with existing NSAIDs in 12,000 patients with rheumatoid arthritis found that the drug is as effective as NSAIDs without injuring the gastrointestinal (GI) mucosa. Merck has also reported promising results with their compound rofecoxib (*Vioxx*).

Investigators recently published results from four phase II studies of the safety and efficacy of celecoxib [*Arthritis & Rheumatism* 1998;41:1591–1602]. A 14-day trial in patients with osteoarthritis and a 28-day trial in patients with rheumatoid arthritis identified doses of celecoxib that were consistently more effective than placebo in treating the signs and symptoms of arthritis. A one-week endoscopic study demonstrated that erosive effects of celecoxib in the stomach are negligible in contrast with the non-selective COX inhibitor naproxen. A fourth study showed that celecoxib, unlike aspirin, has little effect on platelet aggregation.

Also, unlike aspirin, which binds covalently to COX enzymes, marketed NSAIDs as well the investigational COX-2 inhibitors have reversible effects. Researchers have developed compounds that chemically disarm COX-2 instead of just blocking its activity [*Science* 1998;280:1268-70]. Whether these agents will prove more effective than reversibly acting COX-2-selective inhibitors remains to be seen.

Recent laboratory experiments indicate that COX-2 inhibition may be a key factor in staving off colon cancer [*Nature Med* 1998;4:392–93]. Researchers have found high levels of COX-2 in about 90% of colon tumors they examined. Searle reports that the COX-2 gene is overactive in other cancers as well. Genetically engineered cells that make greater than normal amounts of COX-2 are less susceptible to programmed cell death (apoptosis), which normally eliminates mutated or damaged cells. COX-2 might also release free radicals, which can cause mutations, and promote the growth of new blood vessels that carry the nutrients required by the tumor.

New research shows that cyclooxygenases, both COX-1 and COX-2, can induce angiogenic factors needed for the growth and dissemination of colon cancer. This suggests that aspirin and other NSAIDs may work by inhibiting the angiogenesis caused by pro-inflammatory enzymes. The investigators used an *in vitro* model consisting of colorectal cancer cells and endothelial cells separated by a filter and a layer of collagen. They showed that when cancer cells over-expressing COX-2 were used in the model, there was a significant increase in the production of angiogenic factors and in the migration of the endothelial cells into tubular structures (proto-arteries). Aspirin and a selective COX-2 inhibitor (NS-398) reduced this activity [*Cell* 1998;93:705–16].

Preventing cancer may require taking NSAIDs for a lifetime. Selective COX-2 inhibitors seem tailored for such use because they appear safer than marketed NSAIDs. The future looks promising for COX-2 inhibitors. Their only apparent drawback is that, unlike aspirin, they do not lower the risk of cardiovascular disease, because they do not inhibit the clot-promoting effects of the COX-1 enzyme [*Science* 1998;280:1191-92].

Boehringer Ingelheim has marketed a COX-2 selective drug called meloxicam in the United Kingdom since 1996. Indications include rheumatoid and osteoarthritis. In theory, this agent should have a better side-effect profile than other NSAIDs. The safety advantage of meloxicam, however, has been the subject of debate. Competitors suggest that meloxicam may actually be a COX-2 preferential inhibitor rather than a true COX-2 selective inhibitor. The UK Drug and Therapeutics Bulletin (DTB) reported in August that meloxicam is no more effective than existing NSAIDs and shares their unwanted side effects [*Scrip,* August 28, 1998, p 16]. In September 1998, Boehringer Ingelheim strengthened warnings about adverse events.

The results of two large double-blind tolerance trials in patients with osteoarthritis, however, suggest meloxicam is safer than other NSAIDs. MELLISA, which enrolled more than 9,000 patients, randomized participants to either meloxicam or sustained release diclofenac for 28 days. Patients on meloxicam had 32% fewer (13% compared with 19%) GI adverse events than patients receiving diclofenac. Only three patients on meloxicam were hospitalized, for a total of five days, because of adverse events compared with ten patients on diclofenac who spent a total of 121 days in hospital [*Br J Rheumatol* 1998;37:937–45]. SELECT enrolled more than 8,500 patients and compared meloxicam with piroxicam. After 28 days, 33% fewer patients on meloxicam had GI adverse events than those on piroxicam (10% vs. 15%) [*Br J Rheumatol* 1998;37:946–51].

A confounding question about these reports is whether the doses of the two drugs used in each study were equipotent. In MELLISA, differences in efficacy consistently favored diclofenac. Significantly more patients discontinued meloxicam because of lack of efficacy.

The DTB report came as the FDA granted a priority review to celecoxib, Searle's selective COX-2 inhibitor. Searle appears to have a six-month lead on Merck in the race to market. Merck projected a late 1998 NDA filing for *Vioxx*. Earlier in 1998, the arthritis advisory committee said that studies supporting approval of a COX-2 selective inhibitor must show that the new agent has fewer GI side-effects than nonselective NSAIDs.

At a meeting of the American College of Gastroenterology, Merck investigators reported that *Vioxx* has a GI adverse event profile similar to placebo at doses two to four times higher than those that have shown therapeutic benefit. They also reported that the once-daily product has fewer GI side-effects than either ibuprofen or indomethacin. One study in healthy subjects showed that *Vioxx* caused no more GI blood loss than placebo, but subjects on ibuprofen had twice as much blood loss. In another study, again with healthy subjects, *Vioxx* had no more effect on GI permeability than placebo, but indomethacin increased permeability by more than 50% [*Scrip,* October 21, 1998, p 26].

Respiratory Disease

Combination Therapy for Asthma. Glaxo Wellcome is planning to submit an application to the FDA for a new combination product to treat asthma. The combination, *Seretide,* contains the long-acting β-agonist salmeterol and the corticosteroid fluticasone, which are marketed separately as *Serevent* and *Flovent.* It is intended for inhalation. Although the product has received a mixed reaction from asthma experts, Glaxo Wellcome expects *Seretide* to become the "gold standard" of asthma treatment because it works within 24 hours, improves control over other therapies, decreases the need for inhaled steroid, and simplifies dosing. According to a report in *Scrip* [October 23, 1998, p 20], one study shows that *Seretide 50/100* is significantly more effective than *Serevent* 50 μg, *Flovent* 100 μg, or placebo for improving peak expiratory flow.

Substance Abuse

Blocking Glutamate May Help Alcoholics and Drug Addicts. Until recently, scientists studying addiction focused on dopamine. All addictive drugs cause a surge of dopamine, which seems to tell the brain to get more of that stuff. Now, recent work is implicating glutamate, another neurotransmitter, in the addictive learning experience [*Science* 1998;280:2045–47]. The work to date suggests that drug interference with glutamate transmission might be used to treat addiction.

A drug called acamprosate (calcium acetylhomotaurine) is now being used in Europe to treat alcoholism and is under investigation in the US. It was observed in rat brain that acamprosate blocked the ability of glutamate to stimulate electrical signals. A large clinical trial shows that after one year of treatment with acamprosate or placebo, 18.3% of patients receiving acamprosate were still abstinent from alcohol compared with 7.1% of control patients [*Lancet* 1996;347:1438–42].

The pharmacology of acamprosate raises the concern that widespread blockage of brain glutamate receptors can impair learning and memory, and produce hallucinations. Industry scientists have identified safer agents such as dextromethorphan (a medication used widely in cough and cold preparations) that bind only loosely to the N-methyl-D-aspartate (NMDA) glutamate receptor. In rodents, dextromethorphan curtails cocaine-seeking behavior and blocks the development of morphine tolerance. Researchers are also studying other NMDA-receptor antagonists as potential antidotes to morphine tolerance and opiate dependence.

According to *The New York Times* [July 31, 1998, pp C1, C4], the expected arrival of acamprosate in the US in the year 2000 has ignited controversy. Specialists who argue that alcoholics should be treated with counseling alone are pitted against physicians who insist that drugs are important tools. Acamprosate is not a substitute for detoxification but it will help prevent relapse. Also important is that acamprosate does not seem to have any serious adverse effects. Acamprosate is probably safer than disulfiram (*Antabuse*), an alcohol antagonist that can be toxic if a patient consumes a large amount of alcohol while on the drug, and naltrexone, an opioid antagonist that can cause liver toxicity.

Transplantation

New and Important Immunosuppressant on the Horizon. At the end of 1998, Wyeth-Ayerst filed approval applications for its immunosuppressant *Rapamune* (sirolimus). Two key trials in patients undergoing kidney transplantation support the applications [*Scrip,* July 17, 1998 p22]. A trial in the US compared sirolimus with azathioprine, both given in combination with standard therapy—cyclosporine and prednisone—to patients receiving cadaveric or mismatched living donor allografts. Compared with azathioprine, sirolimus reduced acute rejection episodes over the first six months from 24% to 15% in those receiving 2 mg daily and to 10% in those given 5 mg daily. Graft survival and overall survival was excellent in all three groups, but better with *Rapamune* than with azathioprine. *Rapamune* also decreased the need for antibody therapy to treat acute rejection episodes.

A global trial, led by investigators from Nova Scotia, adhered to a protocol very similar to that used in the US trial except that patients were randomized before transplantation rather than after. Among those patients treated with 5 mg sirolimus, 11% experienced acute rejection episodes compared with 19% among those given 2 mg sirolimus and 29% of those receiving only cyclosporine and prednisone.

Wyeth-Ayerst thinks that *Rapamune* will eventually replace cyclosporine because the new agent does not precipitate renal toxicity, which is a serious problem associated with the current market leader. Researchers suggest that initially patients may switch to *Rapamune* after being stabilized on cyclosporine. The addition of *Rapamune* may allow a significant dose reduction of cyclosporine. Pilot studies suggest that *Rapamune* is also effective for patients undergoing heart or liver transplantation. According to *Scrip,* sirolimus blocks an intracellular protein in lymphocytes and prevents the signal cascade that leads to immune system activation and organ rejection.

Women's Health

Combined Hormone Replacement for Postmenopausal Women. The billion-dollar US market for hormone replacement products is dominated by Wyeth-Ayerst's *Premarin* (conjugated estrogens) and has been for many years. *Premarin* should always be used with a progestin to reduce the risk of endometriosis and combination products containing conjugated estrogens and medroxyprogesterone (*Premphase, Prempro*) are now available. A European company, Novo Nordisk, hopes to successfully challenge Wyeth-Ayerst with its newly developed *Activelle,* a continuous combined hormone replacement product [*Scrip,* July 10, 1998, p 18].

Activelle is approved in all European Union countries and is under review by the US FDA. The product contains 1 mg of estradiol and 0.5 mg of norethisterone. Novo Nordisk suggests that the low dose of estrogen will result in a more favorable safety profile, including less breast tenderness. The combination is taken every day rather than sequentially. The advantage of this approach, also used with *Prempro,* is the avoidance of monthly menstrual bleeds. Novo Nordisk is comparing *Activelle* and *Prempro* directly in an ongoing clinical trial.

Also competing in this market is Organon's *Livial* (tibolone), which is a synthetic compound that overlaps the activities of estrogens, progestogens, and androgens, depending on the tissue. According to *Scrip* [October 16, 1998, p 20], tibolone is effective for menopausal symptoms, causes minimal bleeding , and may increase bone density and lower cholesterol.

OTHER INDICATIONS

Modafinil for Sleep Disorders
Therapeutic Potential of Botulinum Toxin
New Strategies for Male Contraception

Modafinil for Sleep Disorders. Narcolepsy, a severe sleep disorder, is characterized by excessive daytime sleepiness and cataplexy—the sudden and temporary loss of muscle tone that can lead to body limpness and collapse. Narcolepsy can be disabling, but the market for drugs to treat the condition is small. Cephalon recently announced that it expects to receive approval to market modafinil (*Provigil*) in the US, where it has received orphan drug status. The drug is already approved in France and the UK [*Scrip*, March 6, 1998, p 18]. Evidence of safety and effectiveness is found in a well-controlled trial in which subjects with narcolepsy received modafinil or placebo daily for nine weeks. Modafinil significantly reduced all measures of sleepiness and was associated with significant improvement in the level of illness [*Annals Neurol* 1998;43:880-97]. Another study reports that *Provigil* significantly improves average scores of wakefulness and daytime alertness. Adverse events are few and mostly rated mild to moderate. *Provigil* seems to be an advance on amphetamines, the standard treatment for this condition, as it has fewer side effects and is less likely to lead to tolerance. Many speculate that the approval of modafinil will result in extensive off-label use by people who seek wakefulness and alertness in the absence of adequate sleep [*The New York Times*, November 3, 1998, pp D1,D8].

Therapeutic Potential of Botulinum Toxin. *The New York Times* (March 10, 1998) reported on the growing interest in the use of botulinum toxin for cosmetic and therapeutic purposes. Botulinum toxin is a potent natural product that blocks the release of acetylcholine. Very small doses of botulinum toxin produce a local paralysis and relieve pain. In 1989, Allergan received permission to market the toxin under the trade name *Botox* for treatment of patients with crossed eyes (strabismus) or involuntary clenched eyelids (blepharospasm). *Botox* does not cure and injections need be given every few months. Growing sales of *Botox* are the result of neurologists and dermatologists prescribing botulinum toxin for nonapproved uses, including other neurological disorders and treatment of facial wrinkles. There are reports that local injections of *Botox* relieve hemifacial spasms, chronic tennis elbow, writer's cramp, tremor, and tics. An ongoing study seeks to assess *Botox's* effectiveness in treating spasticity in patients who have suffered a stroke. The next year or two may bring broader and important indications for botulinum toxin.

New Strategies for Male Contraception. The first clinical trial to assess a new approach to male contraception is underway [*Scrip,* November 4, 1998, p 25] . Participants are receiving a prolactin inhibitor along with testosterone. Previous attempts to develop a male contraceptive have used testosterone alone to inhibit sperm production. Testosterone works by means of a negative feedback mechanism to suppress production of the gonadotrophin hormones, which stimulate spermatogenesis. Use of testosterone alone, however, is effective in only two-thirds of men. The addition of a prolactin inhibitor is based on the understanding that, in the absence of gonadotrophins, prolactin may act as a reserve hormone and maintain spermatogenesis. The investigators believe that if they administer both a prolactin inhibitor and testosterone, they may be able to achieve zero sperm counts in all men. A less robust strategy, effective in about 80% of men, is the combination of testosterone and a progestin. The combination permits the use of a lower dose of testosterone, which may result in fewer adverse effects.

LATE BREAKING REPORTS

Infectious Disease

Zanamivir for Influenza: An Update. A well-controlled trial recruited 455 patients who were 12 years old or older with influenza symptoms of no more than 36 hour's duration. Patients received inhaled zanamivir or placebo for 5 days, and recorded symptoms during and after treatment. Compared with placebo, zanamivir relieved flu symptoms a median of 1.5 days earlier in influenza-positive patients and in patients with fever at study entry. In a high-risk subgroup, zanamivir ameliorated symptoms by a median of 2.5 days, and reduced the development of complications that require antibiotic therapy [*Lancet* 1998;352:1877–81].

Mental Health

Lilly to Extend Prozac's Franchise. *Prozac*'s patent protection will expire by 2004 at the latest, and generic drug manufacturers are poised to market bioequivalent fluoxetine products and sell them at a lower price. Generic competition will savage Lilly's $3 billion market. To protect the franchise, the company announced that it would join with Sepracor to develop the single enantiomer version of racemic fluoxetine, R-fluoxetine [*The Wall Street Journal,* December 7, 1998, pp A1,A8]. The isomer is patent-protected until 2015. There are theoretical reasons to believe that R-fluoxetine may be more effective than racemic fluoxetine, and that it may even have some new uses. Sepracor was founded in 1984 to develop and market isomer-separation technologies to major pharmaceutical companies.

Pain Management

Second COX-2 Inhibitor to Market May Have Competitive Advantage. Searle's COX-2 inhibitor *Celebrex* is likely to be the first to reach the US market, but, according to Merck's CEO, *Vioxx* (rofecoxib) will have a competitive advantage in terms of a pain indication [*Scrip,* December 16, 1998, p 13]. Merck conducted one-year pain studies while Searle, eager to file the first New Drug Application, opted for shorter studies. A FDA panel has recommended approval of *Celebrex* for osteoarthritis and rheumatoid arthritis. Merck is seeking approval for osteoarthritis and acute pain management. Observers think that the pain data for *Vioxx,* which stem from studies in patients with dysmenorrhea, dental pain, and post-orthopedic surgery pain, will be a key marketing advantage. Merck also reported that *Vioxx* caused less gastrointestinal toxicity than ibuprofen in two new six-month safety studies [*Ibid,* p 20]. *Celebrex* has been compared favorably with naproxen or diclofenac in safety studies, but has not been adequately compared with ibuprofen, which some experts consider the safest NSAID on the market.

Boehringer Ingelheim's New Drug Application for the NSAID meloxicam (*Mobic*) to treat osteoarthritis, submitted December 15, may test the limits of FDA's definition of COX-2 inhibitors and their status as a distinct class of drugs [*The Pink Sheet* 1998;60(No51):5]. Meloxicam is about 10 times more selective for COX-2 than COX-1, whereas celecoxib (*Celebrex*) is about 375 times more selective. FDA recently took exception to the promotion of *Relafen* (nabumetone) as a COX-2 selective NSAID; nabumetone is about 12 times more selective for COX-2 than for COX-1. The agency directed SmithKline Beecham to issue a corrective letter noting COX-1/COX-2 specificity profiles are of unknown value in predicting the clinical safety of NSAIDs.

Substance Abuse

Anticonvulsant for Nicotine Addiction. Preclinical studies show that vigabatrin, a drug used in Europe to treat epilepsy, suppresses the addictive effects of nicotine [*The Wall Street Journal*, December 3, 1998, p B9]. Vigabatrin blocks the enzyme that breaks down γ-aminobutyric acid (GABA) and increases brain levels of GABA, which inhibits neural activity and dampens the excessive nerve firing that can lead to epileptic seizures. GABA also lowers dopamine levels in selected parts of the brain. A dopamine surge is thought to underlie the "high " associated with the use of nicotine, cocaine, and other addictive substances. The new work demonstrates that in rats vigabatrin can block the dopamine rush produced by addictive substances. In control animals, nicotine injection doubles the dopamine levels in the "reward centers" of the brain. Vigabatrin given 2.5 hours before nicotine blocks the dopamine rise. Investigators are planning clinical trials. Human studies may be delayed, however, because peripheral vision defects occur in some epilepsy patients who receive vigabatrin. This problem is one reason why FDA has not yet approved the drug. Researchers hope that the low vigabatrin dose needed to overcome nicotine craving may prove safe [*Science* 1998;282:1798–99].

5 Vaccines

INTRODUCTION

Medical history tells us that a single vaccine can save more lives and more money than nearly any other medical intervention. This year there has been a renaissance in vaccine research. Current investigations range from new initiatives for well-recognized infectious diseases to visionary projects on vaccines to prevent autoimmune diseases and cancer. One reviewer, commenting on the pace of vaccine research, observed: ". . . all of a sudden the 1990 dream of a single vaccine given shortly after birth and protective against all major infections seems just a little less far-fetched" [*Nature Med* 1998; 4:475–76].

A recent report reviews the different approaches taken to produce the wide variety of vaccines that meet the requisite standards for safety and efficacy. The author posits that we may catch ". . . a glimpse into the future by considering the scientific rationale for vaccines of the 21st century" [*Nature Med* (Vaccine Supplement) 1998;4:515–19]. The following material highlights new products, some developments in vaccine research, and issues resulting from their use.

NEW PRODUCTS

Intranasal Flu Vaccine for Children
Rotavirus Vaccine Now a Reality
Lyme Disease Vaccine: Ready for the Summer of 1999

Intranasal Flu Vaccine for Children. Inactivated influenza virus vaccine is prepared yearly, with strains chosen on the basis of information provided by a worldwide surveillance network about the strains that are likely to circulate during the upcoming season. Public health officials in the US recommend the vaccine for everyone who is 65 or older as well as for those under the age of 65 who are at particular risk for the complications of influenza. Vaccination rates are poor among high-risk persons under 65 and even worse among high-risk children. Barriers to immunization are the need for yearly injections and the need for two injections of vaccine each season for children under nine years old. Immunization of children not only prevents influenza-virus infection, it also reduces the discomfort and treatment costs of common ear infections that often accompany the primary infection.

The results of a study supported by the National Institutes of Health and Aviron, a biotechnology company, evaluating a new strategy to immunize children against influenzavirus infection is now available [*N Engl J Med* 1998;338:1405–12]. The investigators assigned 288 healthy children who were 15 to 71 months of age to receive one dose, given as a nasal spray, of a live attenuated, cold-adapted trivalent influenzavirus vaccine or placebo. Another 1,314 children received two doses of vaccine or placebo about 60 days apart. The attenuated strains chosen matched the antigens recommended for the inactivated influenzavirus vaccine by the FDA for the 1996-1997 influenza season.

The researchers report that the intranasal vaccine is easy to administer and well tolerated, provoking only mild adverse effects. Culture-positive influenza was significantly less common in the vaccine group than in the placebo group (1.3% vs. 17.9%). Vaccine efficacy against influenza was 93% and it performed equally well in younger and older children. Both the one-dose regimen and the two-dose regimen provided good coverage (89% and 94% effectiveness, respectively) and worked well against both strains of influenzavirus circulating in 1996-1997. Immunized children also had fewer febrile illnesses, including 30% fewer episodes of otitis media. Otitis media developed in more than 20% of placebo recipients who had culture-positive influenza.

The investigators wish to see more widespread immunization of children against influenza. However, decisions about broadening the guidelines for vaccination to include all healthy children need to be made with care. Potential health and economic benefits must be weighed against the cost of implementing a universal program. Some say that immunizing low-risk children against influenza is not cost effective because most children recover quickly from the infection.

In August, Aviron announced the results of a preliminary analysis of data from the second year of a two-year phase III trial of its nasal spray vaccine, *FluMist*. The results suggest that the product provides protection against confirmed influenza resulting from the strains included in the vaccine as well as strains not included, which predominated during that flu season by chance [*Scrip*, August 12, 1998, p 21]. Among more than 1300 children who took part in the study, there were five cases of influenza caused by the strains included in the vaccine and 66 cases caused by a new strain. Only 2% of the children vaccinated with *FluMist* developed influenza; all of the cases were caused by the new strain. In contrast, 13% of the children who received placebo developed influenza. The lead investigator of the phase III trial stressed the importance of *FluMist*'s ability to protect against influenza strains not included in the vaccine formulation [*Scrip*, October 2, 1998, p 21]. Aviron hopes to have their product approved for the 1999-2000 influenza season.

Rotavirus Vaccine Now a Reality. A recent article in *JAMA* observed: "Twenty-five years of dogged, often tedious research into the development of an effective vaccine against a major cause of severe, sometimes lethal diarrhea among children is about to pay off" [*JAMA* 1998;279:489–90]. *JAMA* reported that the US Food and Drug Administration will soon approve the marketing of a vaccine against rotavirus, and the World Health Organization is considering recommending its use in developing countries where the disease more often has a serious outcome. The vaccine is given orally and prevents at least 50% of all rotavirus infections and 80% of severe infections that lead to hospitalization and death.

Rotavirus infection is nearly universal, affecting about 90% of infants and children before the age of three years. The virus attacks the small intestine lining causing multiple episodes of diarrhea and vomiting that can lead to severe dehydration. Approximately 870,000 children die each year because of the infection and most of them from dehydration. Mortality is far less in developed countries where the availability of oral rehydration and other medical care holds the death rate to only 20 to 100 children per year. Even where there is effective treatment, the toll is heavy. An estimated three million cases of diarrhea occur in the US each year, leading to half a million office visits and perhaps as many as 100,000 hospitalizations.

Soon after the discovery of human rotavirus in 1973, public health officials urged researchers to develop a vaccine as soon as possible. The vaccine that emerged after years of research is a considerable technical achievement. It combines the well-established principle of immunization that uses an antigenically-related virus to induce protective antibodies against another virus—the approach taken by Jenner when he used cowpox to immunize against small-pox—with a recent technique that reassorts genes to express the desired neutralizing antibody. An earlier version of the vaccine, based on a rhesus strain rotavirus, provided only limited protection. There are four important glycoprotein serotypes that account for about 95% of all the strains of human rotaviruses detected. The earlier vaccine was effective only in those predominantly infected with rotavirus serotype glycoprotein 3. Thanks to skillful laboratory work, researchers produced a genetically re-assorted tetravalent strain that includes all four of the significant serotypes.

The new vaccine has been effective in five trials. Protection against significant diarrheal illness ranged from 69% to 80%. The vaccine is 75% to 100% effective in preventing severe disease and dehydration. A well-controlled study in Caracas that enrolled 200 infants from a poor urban area, reported that the vaccine reduces severe diarrheal illness by 88% [*N Engl J Med* 1997;1181–87]. The developers of the rotavirus vaccine stress that the goal of the vaccine is to prevent severe disease, not mild infections. The vaccine will be manufactured by Wyeth-Lederle under the name *RotaShield* and be given orally in three doses at ages two, four, and six months, which concurs with existing schedules for vaccinations. The Centers for Disease Control and Prevention's Advisory Committee on Immunization Practices recommended in February that this vaccine be used routinely in full-term infants. Parents need to be alerted that the vaccine can cause fever and irritability.

An economic analysis, reported in 1995, demonstrated that if a vaccine were 50% effective and cost $30 per dose, incorporation of a rotavirus vaccine into routine childhood vaccination schedules would save the US health care system $79 million each year. It would also save the country $466 million through gains in productivity [*Pediatrics* 1995;96:609–15]. Wyeth-Ayerst is pricing the product at $38 per dose for the three-dose series. The company is conducting two US studies to generate more cost-effectiveness data. Anticipating the findings, Wyeth-Ayerst told financial analysts that data from the Centers for Disease Control and Prevention (CDC) show that *RotaShield* would be cost-effective at up to \$58 per dose [*The Pink Sheet* 1998; 60(No36):11–12].

The FDA gave final approval to the oral vaccine at the end of August [*The Wall Street Journal,* September 1, 1998, p B6]. The acting commissioner of the agency said that the new vaccine can prevent the most serious effects of rotavirus in most infants, and even when symptoms of infection do appear, they are milder and do not last as long in immunized infants. FDA's approval letter for *RotaShield* states that Wyeth-Ayerst will perform post-marketing studies in at least 20,000 children as well as additional studies to examine safety in older infants.

Lyme Disease Vaccine: Ready for the Summer of 1999. Lyme disease is of great concern because it affects thousands of people each spring and summer, mostly in the Northeast and Midwest United States. It is caused by a spirochete (*Borrelia burgdorferi*) that is transmitted to people through the bite of infected deer ticks. People typically contract the disease while walking in open fields. It can cause fever, a characteristic rash, and flu-like symptoms. The infection, if recognized, usually responds to the antibiotics amoxicillin and doxycycline. Left untreated, Lyme disease can lead to arthritis, damage to the nervous system, and heart disease.

In May 1998, an advisory committee of the Food and Drug Administration recommended approval of the first vaccine against Lyme disease (*LYMErix*), but expressed concern over its safety and effectiveness, and recommended its use only for people 18 to 70 years of age. The panel also urged SmithKline Beecham to continue testing the vaccine, especially with younger children [*The New York Times,* May 27, 1998, pp A1,6]. Unlike other vaccines, *LYMErix* takes up to a year to establish optimal immunity. The need for additional booster shots has not been studied. Other unanswered questions relate to the safety of the vaccine for patients with arthritis or undiagnosed Lyme disease.

The vaccine is based on a recombinant form of a lipoprotein (OspA) residing on the surface of the spirochete. Studies involving nearly 11,000 people supported approval. A pivotal trial showed that after three doses—one in the winter, a second given a month later, and the third given one year after the first—Lyme disease was confirmed in 13 subjects who received the vaccine and in 61 subjects who received placebo. The data suggest that the vaccine protects about 80% of those who receive all three doses. Two doses protect only about 50% of recipients.

These findings are updated in a recent report in *The New England Journal of Medicine* [1998;339:209–215]. After the first two injections, 22 of 5469 people who received vaccine developed the infection, compared with 43 of 5467 people who received placebo. Following the third injection, given one year later, 16 vaccine recipients acquired Lyme disease compared with 66 of those who were given placebo. The only ill effects of the vaccine were mild or moderate local and systemic reactions lasting a few days after vaccination.

A similar vaccine (*ImuLYME*), developed by a unit of Rhone-Poulenc, is in late clinical trials [*The Wall Street Journal,* May 27, 1998, p A3]. A placebo-controlled study with this vaccine [*N Engl J Med* 1998;339:216–22] involving more than 10,000 people reports results that are similar to those in the *LYMErix* trial. An editorial in *The New England Journal of Medicine* commenting on the two reports says that ". . . an effective, safe, and affordable vaccine for people who live in areas where Lyme disease is endemic would be welcome" [*N Engl J Med* 1998;339:263–64].

SmithKline Beecham is conducting a 36-month follow-up on 1600 participants from the pivotal trial. Another study is examining the persistence of the antibody and the effect of a booster dose. Pediatric trials are also ongoing [*The Pink Sheet* 1998;60(No22):5]. Early results of these new studies suggest that people may have to wait only six months rather than a year after inoculation with *LYMErix* to be protected from the disease. The company said that a study in 800 people shows that three doses over six months is as effective as three doses over one year [*The Wall Street Journal,* September 28, 1998; B4]. If further data analysis supports this observation, it would be good news.

IN THE PIPELINE

Melanoma Vaccine: Early Stages
Multicomponent Malaria Vaccine Fails to Prevent Infection
DNA Vaccines Show Promise
FDA Authorizes Phase III Testing for HIV Vaccine
Other Strategies to Develop a Vaccine for HIV Infection
A Vaccine Against Pneumococcal Meningitis and Bacteremia

Melanoma Vaccine: Early Stages. Malignant melanoma, a skin cancer, is one of the deadliest human cancers. Despite its characteristic resistance to chemotherapy and radiation, melanoma is one of the few human cancers to which host immune responses can be demonstrated. Moreover, the genes encoding melanoma antigens recognized by T-cells have been cloned. Building on these findings, recent reports tell of new approaches to peptide-based therapeutic melanoma vaccination in humans [*Nature Med* 1998;4:269–70].

One report describes the immunization of patients with advanced melanoma using peptide-loaded dendritic cells [*Nature Med* 1998;4:328–32]. These uncommon lymphocytes are regarded as the most potent of all antigen-presenting cells. They evoke immune responses by presenting antigen bound to HLA molecules to T-cells. With knowledge of this property, many scientists see dendritic cells as potential cellular adjuvants for tumor vaccines. Dendritic cells isolated and co-cultured *in vitro* with tumor antigens (e.g., melanoma peptides) and administered as vaccines have been shown to elicit potent anti-tumor immunity in animal models and in preliminary human studies.

Combining knowledge of the relevant target antigens of melanoma with newly discovered means to enhance antigen presentation has led to good clinical responses in patients with malignant melanoma. As a consequence of recent studies showing that dendritic cells are versatile adjuvants that are capable of delivering tumor antigens, clinical trials are now underway. Modification of peptides to enhance HLA binding [*Nature Med* 1998;4:321–27] also offers an exciting new strategy to improve vaccine effectiveness and studies are now in progress.

Scrip [June 3, 1998, p 30] recently reported findings from a study of a polyvalent melanoma vaccine in 38 patients. Mortality at two years was 23% in the vaccine group and 40% in the placebo group. The vaccine was particularly effective when anti-melanoma immune responses were stimulated. Response was enhanced by encapsulating the vaccine into interleukin-2 (IL-2) liposomes [*Lancet* 1998;352:40].

The biotech firm, MediGene, with support from Hoechst Marion Roussel, intends to initiate phase I/II studies using its recombinant adenoassociated virus technology to develop a vector for *ex vivo* malignant melanoma vaccination [*The Pink Sheet* 1998;60(No36):20]. MediGene's trial will use autologous tumor vaccines to induce a specific cytolitic response against tumor cells.

Multicomponent Malaria Vaccine Fails to Prevent Infection. NYVAC-Pf7 is an attenuated vaccinia-virus with seven genes from the malaria-causing protozoan *Plasmodium falciparum* inserted into its genome. Because it is a multicomponent vaccine containing a combination of antigens derived from the different stages of the parasite that occur during the course of the infection, NYVAC-Pf7 offers an immediate solution to the problem of which parasite stage to target.

The results of a phase I/IIa trial of NYVAC-Pf7 in human volunteers were recently reported [*J Infect Dis* 1998;177:1664–73]. The volunteers received either three doses of NYVAC-Pf7 over 26 weeks or a saline control. Four weeks after the third dose they were challenged with infected mosquitoes. Disappointingly, vaccination with NYVAC-Pf7 failed to protect against *P. falciparum* malaria. The only good news was that the time from infection to the appearance of parasites in the blood was significantly longer in vaccinated volunteers than in the control group. Immediate treatment of volunteers who developed parasitemia limited the ability to evaluate protective immunity to subsequent stages of the parasite [*Lancet* 1998;352:1163–64].

DNA Vaccines Show Promise. The development of a safe and effective vaccine against malaria is among the highest priorities of the World Health Organization. On identification of relevant portions of *P. falciparum*, buoyant researchers anticipated a vaccine to follow in short order. However, subsequent vaccine development based on state-of-the-art strategies, such as splicing protozoan genes into vaccinia, infecting cells with a virus to produce *P. falciparum* proteins, administering genetically engineered *P. falciparum* proteins, or relying on peptides derived from the proteins, all failed to promote immune responses sufficient to protect mice against malaria. Only when researchers turned to DNA vaccines did they find the product they sought [*Science* 1997;278:1711–14].

Between 1990 and 1994, the administration of naked DNA encoding a specific protein antigen was shown to induce expression of the protein in mouse myoctes, to elicit antibodies against the protein, and to manifest protection against influenza and malaria that was dependent on CD8+ T-cell responses against the expressed protein. Hundreds of publications have now reported the efficacy of DNA vaccines in animal models of diseases.

DNA vaccines are made of nucleotides that are stitched into a circular piece of bacterial DNA called a plasmid. They contain no protein component. Plasmid DNA is usually introduced to tissue by means of an intramuscular injection. Current thinking reasons that following injection, plasmid DNA is engulfed by myocytes at the site of injection. The host cells take up the foreign DNA, express the viral gene, and make the corresponding viral protein [*Biochem Pharmacol* 1998;55:1151–53]. Viral vectors and liposomes may also be used to transfer DNA into the cell, but at this time the focus is on direct injections.

DNA vaccines can stimulate a cellular immune response. They can also provoke an antibody response (humoral immunity) because the foreign protein expressed by the nucleotide fragment is processed intracellularly and presented to the immune system in the context of the major histocompatibility gene complex (MHC) class I system. Class I molecules are expressed on the surface of virtually all cells, with a profusion on B-cells, T-cells, and platelets. Generally, cellular immunity is better able to challenge viruses and parasites than humoral immunity. Conventional vaccines are processed by the MHC class II system and restricted in expression to B-cells, some monocytes, and activated T lymphocytes. They are usually poor immunogens for cell-mediated immunity. A vaccine that stimulates a cellular immune response could be used to treat patients already infected with human immunodeficiency virus, hepatitis B and C, or herpes simplex virus. It might also be effective against cancer.

DNA vaccines behave like vaccines made from live but attenuated pathogens, rather than subunit vaccines that contain only parts of a pathogen or vaccines made from inactivated pathogens. Inactivated vaccines only stimulate specific antibodies, whereas live, attenuated vaccines stimulate both antibodies as well as killer cells called cytotoxic T lymphocytes (CTLs). While DNA vaccines share this important attribute with live vaccines, they are much less likely than live vaccines to cause the disease they are trying to prevent.

There have been high expectations for DNA vaccines since 1990 when investigators at the biotechnology company Vical announced that naked DNA injected into animal cells prompts the production of foreign proteins. The potential advantages of DNA vaccines first made news in 1993 when research scientists at Merck Research Laboratories showed that injections of naked flu genes could protect mice from lethal doses of influenza A [*Science* 1993;259:1745–49].

Particularly exciting was the observation that the vaccine protected against a flu strain that was wholly distinct from the strain used to develop the vaccine. Even infection with native influenza virus does not provide this broad protection. The DNA vaccine created at Merck against influenza virus uses the nucleoprotein (internal protein) gene of the virus, which is similar across many strains; surface proteins vary from one strain to another.

Today, more than a half-dozen DNA vaccines are in early clinical testing against malaria, HIV infection, influenza, hepatitis B, and cancer. While most of the naked DNA studies are aimed at prevention, the goal of DNA vaccines for cancer is to stimulate the immune system in people who already have neoplasia. The strong CTL response to naked DNA might prove valuable for attacking tumors [*The Scientist*, March 16, 1998, pp 3,12].

Science [1998;282:476–80] reported in October 1998 that vaccination with plasmid DNA encoding a malaria protein designated as PfCSP elicited antigen-specific CD8+ T-cell-dependent cytotoxic T lymphocytes (CTLs) in healthy volunteers. The target of the vaccine is *P. falciparum*-infected hepatocytes. CTLs recognize, lyse, and eliminate parasite-infected cells.

The malaria-naïve participants were randomized to four dosage groups and received three injections of plasmid at four-week intervals in alternate deltoids. This is the first demonstration in healthy humans of the induction of CD8+ CTLs by DNA vaccines. The authors conclude that the study, ". . . provides a foundation for further human testing of this potentially revolutionary vaccine technology."

There are several ways to deliver DNA vaccines. One of the more interesting approaches is the subject of a major business agreement between the broad-based pharmaceutical company Glaxo Wellcome, which has a keen interest in being a player in the vaccine business, and PowderJect Pharmaceuticals, a young company with novel technology. PowderJect technology adheres DNA from a pathogen to gold particles to increase its mass before it is injected through skin using a helium-driven gun that accelerates the particles up to three times the speed of sound. Once injected, the DNA separates from the gold and is incorporated into the skin's antigen-presenting cells, which produce corresponding antigenic proteins that subsequently elicit an immune response. Glaxo Wellcome has licensed PowderJect's hepatitis B prophylactic DNA vaccine and has options to develop ten more DNA vaccines.

FDA Authorizes Phase III Testing for HIV Vaccine. On June 4, 1998, *The New York Times* reported that the FDA reversed its earlier position and gave approval to conduct the world's first full-scale testing of a vaccine to prevent infection with HIV. The vaccine, *Aidsvax,* contains gp 120 a protein from the virus's outer coat that attaches to T-cells to infect them. An FDA panel rejected a petition to test a similar vaccine four years ago. The new vaccine is derived from the two most common strains of HIV instead of the single strain used earlier. The bivalent vaccine is likely to offer broader coverage.

Over the next four years, the trial will recruit and evaluate 5000 American and Canadian uninfected volunteers as well as 2500 volunteers in Thailand, all of whom are likely to be exposed to the virus because of high-risk sexual practices or injection of illicit drugs. Three injections of the vaccine will be given to each volunteer over several months. In the North American arm of the study, two-thirds of the participants will receive the vaccine and the rest will receive a placebo.

Scientists have been sharply divided as to which vaccine to study and even as to whether any vaccine should be fully tested at this time [*Nature Med* (Vaccine Suppl) 1998;4:495–98]. Everyone agrees that *Aidsvax* is safe, as determined in 1200 uninfected volunteers. The vaccine is most unlikely to cause disease because it is made from a fragment of the virus. Although the vaccine induced antibodies in 99% of the participants, its effectiveness is uncertain. Many researchers believe that an effective vaccine must not only induce antibodies, it must also boost the immune system to produce killer T-cells to destroy virus-infected cells. A vaccine under development at the National Institutes of Health appears to induce both neutralizing antibodies and a cytolic-T-cell response but phase III trials are probably one year away.

Central issues in the planning of trials in developing nations include: the obligations of the trial sponsors to make any successful vaccines available to the countries where they are tested, treatment for study participants who become infected, and the nature of the HIV prevention programs that should be included in trials [*Lancet* 1998;351:1789].

In July, *Science* [1998;281:21–22] reported that a meeting in Geneva to set ethical ground rules for AIDS vaccine trials in impoverished nations became very contentious when participants grappled with one question in particular. If a vaccine is tested in a country that cannot afford anti-HIV drugs, and volunteers become infected during the trial, should they be given state-of-the-art treatment? *Science* suggests that the answer could determine the ethical, financial, and scientific viability of the HIV vaccine tests.

The scientific dilemma is that the vaccine under study is unlikely to prevent HIV infection, but it may delay and modify the course of the disease. Therefore, a critical measure of success of the vaccine would be whether, upon infection, it reduces viral replication and better preserves the immune system. However, if participants who become infected soon start taking potent antiretroviral drugs, the researchers will see no effect of the vaccine.

Most of the participants at the meeting in Geneva agreed with the practical argument that people who get infected during an HIV vaccine trial should be offered "the highest attainable" treatment in their locale that can be sustained after the trial ends. An impassioned minority of the panel, however, rejected the idea that participants in trials carried out in underdeveloped countries should be treated differently from participants in developed countries. The first vaccine trial is likely to begin in Thailand and the protocol makes no provision for providing state-of-the-art therapy to all people who become infected.

Other Strategies to Develop a Vaccine for HIV Infection. In most HIV-positive patients, the immune system keeps the infection in check for many years before it progresses, rather abruptly, to AIDS. Why the immune system fails is an urgent question. A piece of the puzzle is now established. Patients whose immune systems still have CD4 T-cells (T helper cells) that specifically recognize HIV proteins seem able to control the infection, while patients who have lost these anti-HIV T helper cells are not. Helper cells seem to keep the virus under control by teaming up with other T-cells called cytotoxic T lymphocytes (CTLs), which destroy virus-infected cells [*Science* 1998; 280:825–26].

Recent work shows that patients who have a strong T helper response against the HIV protein called p24, found in the virus's inner core, have the highest levels of anti-HIV CTLs and the lowest viral levels in their blood. The finding that helper cells specific to p24 promote CTL response is important because envelope proteins that make up HIV's outer coat have been the focus of most unsuccessful efforts at vaccine development. Other recent studies show that four small segments of p24 are most responsible for triggering the immune response. Efforts are underway to determine if these peptides could form the basis of a vaccine to boost the T helpers and CTLs, either in people already infected by HIV or in people at risk of infection.

Another recent report [*Science* 1998;280:1875–79] also comes to the same conclusion that an effective vaccine against HIV must elicit an efficient

HIV-specific CTL response. The author notes that although replication-competent human immunodeficiency viruses attenuated for pathogenicity by selective gene deletion provide protective immunity in non-human primates, the long-term use of such vaccines in humans is suspect. On the other hand, he believes that live-vector based vaccines may be both safe and effective.

Genes encoding viral proteins can be inserted into the genomes of other viruses or bacteria. The recombinant organisms then express the products of the inserted gene. The most extensively studied vaccine vectors are the pox viruses. Organisms created by inserting HIV genes into vaccinia virus—the live, attenuated vaccine virus that has eradicated small pox infection—have elicited HIV-specific cellular and humoral immunity in nonhuman primates. There is concern, however, that even attenuated vaccinia may ignite a serious infection in immunosuppressed AIDS patients. Consequently, interest has turned to other pox viruses with limited *in vivo* capacity to replicate and pose a pathogenic threat for humans. Scientists must still overcome the frustrating obstacle that the immunogenicity of a vector is closely tied to the extent of replication that vector undergoes in the body, and the pathogenicity of a vector is similarly correlated with the extent of *in vivo* replication of that organism. Also of interest are DNA vaccines that can generate HIV-specific CTLs, helper T-cells, and antibodies.

A Vaccine Against Pneumococcal Meningitis and Bacteremia. Scientists presenting at the Interscience Conference on Antimicrobial Agents and Chemotherapy described a new vaccine, developed by the Wyeth Lederle Vaccines unit of American Home Products, against pneumococcus bacteria. In a study of 38,000 children, the vaccine was very successful in preventing pneumococcal meningitis and bacteremia. The study was stopped ahead of schedule because an unblinded interim analysis revealed a high level of efficacy. At the time of the study's unplanned conclusion, there were 22 cases of invasive pneumococcal disease in the control group and none in the treatment group [*Scrip,* October 2, 1998, p 22].

Pneumococcus bacteria are also the leading cause of pneumonia and middle ear infection. Bacterial pneumonia kills more than one million children under five years of age each year in developing countries. Otitis media leads to 30 million visits a year to pediatricians in the US alone. A pneumococcus vaccine is on the market in the US but it does not work in children under two. Their immune systems are probably not sufficiently developed to respond. The new vaccine, which protects against seven strains including the two most serious types, overcomes that problem. "The finding sets the stage for the vaccine to be added to the list of immunizations given routinely to infants and toddlers during the first two years of life" [*The Wall Street Journal*, September 28, 1998, p B4]. The company expects to submit an application for FDA approval of the vaccine in late 1998.

OTHER ISSUES

Vaccine Liability and Safety
Activists Challenge Safety of Hepatitis B Vaccination Effort
CDC Recommends Major Tuberculosis Vaccine Effort

Vaccine Liability and Safety. A recent editorial [*Arch Pediatr Adolesc Med* 1998;152:7–10] observed: "In this country, vaccine safety and liability are inexorably intertwined." Young parents today, thanks to extraordinarily effective vaccines, have never seen the dreaded consequences of childhood diseases that raged earlier in the century. They only hear reports of dreadful illness in children who recently received a vaccine. This one-dimensional message has created powerful anti-vaccine movements in many developed countries.

Controversy over the safety of pertussis vaccine provides a rich example of the problem. Of the vaccine-preventable diseases, pertussis rivals most others in importance and severity among young children in the developing world. Millions of cases and hundreds of thousands of deaths occur each year. Complications are common. Because the disease is so serious and so difficult to treat, prevention is paramount. Whole-cell vaccines, whether monovalent or in diphtheria-tetanus-pertussis (DTP), have been important in the control of pertussis.

The story of anti-vaccine sentiment started in the US with the 1982 award-winning television documentary *DPT Vaccine Roulette,* which displayed severely neurologically impaired children whose conditions were claimed to be vaccine-related. The media frenzy that followed led to the filing of hundreds of lawsuits against vaccine companies alleging DTP-related adverse effects. As a result, prices of vaccines soared and some manufacturers ceased production, thereby creating a critical shortage. Only the passage of the National Childhood Vaccine Injury Act of 1986, which indemnified the industry, averted long-term public health consequences. A recent report relates the impact of anti-vaccine movements on pertussis control in the US, UK, and other European nations [*Lancet* 1998;351:356–61].

The attention drawn by the DTP vaccine is not unexpected in light of its transient local and systemic reactions, and serious but rare adverse events. DTP is given early in infancy when genetic and developmental disorders first become apparent. Therefore, it is easy to confuse cause and effect when vaccine-related adverse events after immunization occur in children who are later diagnosed with such conditions.

Even today, anti-vaccine movements remain strong in many parts of the world. Another example of their impact was seen after publication of an ill-considered paper in *The Lancet* linking immunization with the measles/mumps/rubella (MMR) vaccine to the development of bowel disease and autism in 12 British children [*Lancet* 1998;351:637–41]. Fortunately, *The Lancet* had the wisdom to invite a commentary on the work by scientists at the US Centers for Disease Control and Prevention (CDC). They presented evidence that the methodology used by the investigators was flawed and that the adverse events are coincidental rather than causal [*Lancet* 1998;351:1327–28]. Britain's Chief Medical Officer and scientists from the World Health Organization also weighed in against the report.

Despite the efforts to put the article in perspective, it has already had repercussions. A suggestion in the report that it might be safer to give the components of the vaccine separately resulted in a run on individual vaccines and led to severe shortages. The alarm also spread across the Atlantic causing parent groups and policymakers in the US to clash over MMR vaccination. Autism advocate groups demanded that the government appropriate one billion dollars annually to the department of Health and Human Services to support research into the link.

A positive outcome of the fear and frenzy over childhood vaccines is the establishment of a surveillance system requiring that all vaccination and medical records in the US are computerized, linked, and studied for possible association [*Nature Med* (Vitamin Supplement) 1998;4:478–79].

Activists Challenge Safety of Hepatitis B Vaccination Effort. The World Health Organization estimates that hepatitis B virus (HBV) infects 350 million people, most of whom live without symptoms. In a fraction of cases, however, infection leads to liver failure or liver cancer. The complications kill each year an estimated one million people around the world and about 4000 in the United States. In the 1980s, health officials in the US and Europe sought to reduce this toll by requiring the immunization of high-risk adults including healthcare workers. In 1991, this mandate was extended to all newborns in an effort to eradicate HBV.

Science [1998;281:630–31] now reports that these efforts are being stalled by a small number of vaccinated people who claim to have experienced serious adverse effects covering a range of autoimmune and nervous system disorders. Already, activists are demanding compensation from governments and manufacturers or insisting that mandatory vaccination be stopped. Health officials queried by *Science* say they have no evidence that autoimmune diseases are appearing at a higher rate among people who received the vaccine. While dismissing safety concerns, health officials worry that adverse publicity alone could interfere with immunization efforts.

Public health officials must take the claims of injury seriously. Epidemiological investigations of the link between hepatitis B vaccination and multiple sclerosis (MS)—the most publicized concern—have already begun and some data may be available in 1999. More than 20,000 adverse-reaction reports have been filed with the FDA, including 111 cases of MS. The agency says that there is no evidence that the cases were actually caused by the vaccine. Critics say that the FDA may be overlooking a possible biological mechanism. They suggest that a hepatitis B surface protein used as an antigen in the recombinant vaccine may provoke an autoimmune attack on a similar protein in tissues of a genetically susceptible group of vaccine recipients. This is an unproved but plausible hypothesis.

CDC Recommends Major Tuberculosis Vaccine Effort. In August 1998, the Centers for Disease Control and Prevention (CDC) issued a report calling on government, academic, and corporate researchers to pool their intellectual resources to develop a new generation of vaccines against tuberculosis (TB) [*Nature Med* 1998;4:1097]. Despite progress in the treatment and control of TB, the report concludes that eliminating TB as a public health threat will ultimately require an effective vaccine. Worldwide, TB kills approximately three million people per year.

The only TB vaccine in widespread use today is bacille Calmett-Guerin. This vaccine provides protection from some childhood forms of TB but does not prevent the development and spread of the more common adult disease. While several potential TB vaccines to prevent infection are in development, the CDC has asked researchers to focus efforts on the more elusive goal of developing an effective post-infection vaccine.

LATE BREAKING REPORTS

New Products

FDA Clears Lyme Vaccine. In December, *The New York Times* [December 22, 1998, p A16] reported the approval of *Lymerix,* the first vaccine against the tick-borne infection. The agency was cautious in recommending use of the vaccine. It noted that three injections carefully timed over a year are required for maximum effectiveness, that there is no evidence of effectiveness in children under 15 years old, and that there is no safety data for people with rheumatoid arthritis and certain heart conditions.

Other Issues

Pediatricians Advise Against Oral Polio Vaccine. In December 1998, the American Academy of Pediatrics issued a statement that advises pediatricians and other health care professionals to avoid the use of oral live-virus polio vaccines in infants and to rely on injections to immunize them against the disease. The recommendations call for the use of injections of inactivated polio vaccine for the first two doses at two and four months after birth. Additional doses for children between 6 and 18 months and between 4 to 6 years may be given as either the injection or the oral preparation. The new policy's aim is reduce the rare incidence of polio associated with the oral vaccine.

6 Biotechnology

New Products

Platelet-Derived Growth Factor (PDGF) for Diabetic Foot
  Ulcers
Herceptin, a Monoclonal Antibody for Breast Cancer
Infliximab (*Remicade*) for Crohn's Disease
Palivizumab (*Synagis*) Prevents RSV Disease in Children
Monoclonal Antibodies to Prevent Transplant Rejection
Vitravene: First Antisense Agent Clears FDA Panel
Advisory Committee Supports Approval of Stem-Cell
  Growth Factor
FDA Approves *Enbrel* for Rheumatoid Arthritis

Platelet-Derived Growth Factor (PDGF) for Diabetic Foot Ulcers.
Complications of foot ulcers—gangrene, infection, and failure to heal—are
the leading cause of hospitalization for people with diabetes and result in
67,000 lower extremity amputations each year. Routine foot inspection and
preventive care—wound healing and debridement, controlling infections,
relieving pressure—can minimize foot problems. The latest tool for the treatment of lower extremity diabetic ulcers is a recombinant growth factor, PDGF,
to promote healing of the affected area [*Med Letter* 1998;40:73–74].

Growth factors act locally to repair wounds. They attract immune cells
to fight infection, stimulate production of connective tissue, create a new
supply of blood vessels, and promote remodeling. They aid in the formation
of granulation tissue and re-epithelialization. Becaplermin is a recombinant
human platelet-derived growth factor (rhPDGF-BB). *Regranex* is a topical
gel containing becaplermin, indicated for the treatment of deep diabetic
neuropathic foot ulcers that have adequate blood supply. The product is an
adjunct to, not a substitute for, diligent preventive care. Ortho-McNeil has
stressed its plans to market *Regranex* with a broad wound management campaign.

Used properly, *Regranex* increases the incidence of complete healing
of diabetic ulcers. One well-controlled trial compared daily application of
becaplermin gel with placebo gel, in 118 patients. After 20 weeks, nearly half
the patients receiving active treatment achieved complete wound healing,
compared with 25% of patients receiving placebo. *Regranex* also reduces
wound size and the rate of recurrence of ulcers [*J Vasc Surg* 1995;21:71–81].

Herceptin, a Monoclonal Antibody for Breast Cancer. Scientists attending
the annual meeting of the American Society of Clinical Oncology in May

1998 learned of promising results from pivotal trials evaluating the safety and effectiveness of the humanized monoclonal antibody trastuzumab (*Herceptin*), in women with a certain type of breast cancer. In up to 30% of all breast cancer cases in the US, a mutated oncogene overproduces a cell surface growth factor receptor called HER-2. Binding of growth factors to this surface receptor sends a signal to the nucleus to initiate cell division. Breast cancer patients whose tumors overproduce HER-2 have worse prognoses and shorter life expectancies. About 20% of ovarian cancer cases involve the same genetic defect.

Genentech's *Herceptin* binds to HER-2 and prevents signaling. In a phase III trial, women with previously treated metastatic breast cancer received *Herceptin* in combination with chemotherapy—paclitaxel (*Taxol*) or doxorubicin (*Adriamycin*) plus cyclophosphamide—or chemotherapy alone. With the antibody, the median time to disease progression was increased by several months. About 28% of those in the chemotherapy plus *Herceptin* group showed no evidence of tumor progression at one year compared with 14% of those who received chemotherapy alone. Adding *Herceptin* increased the complete or partial response (> 50% tumor shrinkage) from 32% to 49%.

Combining the antibody with paclitaxel produced the most striking results. With paclitaxel alone, the overall response rate was 16%. When *Herceptin* was added, the overall response rate was 42%. Combining *Herceptin* with doxorubicin plus cyclophosphamide increased the overall response rate from 43% to 52%. A second phase III trial evaluated *Herceptin* as monotherapy in women who had relapsed following treatment with at least one regimen for metastatic disease. The overall response rate was 16% and the median duration of response was 9 months [*Scrip*, September 2, 1998, p 19].

About half of the patients treated with *Herceptin* developed chills, fever, pain, nausea, and headache after the first dose. These side effects were generally mild, and were less likely to occur with subsequent infusions. Cardiotoxicity is the only serious safety concern. In the combination therapy trial, 27% of women treated with *Herceptin* and doxorubicin plus cyclophosphamide manifested toxicity, compared with just 6% of those on doxorubicin plus cyclophosphamide alone. With *Taxol*, the respective outcomes were 12% and 2%. For those receiving only the antibody, the incidence was only 5%. Leukopenia, anemia, diarrhea, abdominal pain, and infections were also more frequent with *Herceptin* plus chemotherapy compared with chemotherapy alone [*Scrip*, September 30, 1998, p 20].

In September, *The New York Times* [September 3, 1998, pp A1, A18] reported that an FDA advisory panel voted unanimously to recommend the use of *Herceptin* in combination with *Taxol* for first-line treatment of metastatic breast cancer when tumors overexpress the HER-2 growth factor receptor. The advisory group also supported the use of *Herceptin* alone for second- or third-line therapy.

Panel members agreed that compared with *Taxol* alone, the clinical benefit of adding *Herceptin* outweighs the increased incidence of cardiotoxicity. The panel voted not to recommend *Herceptin* in combination with anthracycline chemotherapy—doxorubicin or epirubicin. The majority concluded that the risk of cardiac dysfunction outweighs the modest additional benefit provided by the antibody. Proposed labeling recommends pretreatment evaluation of a patient's heart condition and continuous heart monitoring during therapy. The drug should probably not be used for patients with heart failure [*The Pink Sheet* 1998;60(No36):21–22].

After only a few weeks of deliberation, FDA followed the panel's advice and approved *Herceptin,* but with fewer restrictions than recommended by the advisory panel. At the urging of an advocacy group that sought to assist the maximum number of cancer patients to obtain reimbursement for therapy, the approved label does not rule out co-administration of *Herceptin* with anthracyclines, and lists no known contraindications [*The Pink Sheet* 1998; 60(No40):4].

Herceptin and a HER-2 diagnostic kit (*HercepTest*) were marketed in October. The drug costs about $18,000 per course of treatment. *Herceptin,* added to *Taxol* therapy, nearly triples the cost of treatment. *Herceptin* is the second monoclonal antibody to reach the US market for the treatment of cancer. In 1997 FDA approved *Rituxan* (rituximab), a chimeric murine/ human monoclonal antibody directed against the CD20 antigen found on the surface of normal and malignant B lymphocytes. *Rituxan* is indicated for the treatment of patients with relapsed or refractory low-grade, CD20-positive, B-cell non-Hodgkin's lymphoma.

Infliximab (Remicade) for Crohn's Disease. Crohn's is a chronic, debilitating, and incurable inflammatory bowel disease, affecting approximately 100,000 Americans and often requiring surgery. Treatment is empirical—steroids and antibiotics—and falls well short of ideal. A more specific approach is now available.

At the end of December 1997, Centocor filed a biologics license application (BLA) with the FDA for its chimeric anti-tumor necrosis factor (TNF) monoclonal antibody infliximab (*Remicade,* formerly called *Avakine*) for the treatment of Crohn's disease [*Scrip,* January 7, 1998, p 10]. TNF-α is a cytokine associated with overstimulation of the immune system in many inflammatory diseases. Infliximab acts early in the inflammatory cascade, neutralizing TNF-α. It binds soluble and cell-bound TNF, thereby eliciting complement, which then lyses and kills TNF-expressing cells. In one study, 82% of patients who had failed to respond to standard therapy achieved a significant improvement in disease activity at four weeks after a single infusion of infliximab and nearly half achieved disease remission [*N Engl J Med* 1998;337:1029–35]. Following four additional infusions given eight weeks apart, infliximab maintained the initial treatment response.

On May 28, 1998, an FDA advisory panel unanimously recommended approval of infliximab to relieve the symptoms and improve the condition of people with moderate to severe disease in which standard therapy is not adequate [*The New York Times,* May 29, 1998]. The panel called on Centocor to continue to study the drug to determine its long-term safety and effectiveness. There is concern that extended treatment may increase the risk of lymphoma. Another study showed that infliximab is effective in patients with draining fistulae—painful channels that open between the bowel and the skin, causing drainage of mucous and/or fecal material [*Scrip,* June 3, 1998, p 25]. About 30% of patients with Crohn's disease develop fistulae.

In August, Centocor received approval to market *Remicade* as a short-term treatment for patients with moderate to severe Crohn's disease [*The Wall Street Journal,* August 25, 1998, p B5]. The FDA suggests that the use of *Remicade* be limited to patients in whom conventional therapy is inadequate, and for the treatment of patients with fistulizing Crohn's disease. Patients with fistulae will require three infusions, at weeks zero, two, and six, while patients without this complication will likely need only one infusion.

Infliximab is the first drug developed primarily to treat this uncommon but debilitating bowel disease. Crohn's disease is a niche indication, and drugs to treat the disease qualify for the financial incentives of the Orphan Drug Act. Centocor hopes that *Remicade* will also be approved for the treatment of rheumatoid arthritis, which would open a much larger market. The company plans to file a regulatory submission with the FDA by the end of 1998.

Efforts to further develop *Remicade* were slowed in November. Centocor confirmed it had sent a letter to health care professionals warning that during one study several patients with Crohn's disease experienced adverse reactions [*The Wall Street Journal*, November 22, 1998, B6]. In the small trial, patients who had received an earlier version of infliximab several years before were re-treated with the current formulation of *Remicade*. Ten of 40 patients developed delayed reactions to the drug, including rashes and flu-like symptoms. Six patients required hospitalization. Symptoms uniformly resolved within a few days. Centocor representatives said that the side effects occurred because patients in the trial had taken the old version, which led to an immune reaction when those same patients took the new formulation. The FDA did not seem unduly alarmed. Nevertheless, the new findings support concerns that repeated use of *Remicade* might stimulate antibodies against the drug, which can limit its effectiveness.

Palivizumab (Synagis) Prevents RSV Disease in Children. For the first time, FDA has approved the use of a monoclonal antibody for an infectious disease—respiratory syncytial virus (RSV) disease—in pediatric patients at high risk [*Pharmacy Today*, August 1998, p 6]. Palivizumab (*Synagis*) binds to the F protein on the surface of the virus and keeps it from infecting cells. The new agent prevents serious lower respiratory tract disease caused by the virus and joins *RespiGam* (RSV immune globulin), a polyclonal antibody, as the only drugs approved for the prevention of RSV disease. Because of palivizumab's ease of administration—an intramuscular injection given monthly during the RSV season—it is expected to replace *RespiGam*.

Safety and efficacy were established in children aged 24 months or younger. The pivotal trial reported that hospitalizations for RSV disease occurred in 4.8% of patients receiving palivizumab, compared with an incidence rate of 10.6% among those receiving placebo [*Pediatrics* 1998; 102:531–37]. Whether *Synagis* is effective and safe for the treatment of established RSV disease has not been determined. A full course of treatment is expected to cost about $4,500, compared with $5,000 for *RespiGam*.

Monoclonal Antibodies to Prevent Transplant Rejection. Two new mouse/human monoclonal antibodies—basiliximab (*Simulect*) and daclizumab (*Zenapax*)—that bind to the interleukin-2 (IL-2) receptor on T-lymphocytes and prevent acute renal transplant rejection are now available. The new agents block IL-2-mediated activation of T-lymphocytes with minimal decreases in the number of circulating T-cells. Both drugs are used with cyclosporine (*Sandimmune, Neoral*) and corticosteroids [*Med Letter* 1998;40:93–94]. A mouse anti-CD3 monoclonal antibody called muromonab-CD3 (*Orthoclone OKT3*) has been available for many years.

A pivotal study enrolled 260 patients undergoing a first cadaveric renal transplant. It demonstrated that the addition of daclizumab to cyclosporine, prednisone and azathioprine before and once every week after transplantation, for four weeks, lowers the rate of acute rejection at six months from 35%, in the group receiving immunosuppressive therapy alone, to 22% [*New Engl J Med* 1998;338:161–65]. A well controlled trial in 376 patients treated with cyclosporine and corticosteroids for a first cadaveric renal transplant reported that two doses of basiliximab, one on the day of transplantation and the other four days later, reduced the incidence of acute rejections at six months from 44% to 30%, compared with cyclosporine and corticosteroids alone [*Lancet* 1997;350:1193–98]. Clinical studies also show that basiliximab and daclizumab have far fewer side effects than muromonab-CD3, and, unlike the mouse antibody, they do not evoke neutralizing antibodies.

Medical Letter consultants conclude: "Addition of basiliximab or daclizumab to a prophylactic anti-rejection regimen can decrease the incidence of graft rejection in the first six months after renal transplantation, but has little effect on graft survival rates after one year." They add that the new agents are tolerated much better than muromonab-CD3. Whether they are as effective as muromonab is not established.

Vitravene: First Antisense Agent Clears FDA Panel. On a split vote, an advisory panel recommended that the Food and Drug Administration approve Isis Pharmaceutical's fomivirsen (*Vitravene*) for the treatment of cytomegalovirus (CMV) retinitis [*The Pink Sheet* 1998;60(No30):5–6]. Fomivirsen, a chain of 21 oligonucleotides, is the mirror image of a section of CMV RNA. It binds to CMV's messenger RNA and inhibits replication of the virus. The drug is injected monthly, directly into the vitreous humor of the affected eye.

Because of the limited data there was sentiment among some members of the panel to approve the drug for use only when other drugs failed, but the majority concluded there was no need to restrict use of the drug in that way. Indeed, there is evidence to support the use of fomivirsen in both newly diagnosed patients and patients with advanced retinitis to delay disease progression, but it is not robust.

The underlying problem is that there were only 330 patients in the database and not all of them met FDA's evaluation criteria. Both Isis and the FDA expected that more patients would enroll in the trials. However, because of the success of highly active antiretroviral therapy to prevent opportunistic infections in patients infected with HIV, and competition from other clinical trials, expectations were not met [*Scrip*, July 29, 1998, p 22]. The increased use of combinations of potent anti-HIV drugs has changed the status of CMV retinitis from an orphan disease to a rare disease. Other treatments for CMV retinitis are intravenous and oral ganciclovir (*Cytovene*), intravenous foscarnet (*Foscavir*), injectable cidofovir (*Vistide*), and an ocular implant containing ganciclovir (*Vitrasert*). All are more toxic than fomivirsen and susceptible to cross-resistance.

In August, the FDA gave Isis final approval to market *Vitravene*. The agency, however, did not heed its panel's recommendation that no restrictions be put on the use of *Vitravene*. The anti-sense compound is indicated as second-line therapy for patients who are intolerant or have a contraindication to other treatments or who were insufficiently responsive to previous treatments. Labeling warns that *Vitravene* should not be used in patients who have been treated within the past two to four weeks with cidofovir, because of the risk of exaggerated ocular inflammation. The agency cleared the drug in just five months after receiving the application. The product will be co-marketed by Ciba Vision, the eye-care unit of Novartis [*The Pink Sheet* 1998;60(No35):27].

Advisory Committee Supports Approval of Stem-Cell Growth Factor.

Intensive chemotherapy is toxic not only to tumor cells but to bone marrow as well. Bone marrow transplantation is used as a rescue to reconstitute the immune system. Autologous transplantation of stem cells is an alternative. Before treatment, patients undergo apheresis to extract sufficient stem cells from peripheral blood to assure the success of transplantation. The target number ranges from three to five million stem cells per kg total body weight, depending on treatment center. Transplanting less than one million cells per kg is deemed inadequate.

In July, FDA's biological response modifiers advisory panel voted 10 to 1 to recommend the approval of Amgen's *Stemgen* (ancestim), a blood cell growth factor, for use in the treatment of patients with cancer who receive autologous stem cell transplants [*Scrip*, August 5, 1998, p 24]. The panel concluded that *Stemgen*, added to Amgen's *Neupogen* (filgrastim; granulocyte colony stimulating factor) increases the proportion of patients able to produce sufficient stem cells for transplantation.

Amgen told the panel that in a 200-patient breast cancer study, 60% of the patients receiving *Stemgen* reached the target level of stems cells, compared with 46% of those who received only filgrastim. The company, however, did not provide sufficient evidence to convince the advisory panel to allow the claim that *Stemgen* reduces the number of apheresis procedures to achieve target levels. Because apheresis costs more than $2000 per procedure, Amgen sought this claim to demonstrate cost effectiveness.

In considering the approval of *Stemgen,* the FDA must also weigh its adverse effects. The trials show that the growth factor induces mast cell degranulation, which leads to injection site reactions and sometimes to severe systemic allergic-like reactions. In the pivotal study, *Stemgen* produced injection site reaction in 92% of patients, compared with an incidence of 10% for the patients in the control arm. Respiratory symptoms were observed in 28% of *Stemgen* patients and 16% of control patients.

FDA Approves Enbrel for Rheumatoid Arthritis. Rheumatoid arthritis affects 2.5 million Americans. Few drugs have shown consistent effectiveness against the disease. Patients usually move from one drug to another and suffer an array of side effects as joints degenerate. In September 1998, an FDA advisory committee recommended the approval of Immunex's *Enbrel* (entanercept) to relieve symptoms and slow progression of severe rheumatoid arthritis. It is probably the safest drug ever approved for this indication [*The Wall Street Journal,* September 17, 1998, p B21].

The panel stopped short of endorsing *Enbrel* for all patients. Rather, it recommended its use, either alone or in combination with methotrexate, when other therapy has failed. Analysts speculate that the approved indications for *Enbrel* cover about 30% of patients with rheumatoid arthritis. Panel members agreed that indications could be expanded to include first-line therapy if Immunex can provide data showing long-term safety.

Tumor necrosis factor (TNF) is a pro-inflammatory cytokine implicated in rheumatoid arthritis, septic shock, and other medical disorders. *Enbrel* is a recombinant fusion protein that consists of the soluble TNF receptor (TNFR) linked to the Fc portion of human IgG1. *Enbrel* competitively inhibits TNF binding to cell-surface TNFR. *Enbrel's* only common side effects are a skin reaction at the site of injection and mild upper respiratory tract symptoms. There are no dose-limiting toxic effects and no antibodies to *Enbrel* have been detected in serum samples.

In July 1997, researchers reported the results of a multicenter placebo-controlled phase II study that enrolled 180 patients with refractory rheumatoid arthritis [*N Engl J Med* 1997;337:141-47]. The patients were randomized to receive subcutaneous injections of placebo or one of three doses of *Enbrel,* twice weekly for three months. The clinical response was measured by changes in composite symptoms of arthritis according to standardized criteria.

Treatment with *Enbrel* resulted in significant reductions in disease activity in a dose-dependent manner. The greatest effect was seen at a dose of 16 mg per square meter of body surface area. Among those receiving the maximum dose, 75% had improvement of 20% or more in symptoms, as compared with 14% in the placebo group. The mean percent reduction in the number of tender and swollen joints at three months was 61% among those receiving the highest dose of *Enbrel,* as compared with 25% of those receiving placebo injection. Cessation of therapy was associated with an increase in disease activity, suggesting that *Enbrel* must be given continuously for sustained effect. A six-month study compared 59 patients on both *Enbrel* and methotrexate with 30 patients on methotrexate and placebo. Enrolled subjects had failed to respond to an average of three disease-modifying drugs and had advanced disease. Seventy one percent of the patients in the combination arm had an improvement of at least 20% at six months; twenty-seven percent of those treated only with methotrexate had achieved the same results at six months [*The Pink Sheet* 1998;60(No38):7–8].

The researchers speculate that soluble cytokine receptors may exhibit less immunogenicity compared with other TNF-neutralizing agents, such as monoclonal antibodies. Patients receiving monoclonals may form antibodies that neutralize the therapeutic agent, limiting its long-term usefulness or causing allergic reactions on re-treatment. Soluble cytokine receptors or receptor-Fc fusion constructs containing only human amino acid sequences may eliminate that concern.

In September, *Scrip* [September 19, 1998, p 19] reported that *Enbrel* had shown positive results in a pivotal phase III trial. In the study, 234 patients with severe rheumatoid arthritis who had failed to respond to at least one disease-modifying anti-rheumatic drug (DMARD) were treated for six months with twice-weekly injections of 10 mg or 25 mg *Enbrel* or placebo. Significant improvement in symptoms was observed after three and six months of therapy with either dose of *Enbrel,* compared with placebo. The findings mirrored the results of the earlier phase II trial.

In November 1998, the FDA announced the approval of *Enbrel* for the treatment of patients with moderate to severe rheumatoid arthritis who have had an inadequate response to one or more disease-modifying drugs [*The Wall Street Journal,* November 3, 1998, pp A3,A6]. FDA cautions that *Enbrel* is not for patients with osteoarthritis. Treatment with *Enbrel* requires self-injection twice a week at a cost of $220 per week. Immunex and American Home Products will jointly market the new agent. Rapid uptake by the market is likely because of heavy promotion and because many experts are impressed with the effectiveness of *Enbrel* and surprised by its unusually clean side-effect profile.

IN THE PIPELINE

Telomeres, Telomerase, Aging, and Cancer
Nerve Growth Factor for Corneal Ulcers and Diabetic
    Neuropathy
Replication-Competent Viruses for Tumors
P53-Based Strategies to Keep Cancer in Check
Blocking Oncogenes
Monoclonal Antibodies for the Treatment of Cancer
Matrix Metalloproteinases (MMPs) for the Treatment of Cancer
New Therapies to Prevent Diabetic Retinopathy
A Role for Pro-inflammatory Cytokines in Heart Failure?
Administering the Products of Biotechnology
Replenishing Blood Components
Small Molecule Drugs Substituting for Large Ones
Leptin: The Antiobesity Hormone
Leptin Triggers Angiogenesis
A New Target for Anti-HIV Therapy
The Search for Effective Strategies against Septic Shock
Monoclonal Antibody to CD4 in Chronic Severe Asthma
Pharmacologic Manipulation of Gene Expression

Telomeres, Telomerase, Aging, and Cancer. Telomeres—sequences of six DNA bases replicated thousands of times—are found at the ends of chromosomes. In normal somatic cells, which do not express the enzyme telomerase, telomeres shorten by about 200 basepairs of DNA from each chromosomal end each time the cell divides. After a fixed number of cell divisions, the progressive loss leads to senescense and cell death. Telomeres of long-lived germ cells, which do express telomerase, do not shorten during cell division. About 85% of cancer cells have telomerase activity, which perhaps accounts for their "immortality." These findings suggest that telomerase protects chromosomal ends from fraying during cell division and increases the life-span of a cell.

In January 1998, Geron Corporation announced that their scientists had extended the life span of normal human foreskin fibroblasts and retinal pigment epithelial cells by genetically engineering the cells to express telomerase. The company reported that the cells, which normally senesce at 50 to 55 divisions, had divided more than 100 times. Important to note is that the activation of telomerase in these cells did not transform them into cancer cells. This technique could lead to improved therapy for chronic skin ulcers or macular degeneration by local treatment with cultured skin cells or retinal pigment epithelial cells, respectively, engineered to express telomerase. The development of telomerase inhibitors may be an effective approach to the treatment of diseases of aging (e.g., atherosclerosis, osteoporosis) and cancer. While there is considerable interest in this avenue of research, there is also concern that cancer cells treated to suppress telomerase activity may recruit an alternative mechanism for lengthening telomeres. About 5% of tumors have no detectable telomerase activity but nevertheless have long telomeres and long life [*Lancet* 1998;351:1186].

Nerve Growth Factor for Corneal Ulcers and Diabetic Neuropathy. Corneal ulceration is an important reason for loss of vision. Herpes simplex virus is the leading cause of corneal ulceration in the US. Corneal ulcers can also result directly from loss of the sensory innervation of the cornea, the consequence of some ocular or systemic diseases such as diabetes or multiple sclerosis, or injuries such as a chemical burn. This condition is called corneal neurotrophic ulceration. Although uncommon, these ulcers have devastating effects on the cornea.

Nerve growth factor (NGF), a polypeptide discovered in 1986, is integral to the growth and development of the nervous system, and obligatory for the survival of sympathetic and sensory neurons. In a recently published paper, investigators report the dramatic healing effects of topically applied recombinant human NGF in 12 patients (14 eyes) with neurotrophic corneal ulcers [*N Engl J Med* 1998;338:1174–80]. Corneal healing began two days to two weeks after the initiation of rhNGF therapy. All patients had complete healing of corneal ulcers after ten days to six weeks and visual acuity increased progressively during treatment.

A commentary on the report pointed out that the findings are provocative because they extend the function of NGF to a possible role in modulating and promoting corneal wound healing [*N Engl J Med* 1998;338:1221–22]. "Nerve growth factor may affect the healing of simple corneal abrasions, ulcers, and injuries as well as influencing the postoperative course of cornea transplantation and photorefractive surgery, in which the regeneration of nerves facilitates corneal healing."

Another important application of rhNGF is in the prevention and treatment of diabetic neuropathy. At this time, only palliative treatment is available.

Recently reported, though, were the results of the first randomized placebo-controlled trial of rhNGF [*Neurology* 1998;51:695–702]. Two hundred and fifty patients with symptomatic diabetic neuropathy received placebo or one of two doses of rhNGF three times a week for six months by means of self-administered subcutaneous injection. Patients treated with active drug experienced an improved response to heat and cold. Among those receiving rhNGF, 75% reported symptom improvement, compared with 49% among those receiving placebo. Patients with early, less severe neuropathy seemed to respond better and sooner to rhNGF than those with established neuropathy.

Conclusions of the study were clouded, however, because an injection site reaction to active drug but not to placebo was observed and led to the unblinding of the investigators and even some patients. A phase III study, now underway, has corrected the problem by making the placebo a hypertonic solution. A report at the International AIDS Conference in Geneva showed that rhNGF may also be effective in the treatment of HIV-related neuropathy [*Lancet* 1998;352:1039].

Replication-Competent Viruses for Tumors. Scientists are developing viruses that wreak havoc on cancer cells but are naturally harmless to normal tissue or genetically altered to make them so. Up to now, investigators have identified about half a dozen of these tumor-killing viruses. Interest is especially keen in reoviruses because they are apparently harmless in people [*Science* 1998;282:1244–46].

One research team found that a particular reovirus thrived best in cancer cells that have epidermal growth factor (EGF) surface receptors. Later work showed that it was not the EGF receptor per se that was important, but the signaling pathway the receptor activates when it binds the growth factor. This team now reports that what enables the virus to thrive is a particular component of that pathway, the protein made by the *ras* gene. To replicate, the virus needs the Ras protein because it blocks the activity of another protein that would otherwise prevent the synthesis of viral proteins. Recognizing that *ras* is one of the oncogenes that can, when activated, spur cancer cell growth, the investigators deduced that the virus would probably replicate readily in tumors that have an overactive *ras* gene. Such tumors include some colon, pancreatic, and lung cancers. Studies show that the virus partially or completely shrinks tumors in up to 80% of immune-deficient mice implanted with human glioblastoma cells with high levels of Ras protein. These investigators also report that the virus kills cultured cells derived from breast, prostate, and pancreatic cancers, but none of the noncancerous cell lines with low *ras* activity [*Ibid*].

Researchers are also studying the potential of selectively replication-competent herpes simplex virus (HSV) as a cytotoxic agent in the treatment of malignant brain tumors [*Nature Med* 1997;3:1323]. HSV mutant 1716, which is only capable of replication in proliferative cells, is safe when inoculated directly into the brain of rodents and shows good anti-tumor activity in xenograft models. A phase I study in patients with glioblastoma who had failed conventional treatments shows no adverse outcomes after direct injection of the selective strain of HSV. Fear that the replication-competent virus might cause encephalitis was laid to rest [*Nature Med* 1998;4:133]. The authors conclude: "We . . . believe that progression to human trials of 1716 is totally justified in patients whose disease offers no prospects of even modest survival and who are fully informed of the experimental nature of the procedure."

On the horizon are oncolytic viruses that not only kill cancer cells but also carry genes that make the cells more susceptible to radiation or chemotherapy. The early work of one research team provides an example. The investigators have added the rat gene for the protein cytochrome P-450, a drug metabolizing enzyme, to the genome of a herpesvirus. Cytochrome P-450 converts cyclophosphamide, widely used for cancer chemotherapy, to its active form. As the virus spreads through a tumor, it not only kills the cells directly, but also makes them susceptible to cyclophosphamide [*Science* 1998;282:1244–46]

P53-Based Strategies to Keep Cancer in Check. *P*53, a tumor suppressor gene, and its protein are central to the body's defense against cancer. About 40% of all cancers contain *p*53 mutations. Mutations occur even more frequently in lung and colorectal cancers. In other types of cancer, the *p*53 protein seems normal but inactivated. Human papilloma virus, which causes cervical cancer, produces a protein that inactivates *p*53 in about 90% of these cancers. More than one-third of soft-tissue sarcomas have normal but inactive *p*53. Taken together, lack of properly functioning *p*53 is linked to 50% to 60% of all cancers.

The most direct way to correct deranged *p*53 is to use gene therapy techniques to put an unmutated *p*53 gene into tumor cells that lack its activity. Researchers have tested direct injection of a modified retrovirus containing a normal *p*53 gene into tumor cells of patients with lung cancer whose tumors carry mutant *p*53 genes. Treatment triggers apoptosis but, as yet, there is no clinical evidence of benefit. Other researchers are using an adenovirus as the vector to carry the *p53* gene into tumor cells.

Onyx Pharmaceuticals has a different way to use genetically engineered viruses to kill *p53*-deficient cancers. Researchers have constructed viruses that replicate and kill cells that do not have functioning *p53*, but do not affect other cells. Ordinarily, when a virus infects a cell it turns off *p53*. Adenoviruses accomplish this by producing a protein that binds to and inactivates *p53*. The engineered adenovirus lacks the gene for that protein. The virus cannot inactivate *p53* and quickly dies. In tumor cells that lack functioning *p53*, however, the virus replicates, takes over the cells, and kills them [*Chem Eng News*, February 1998, pp 38–41].

A phase II trial of a modified adenovirus in a small group of patients with advanced head and neck cancer shows promising results. Ten patients were given the virus as well as cisplatin and 5-fluorouracil (5-FU). All patients responded to treatment. Two patients had complete regression of their cancers and seven had significant shrinkage (50% or more) of their tumors. With cisplatin and 5-FU alone, only 35% of head and neck cancer patients responded with significant shrinkage [*The Wall Street Journal*, May 19, 1998, p A18].

Blocking Oncogenes. Scientists have identified more than 20 defective genes that result in the unbridled growth of tumor cells. In 1978, researchers discovered an oncogene in rats and named it *ras*, for rat sarcoma. We now know that defective *ras* genes play a central role in as many as 30% of human tumors, including half of all colon cancers, 90% of pancreatic tumors, and 25% of lung cancers.

In health, the *ras* gene makes Ras, a protein that sits near the inner surface of all cells and acts as a relay station for cell division. Growth hormones in the circulation, when necessary, signal the protein to direct the cell's nucleus to start multiplying. In the absence of chemical signals, the Ras protein is quiescent and the cell refrains from dividing. In cancer, however, a mutation in the *ras* gene turns the Ras protein into a killer. "Stuck in the 'on' position, the Ras protein continuously conveys a phantom message telling the cell to divide and multiply" [*The Wall Street Journal*, May 6, 1998, pp A1,12].

In 1990, researchers found a helper protein, farnesyl transferase, that the *ras* gene needs to transmit messages. This discovery ignited a search for inhibitors of farnesyl transferase that is ongoing [*Chem Eng News*, April 20, 1998, pp 67–69].

One drug company, stimulated by research findings in the early 1990s, took a different tack in developing anti-Ras drugs. It seems that a bit of protein on the surface of cells, called epidermal growth factor (EGF) receptor, acts as a chemical gatekeeper. The receptor gets signals from growth hormones indicating it is time for cells to divide, then sends the message to Ras, which relays it to the cell nucleus. Lung, prostate, and brain tumor cells have as many as one hundred times the number of EGF receptors as normal cells. Pfizer has announced it has a drug that can block the EGF receptor selectively.

Monoclonal Antibodies for the Treatment of Cancer. Upon the first synthesis of monoclonal antibodies (MABs), more than 20 years ago, observers believed that these "magic bullets" would resolve a host of human diseases, particularly cancer. The extraordinary research efforts to develop safe and effective MABs against cancer did not bear fruit until 1997. The first anti-cancer MAB approved by the FDA was rituximab (*Rituxan*), for use in the treatment of low-grade non-Hodgkin's lymphoma (NHL). The FDA supports the use of the drug for patients with follicular lymphoma who are resistant to chemotherapy or are in their second or subsequent relapse after chemotherapy. Follicular lymphoma is a type of B-cell lymphoma, an unusual cancer because it proliferates slowly. Indolent NHL accounts for about 40% of all NHL, and NHL accounts for about 85% of all lymphomas. Indolent lymphoma is incurable and patients have less than a 50% chance to live ten years after diagnosis. Chemotherapy and other treatments have no significant effect on survival.

Rituximab binds to the CD20 antigen found on the surface of B-lymphocytes and activates the immune system to attack malignant cells and induce apoptosis. Roche Laboratories hopes that rituximab, administered with chemotherapy, can slow or even stop disease progression. The company reports that one study shows complete remission in 60% to 65% of patients with indolent follicular lymphoma when treated with chemotherapy and rituximab.

MABs can also be used to deliver cytotoxic molecules to enhance the specificity of chemotherapy or radiotherapy. Another antibody in development for NHL is *Bexxar*—iodine-131 tositumomab. This investigational agent also acts at the CD20 site on B-cells, but differs from rituximab in that the antibody is linked to radiolabeled iodine. The company developing *Bexxar* hopes that it will deliver radiation and activate the immune system at the same time [*Scrip,* October 28, 1998, p 25]. A recent article in *Nature Biotechnology* [1998;16:1000–01] compares and contrasts *Rituxan* and *Bexxar*.

Matrix Metalloproteinases (MMPs) for the Treatment of Cancer. Matrix metalloproteinases are a family of enzymes that degrade collagen and proteoglycans, which are required components of the extracellular matrix. They hold cells together inside tissues and make room for new cellular growth. While MMPs are very important in fetal development, ovulation, and wound healing, excess production when there is no biological need can lead to disease. In cancer, MMPs break down the matrix of healthy tissue allowing a tumor to proliferate, they loosen tissue structure permitting cancer cells to break away and migrate, and they help provide space for new blood vessels to grow as the extracellular matrix degrades.

The most advanced MMP inhibitor in clinical development is British Biotech's marimastat, followed by Agouron's AG 3340 and Bayer's BA 12-9566. The major side effect with MMP inhibitors is joint pain. This problem has been seen with AG 3340 but not with the Bayer compound. Both drugs have stayed the progression of tumor growth after oral administration in some patients [*Scrip,* July 3, 1998, p 20].

New Therapies to Prevent Diabetic Retinopathy. Diabetic retinopathy is the leading cause of blindness among the working-age population in developed countries. Intensive monitoring and control of blood glucose levels slows progression, but tight control is difficult to maintain and increases the risk of hypoglycemia. Lisinopril (*Zestril*), an ACE inhibitor, also seems to decrease the progression of retinopathy, at least in patients with type 1 diabetes [*Lancet* 1998;351:28–31].

Advances in understanding how hyperglycemia may damage blood vessels in the eyes have suggested new prevention strategies [*JAMA* 1998; 278:1480–81]. Of particular interest are drugs that inhibit the formation of glycosylated proteins and lipids, collectively called advanced glycosylation end products (AGEs). Because of their high glucose levels, patients with diabetes have excess levels of these end products. A cellular binding site receptor for AGE, called RAGE, is highly expressed in retinal tissue. The binding of AGE to RAGE probably mediates the damage to blood vessels in the retina. Preclinical studies using aminoguanidine, a drug that inhibits the formation of AGE, have been encouraging. A US company, Alteon, is developing pimagedine and other AGE inhibitors.

RAGE is a protein that is linked to the surface of cells by a transmembrane component. Researchers have developed a soluble form of RAGE without the transmembrane component. Soluble RAGE retains its high affinity for AGE and may offer an effective therapy against retinopathy and, perhaps, other diabetic complications.

Levels of vascular endothelial growth factor (VEGF) are abnormally high in the retina of patients with diabetes. VEGF activates protein kinase C (PKC) in the retina and the excess PKC activity leads to increased intraocular vasopermeability. Drugs that inhibit PKC activity may prevent the macular edema of diabetic retinopathy.

A Role for Pro-Inflammatory Cytokines in Heart Failure? Heart failure is a complex neurohumoral and inflammatory syndrome characterized by fatigue, shortness of breath, congestion, and cachexia. Symptoms relate to inadequate tissue perfusion, fluid retention, and neurohumoral reactions. Despite significant progress in the prevention and treatment of cardiovascular disease in the past 20 years, surveys indicate that the incidence and prevalence of chronic heart failure have been increasing steadily in recent years, particularly in the elderly [*Circulation* 1998;97:292–89].

A recent report reviews the evidence suggesting that pro-inflammatory cytokines—interleukin-1 (IL-1), IL-2, IL-6, and tumor necrosis factor (TNF)—play an important role in cardiac depression and heart failure [*Am Heart J* 1998;135:181–6]. The authors suggest that the use of monoclonal antibodies directed against specific cytokines may block the progression of heart failure.

Administering the Products of Biotechnology. Many of the drugs developed by the biotechnology segment of the pharmaceutical industry are macromolecules that show little or no activity after oral administration and are usually given by intravenous infusion or subcutaneous or intramuscular injection. Delivering proteins is a challenge because of their large size and fragile three-dimensional structure, which must be maintained for biological activity. Proteins, peptides, and other macromolecules are poorly absorbed from the gastrointestinal (GI) tract, degraded by enzymes in the GI tract, or both. Noninvasive administration—intranasal solutions, skin patches, needleless injection devices—have had some success. The leading strategy today seems to be delivery by inhalation, a route of administration well established for the treatment of asthma and other respiratory diseases. Technology has progressed so that now inhalation can be used to deliver proteins and peptides systemically. Among the drugs under investigation are calcitonin, growth hormone, insulin, interferon-alpha, and somatostatin [*Nature Biotech* 1998; 16:141–43].

The potential ways to deliver protein drugs to the lungs are dry powder aerosols, liquid aerosols, and hydrofluorocarbon propellant aerosols. Delivered by dry powder aerosols, most peptides and proteins are water soluble and quickly dissolve in the fluid layer on the surface of the lung before moving through the thin alveolar barrier to the circulation. A challenge facing dry powder aerosol preparations is the tendency of fine powder particles to stick together forming clumps that may impact the oral cavity and never reach the lungs. Dura Pharmaceuticals has developed an inhalation system that uses mechanical energy to aerosolize and disperse powdered medication. Their first product, albuterol in a pocket-sized inhaler, is under review by the FDA. In September [*Scrip*, September 30, 1998, p 9], Eli Lilly and Dura announced they would collaborate on the development of pulmonary delivery technology for insulin using Dura's *Spiros* system. NovoNordisk and Aradigm are also merging their efforts to develop an inhaled insulin product.

Inhale Therapeutic Systems has designed a device that uses sonic velocity compressed air to aerosolize the powder. The deagglomerated particles form a cloud in a holding chamber (spacer). And the patient then inhales the cloud with one, slow deep breath. There is no need for a patient to coordinate aerosolization and inhalation as is the case for metered-dose inhalers.

A report in *The Wall Street Journal* [June 17, 1998] described the first clinical trials designed to demonstrate that inhaled insulin is effective to control glucose level in diabetic patients. Pfizer is developing the product using dry-powder technology developed by Inhale. Studies suggest that the bioavailability of inhaled insulin in humans is about 20%.

The trials enrolled 121 people with type 1 or 2 diabetes and found that inhaled insulin, taken before meals, controlled blood-glucose levels just as well as injections of insulin, and without additional side effects. Patients in the study, however, had to take one injection of long-acting insulin at bedtime because the inhalation device delivered only short-acting insulin. Another study showed that at doses of subcutaneous insulin and inhaled insulin that comparably reduce elevated levels of glucose after a meal in type 2 diabetics, reproducibility of inhaled insulin, even in patients inexperienced in the use of an inhaler, is as good as that of subcutaneous insulin. Observers say that Pfizer and Inhale are ahead of their competitors in the race to develop the first product that can reliably deliver insulin by inhalation [*Scrip*, June 19, 1998, p 21].

Attendees at the annual meeting of the European Association for the Study of Diabetes in September 1998 learned of the results of a recently completed phase II trial evaluating Inhale/Pfizer's inhaled insulin. The study showed that the combination of inhaled insulin, taken before meals with a sulfonylurea and/or metformin, improves glycemic control in type 2 diabetics who have failed oral therapy alone. Patients randomized to their usual oral agent(s) had an average lowering of glycosylated hemoglobin of 1%, to 9.8%. In contrast, patients assigned to their usual drug(s) along with inhalations of insulin had an average lowering of 2.3%, to a level of 7.5% [*Scrip*, September 30, 1998, p 25].

Another interesting approach is an injectable biodegradable system that provides slow release of active ingredient over time [*Science* 1998;281:1161–62]. Clinical trials have been started with the *ProLease* biodegradabe microsphere delivery system for proteins and peptides. The system is a drug powder composed of polymeric microspheres containing a protein in a polymer matrix that can be injected in an aqueous diluent through a narrow-gauge needle. Following injection of the microspheres, the encapsulated protein is released by a complex process involving hydration of the particles, dissolution of the drug, drug diffusion through water-filled pores within the particles, and polymer erosion.

Recombinant human growth hormone (rhGH) has been formulated into microspheres (*ProLease hGH*). Clinical testing began with a study in growth-hormone deficient adults. Serum levels of hGH remained above baseline for a median of 23 days after administration of the product. *ProLease hGH* also increased levels of insulin-like growth factor I and insulin-like growth factor-binding protein. Injections were well tolerated and no antibodies to rhGH were detected. Clinical testing of *ProLease hGH* in growth-hormone deficient children is under way.

Replenishing Blood Components. Surveys suggest that between 10 and 14 million units of donor blood and more than 8 million units of donor platelets are transfused each year in the US. Another 7 million units are needed to obtain other blood products such as clotting factors. The need for safe and affordable blood and the financial windfall from successful products has catalyzed the development of substitute or artificial blood products [*Scrip Magazine*, July/August 1998;39–41].

Until recently, development of blood substitutes concentrated on modified hemoglobin solutions and perfluorocarbons. More recently, researchers have introduced cytokine-based products to stimulate the patients' own production of red blood cells. Erythropoietin (epoetin, *Epogen*) is widely used to prevent anemia in patients with renal disease who require dialysis. It has also been approved to treat anemia in patients with HIV infection and in those undergoing cancer chemotherapy. Colony stimulating factors that enhance the production of white cells have been available for some time and are used extensively in patients undergoing chemotherapy.

Now, there is a great deal of interest in products that can replenish blood platelets. Because of the lack of a platelet growth factor, chemotherapy often has to be interrupted to allow platelet levels to recover. A reduction in platelets—thrombocytopenia—can lead to uncontrolled bleeding. A failure of bone marrow to produce a sufficient number of platelets is seen in patients with leukemia, lymphoma, and aplastic anemia, in patients with certain viral infections, and after chemotherapy and radiotherapy. The condition may also be inherited or drug induced. Approximately 1.3 million platelet transfusions take place each year in the US, about half of which are given to patients with cancer. An estimated 18 million units of platelets are transfused worldwide each year with 70% to 80% given to oncology patients. Donated platelets, however, have serious drawbacks and often precipitate complications that require careful monitoring.

Researchers are trying to get around the problems associated with platelet transfusion by developing products that will stimulate the patient's own platelet production. One of these cytokines is interleukin-11 (IL-11), which enhances the growth of megakaryocyte progenitor cells. A recombinant version of the protein, *Neumega,* is approved in the US to increase platelet count and decrease the need for platelet transfusions in patients with severe thrombocytopenia caused by chemotherapy for nonmyeloid malignancies [*Med Letter* 1998;40:77–78].

Another strategy is based on thrombopoietin, the chief regulator of megakaryocyte development [*N Engl J Med* 1998;339:746–54]. Megakaryocytes are the giant cells of bone marrow; platelets are released from their cytoplasm. Two forms of thrombopoietin have been studied in clinical trials. One, called recombinant human thrombopoietin, is a full-length polypeptide. The other, a truncated protein containing only the receptor-binding region, which is chemically modified by the addition of polyethylene glycol (PEG), is called PEG-conjugated recombinant human megakaryocyte growth and development factor (PEG-rHuMGDF). The biological activity of the two forms of thrombopoietin is thought to be similar.

In August, Amgen announced that it would discontinue phase III trials of PEG-rHuMGDF to improve the yield and efficiency of platelet collection for transfusion from healthy volunteer donors. To the disappointment of the investigators, treatment led to the development of neutralizing antibodies and thrombocytopenia in some volunteers. The paradoxical thrombocytopenia may be explained by neutralizing antibodies produced against PEG-rHuMGDF that bind to and inactivate MGDF naturally present in the body.

Amgen said it would continue to study the drug for other indications. One month later, however, the company decided to pull the plug on the entire development plan for MGDF [*The Wall Street Journal*, September 14, 1998, p B11]. Amgen's decision to abandon the project followed reports that some cancer patients also developed neutralizing antibodies and low platelet counts.

Small Molecule Drugs Substituting for Large Ones. A dream shared by pharmaceutical researchers around the world is the development of small molecules that mimic the effects of proteins such as recombinant insulin and many other recently developed products of biotechnology. Protein drugs seem to mold themselves to the complex contours of target molecules and activate receptors that seem virtually inaccessible. Small molecules appear not to have enough contact points. Now, recent work by drug company scientists shows that the task is difficult but not impossible. They report the discovery of a small molecule that activates the receptor for granulocyte-colony-stimulating factor (G-CSF), a cytokine commonly used to boost the immune system in patients undergoing chemotherapy [*Science* 1998;281:257–59].

Although the new drug works in mice but not in humans, the discovery is widely hailed as proof of principle—the right small molecule can substitute for a protein drug. The groundbreaking work will catalyze the drug industry's search for protein-mimicking drugs. The first steps have already been taken. In the past two years, two research teams have shown that peptides could activate receptors for thrombopoietin and erythropoietin. Although peptides cannot be given orally, the findings are an important advance [*Science* 1998;281:150–51].

Leptin: The Antiobesity Hormone. Leptin is the protein product of the ob gene and is known to block hunger by affecting the hypothalamus. Its potential as a weight-reducing drug, however, has been debated because obese patients have higher levels of leptin than do normal-weight people. Obesity has also been linked to leptin resistance and defects in the leptin receptor and its signaling pathways. The first trials with leptin, reported in 1997, showed that low doses result in only modest weight loss and higher doses are not well tolerated [*Scrip,* September 18, 1998, p 19].

A meeting report in *JAMA* [1998;280:869–70] notes that leptin received a lot of attention at the American Diabetes Association's Scientific Session in June 1998. Investigators presented evidence from phase I and II clinical trials showing that Amgen's recombinant methionyl human leptin has an acceptable safety profile and causes dose-dependent weight loss. Recombinant methionyl human leptin is a synthesized form of the natural hormone.

In a multicenter study, 53 lean subjects with a body mass index (BMI) of less than 27.5 kg/m^2, and 70 moderately obese patients with a BMI of at least 27.5 kg/m^2, received daily subcutaneous injections of leptin or placebo. All participants were asked to adhere to a weight-reduction diet. Treatment was tolerated well and average weight loss after one month ranged from 0.4 kg for those receiving placebo to 1.9 kg for those receiving the highest dose of leptin, 0.3 mg/kg per day. Sixty of the obese patients continued on protocol for another five months. At the end of that period, average weight loss ranged from 0.7 kg for those taking the lowest dose of leptin, 0.01mg/kg per day, to 7.2 kg for those taking the highest dose. While not everyone given leptin lost weight, a follow-up report presented at the International Congress on Obesity in Paris said that the weight loss caused by recombinant leptin is predominantly due to fat loss.

Additional clinical testing to determine leptin's potential role in treating obesity is now being planned and will span several years. Diabetes experts are interested in leptin because obesity is the major barrier to effective treatment and control of type 2 diabetes. For these patients, a weight loss of only 5% of body weight significantly improves insulin sensitivity.

Leptin Triggers Angiogenesis. Researchers have linked two of the hottest biomedical research areas—angiogenesis and leptin. An adequate blood supply is needed for the complex endocrine function that regulates body weight. Leptin appears to meet that need by provoking angiogenesis. Leptin may also spur blood vessel growth in the maturing egg and early embryo, and in healing wounds [*Science* 1998;281:1582].

The successful engineering of cultured cells to make the cell surface receptor (OB-Rb), through which leptin acts, fortuitously led to current research. OB-Rb is expressed primarily in the hypothalamic region of the brain. Subsequently, investigators used monoclonal antibodies specific for the intracellular domain of OB-Rb to confirm that the cells actually contained the receptor. By chance, they selected ordinary endothelial cells as a negative control. To their surprise, the controls were also positive, indicating that endothelial cells naturally contain the leptin receptor. Following this lead, the researchers found that leptin causes cultured endothelial cells to aggregate and form tubes that resemble the early stages of blood vessels. They then ran a standard test to detect angiogenic activity and showed that leptin causes new blood vessels to form in the corneas of rats [*Science* 1998;281: 1683–86].

Another research team has discovered that leptin is also made in human ovarian follicles, which is where eggs mature until they are ready to be released and fertilized. The protein is also packaged in parts of the egg that develop into cells responsible for forming the placenta. Wound healing also depends on blood vessel growth and investigators have learned that healing is slow in leptin-deficient mice but accelerated when leptin is applied. Like other angiogenic factors, leptin may also be deployed by some cancers to develop new blood vessels.

A New Target for Anti-HIV Therapy. T-20, a synthetic 36-amino-acid peptide that corresponds to residues in the extracellular portion of a receptor (gp41) of the HIV envelope glycoprotein, inhibits HIV entry into host cells [*Nature Med* 1998;4:1302–07]. This is the first demonstration of potent antiretroviral activity directed against a target other than reverse transcriptase or protease. T-20 is thought to interfere with the conformational change in gp41 that is triggered by the binding of the HIV envelope glycoprotein to the host cell CD4 receptor and chemokine co-receptor. Thereby, T-20 prevents fusion of viral and host cell membranes.

The researchers reported dose-response activity in all 16 HIV-infected patients treated with T-20, with a two log reduction in plasma HIV RNA at the highest dose. This level of activity is equivalent to that of the most potent drugs in the three classes of anti-HIV agents now in clinical use—nucleoside reverse transcriptase inhibitors (RTIs), non-nucleoside RTIs, and protease inhibitors.

A commentary in the same issue of *Nature Medicine* [1998;4:1232–33] cautions that much more study is needed to assess the usefulness of T-20. Tolerance to long-term T-20 therapy and durability of T-20 activity are not yet known. The 36-amino-acid peptide is not absorbed and must be given by injection. At this time, the drug is likely to be considered only for people who have exhausted more convenient options. The study raises two key questions. "First, if a complicated peptide shows this level of potency, could a smaller molecule with more desirable pharmacologic characteristics (oral bioavailability and central nervous system penetration) be designed with similar activity? Second, are there other essential interactions of HIV proteins with the host cell that can be interrupted with small molecule ligands?"

The Search for Effective Strategies against Septic Shock. Sepsis is a dangerous, often life-threatening, immune response to infections due to gram-negative, gram-positive, and fungal organisms. There are about a half million cases of sepsis each year in the US. About half develop septic shock—hypotension refractory to fluid resuscitation, activation of the clotting cascade, and organ or system dysfunction. Septic shock is the most common cause of death in intensive care units. Estimates of mortality range from 40% to 70%, despite the availability of potent antibiotics and intensive supportive care.

Advances in our understanding of the pathogenesis of sepsis has led to the development of a host of immunomodulating strategies that can, in principle, be used irrespective of the infecting organism. Repeatedly, however, hopes raised by studies in laboratory animals have been dashed in clinical trials. The latest disappointment comes from a controlled trial of a monoclonal antibody to human tumor necrosis factor (TNF), a pro-inflammatory cytokine. Investigators randomly assigned 1879 patients to either a single infusion of the monoclonal antibody or placebo. The main endpoint was the rate of all-cause mortality at 28 days. They found that 40% of patients who received the antibody and 43% of patients who received placebo died at 28 days. They concluded, as have others before them, that TNF blockade alone is not sufficient to improve survival [*Lancet* 1998;351:929–33].

The results are both disappointing and frustrating. Many scientists see TNF as a principal mediator of sepsis and septic shock. Administration to laboratory animals provokes all the manifestations of sepsis and septic shock. Anti-TNF antibodies protect animals from death caused by endotoxins as well by gram-negative and gram-positive bacteria. So, why do anti-TNF strategies fail in humans?

In the same issue of *Lancet,* a report from investigators studying the relationship of anti-inflammatory cytokine profile and mortality in patients with fever caused by an infection provides a possible reason for the poor showing of anti-TNF strategies. The researchers found that levels of interleukin 10 (IL-10), an anti-inflammatory cytokine, were twice as high in patients succumbing to their illness than in survivors. Further, patients with high IL-10 levels were significantly more likely to die, irrespective of TNF levels. Furthermore, IL-10 was higher and TNF lower, on average, in patients who died than in those who survived. The median ratio of IL-10 to TNF was 6.9 in those who died compared with 3.9 in those who survived. The findings are consistent with the experience that immunosuppression increases the risk of death from infection.

The investigators conclude: "An anti-inflammatory cytokine profile of a high ratio of IL-10 to TNF is associated with fatal outcome in febrile patients with community-acquired infections." They cautioned against the use of pro-inflammatory cytokine inhibition in patients with sepsis [*Lancet* 1998;351:950–53]. Blocking the action of TNF may force the circulating cytokine profile into an anti-inflammatory direction that results in exacerbation of systemic disease and adverse outcome in febrile patients.

One way to explain the seeming duality of TNF is to recognize that severe infection involves both a pro-inflammatory and an anti-inflammatory response and that TNF can be both friend and foe [*Lancet* 1998;351:922–23]. Its administration reproduces virtually all the toxic effects of endotoxins and bacteria, but in certain infections TNF is an essential part of the body's defenses. Under certain circumstances anti-TNF strategies may provide benefit to patients with sepsis. At this time, however, we cannot define those circumstances.

Monoclonal Antibody to CD4 in Chronic Severe Asthma. Asthma is characterized by bronchial inflammation with increased numbers of airway eosinophils and activated T-lymphocytes. Eosinophil activation is enhanced by an array of cytokines produced by CD4 T-cells. Inhaled steroids are effective treatment for asthma but when they start to fail, physicians must resort to oral steroids and then to immunosuppressants such as methotrexate or cyclosporine. An alternative approach is therapy with monoclonal antibodies, which allows specific cellular or mediator targeting. With this in mind, investigators designed a randomized placebo-control trial to assess the safety and efficacy of a single dose of a chimeric human/macaque monoclonal antibody to CD4, called keliximab, in 22 patients with severe corticosteroid-dependent asthma [*Lancet* 1998;352:1109–13]. Patients continued to receive prescribed medication during the trial.

Those who received 3 mg/kg keliximab had a significant improvement in morning and evening peak expiratory flows compared with those assigned to placebo. These changes were accompanied by a decrease in symptom score, although the benefit did not reach statistical significance. And there were no differences in measures of forced expiratory volume in one second (FEV_1). There were no serious adverse effects related to treatment. The results raise the possibility that T-cell-directed treatment for severe asthma may be an alternative approach.

Pharmacologic Manipulation of Gene Expression. Information about the biochemical and genetic bases of inherited diseases abounds, but there has been less progress in the development of therapies. Treatment for some congenital metabolism errors relies on restricted dietary intake of certain food components (e.g., phenylketonuria). Pharmacological prevention of toxic metabolite formation has shown promise for the treatment of a form of tyrosinemia. The disorder is characterized by an excess of tyrosine, which results from a deficiency of fumarylacetoacetase. This enzyme is the final one in the tyrosine catabolic pathway. The metabolism of tyrosine by 4-hydroxyphenylpyruvate dioxygenase leads to the formation of hepatotoxic metabolites. Inhibition of this enzyme by 2-(2-nitro-4-trifluoromethylbenzoyl)-1,3-cyclohexanedione markedly improves the course of the disease [*J Inher Metab Dis* 1998;21:507–17]. In other disorders, treatment aims to correct the primary defect directly. One example is the administration of glucocerebrosidase to patients with Gaucher disease.

Still another strategy uses drugs to increase the expression of a gene that is functionally related to the defective gene causing the disease. Pharmacologic induction of the expression of redundant genes has been applied to the treatment of several disorders. Cytotoxic agents such as 5-azacytidine and hydroxyurea have been shown to induce production of fetal hemoglobin in patients with sickle-cell disease or β-thalassemia. The agent 4-phenylbutyric acid (4-PBA) has been used to promote expression of the aberrant transporter gene in cystic fibrosis. Now, 4-PBA has been applied to the treatment of X-linked adrenoleukodystrophy (X-ALD), a genetic disorder popularized by the film *Lorenzo's Oil.*

The new study [*Nature Med* 1998;4:1261–68] shows that 4-PBA promotes the expression of a peroxisomal protein that is functionally related to the defective peroxisomal protein in X-ALD. The induction corrects the metabolism of very-long-chain fatty acids and prevents their accumulation in the brain. A commentary on the work observes: "These exciting new data should promote the clinical investigation of 4-PBA efficacy in X-ALD patients who have been bereft of any treatment . . . . Furthermore, these findings tempt one to speculate about other inherited metabolic diseases that might be responsive to this form of pharmacologic gene therapy" [*Nature Med* 1998;4:1245–46].

THERAPEUTIC STRATEGIES

Antisense

Antisense Technology in the Clinic. Many diseases can be viewed as the result of inappropriate or excess production of a particular protein. Antisense drugs consist of oligonucleotides and are designed to block the production of selected proteins by targeting the messenger RNA (mRNA) involved in their synthesis [*Biochem Pharmacol* 1998;55:9–19]. Oligonucleotides are short synthetic pieces of nucleic acids, typically 15 nucleotides long, that have a mRNA-targeted complementary base sequence. The drug recognizes and binds to the mRNA, and the enzyme RNase H then cleaves the bound mRNA. The efficacy of an antisense agent depends on its binding affinity and resistance to nuclease activity, as well its ability to promote the breakdown of the bound mRNA.

Research scientists recognized that the structure of ordinary oligonucleotides, with phosphodiester links, required modification to be useful because these compounds are quickly broken down by nucleases. The first generation agents survived nuclease attack by having phosphorothioate groups between the bases rather than phosphodiester linkages. This modification, however, reduced the binding affinity to mRNA, increased nonspecific protein binding, and caused dose-limiting thrombocytopenia. Second-generation agents, chemically modified to overcome some of the problems associated with phosphorothioate derivatives, are now entering the clinic and appear to have improved safety [*Scrip*, October 21, 1998, pp 24–25].

One strategy that has allowed a reduction in phosphorothioate content and increased the potency of the compounds is the incorporation of 2'-methoxyethyl substituted ribonucleosides at appropriate positions. Ribozymes work in a manner similar to antisense oligonucleotides. They are made from RNA but have two arms that bind to the target mRNA as well as a catalytic core. They cleave the bound mRNA without the need for RNase H.

A research news report in *Science* [1997;276:1192–93] noted that early clinical studies are showing promise. Investigators have reported that ISIS 3521, a 20-base oligonucleotide, stopped the spread of ovarian cancer in 3 of 17 patients. Another Isis antisense oligo, when injected locally, blocked replication of cytomegalovirus (CMV) and benefited patients with HIV infection who had developed CMV retinitis.

The most exciting results are from a phase II trial of ISIS 2302 as a treatment for Crohn's disease [*N Engl J Med* 1996;334:316–18]. The antisense compound inhibits the synthesis of the cell adhesion protein ICAM-1 that promotes inflammation. After one month of treatment, 7 of 15 patients achieved remission compared with none of five patients taking placebo. Another potential breakthrough is the development of antisense oligos to correct a genetic defect in patients with thalassemia, a hereditary form of anemia.

Reviews in *Chemical Engineering News* [June 2, 1997, pp 35–39] and *Nature Biotechnology* [1997;15:519–24] have also highlighted clinical advances with antisense oligos. They report that investigators have seen encouraging results in a study of patients with lymphoma treated with an antisense compound called G3139. The oligo binds to mRNA produced by the BCL-2 gene. When turned on, this gene seems to help cancer cells avoid death caused by conventional anticancer drugs. An uncontrolled trial shows that in patients with relapsing non-Hodgkin lymphoma, BCL-2 antisense therapy leads, in some cases, to an improvement of symptoms, tumor response, and down-regulation of the BCL-2 protein [*Lancet* 1997;349:1137–41]. More recent developments have been summarized in *Scrip* [October 21, 1998, p 24].

In February 1998 Isis filed a New Drug Application for fomivirsen (ISIS 2922) as a treatment for HIV-related cytomegalovirus (CMV) retinitis, a condition that often leads to blindness. This is the first FDA filing of an antisense drug [*Scrip*, April 10, 1998, p 21]. A few months later, the product received FDA approval. The proposed dosing regimen calls for direct injection into the vitreous humor on days one and five followed by monthly maintenance doses. Clinical trials indicate that intraocular injections of fomivirsen delay the progression of CMV retinitis in patients with advanced disease as well as in patients with newly diagnosed and previously untreated CMV retinitis.

Isis has several other compounds in clinical trials. Most advanced is ISIS 2302, the antisense inhibitor of ICAM-1, in a pivotal trial for Crohn's disease and in phase II trials for renal transplant rejection, rheumatoid arthritis, psoriasis, and ulcerative colitis. A hurdle for antisense therapy is the high cost of producing specifically targeted genetic analogs.

APOPTOSIS

Restoring a Cell's Ability to Die. Research during the past 25 years has revealed that animal cells are armed with the genetic machinery to die a natural death. The 20,000 publications on cell death within the past five years are evidence of the extraordinary interest in the topic. It seems that each cell can release a set of proteins that can kill it from within. Once released, these proteins systematically direct other molecules to attack the cell and destroy it. This characteristic is called programmed cell death or apoptosis. Apoptosis plays crucial roles in development, health maintenance, and disease initiation and progression [*JAMA* 1998;279:300–07].

Both too much and not enough apoptosis can be catastrophic. Cancers are resistant to chemotherapy and radiation because they fail to respond to apoptotic signals. In Parkinson's disease, Alzheimer's disease, or in the oxygen deprivation caused by stroke, excess apoptosis may kill brain neurons.

About seven years ago, researchers found a family of protein-cleaving enzymes known as caspases (cysteine-containing aspartate-specific proteases) that are central to apoptosis [*Science* 1998;280:32–34]. Initiator caspases are activated in response to signals indicating that the cell has been stressed or damaged or has received instructions to die. Cytochrome c, a mitochondrial protein, can also trigger cell death by binding to a protein called apoptotic protease activating factor-1 (Apaf-1), which activates an initiator caspase. Initiator caspases clip and activate another family of caspases, which go on to cut key proteins in the cell. Activation of a caspase can result in a cascade of proteolysis with active caspases cutting and activating more caspases.

The extraordinary activity of caspases to direct the destruction of cells means that there must be robust systems to keep caspases in check when there is no need for a cell to die. Two proteins that contribute to keep caspases and apoptosis under control are Bcl-2 and Bcl-x. They both block the release of cytochrome c from mitochondria. Bcl proteins may also bind directly to Apaf-1 to prevent caspase activation. Excess Bcl-2, however, can turn normal cells into cancer cells that resist apoptosis. Proteins called inhibitors of apoptosis (IAPs) also slow or eliminate cell death, by directly inhibiting caspases.

The pharmaceutical industry is hopeful that what we are learning now about caspases will lead to better therapies for cancer and other diseases. Researchers have recently found that cancer cells that do not heed instructions to die have high levels of a protein they call survivin. Survivin, structurally related to IAPs, probably inhibits caspases. A therapeutic strategy to inactivate survivin may make cancer cells more susceptible to conventional treatment.

On the face of it, reducing apoptotic activity would seem to be a way to ameliorate neurodegenerative damage and disease, but most experts are worried about the consequences of turning down this vital process. However, there may be other ways to address the problem. One study shows that transgenic mice with extra IAP proteins lose fewer neurons when a stroke is induced; IAPs may protect some neurons from apoptosis [*Science* 1998;280:33]. Other examples of potentially useful neuroprotective strategies are cited in another recent report [*J Clin Invest* 1998;101:1809–10].

Investigators from several institutions have reported the creation of a knockout mouse that lacks caspase 9 [*Cell* 1998;94:339–52]. Many of the study animals died perinatally with severe malformations of the brain due to a reduction of apoptosis in the proliferative neuroepithelium. This finding points to an essential role for caspase 9 and is a major step in establishing links between particular caspases and specific tissue damage.

A recent issue of *Science* [1998;281:1283,1298–99,1301–26] was largely devoted to a major multi-authored review of apoptosis and strategies for modulation. One article concerns the role of apoptosis in neuronal death resulting from stroke. When the blood supply to part of the brain is blocked, neurons in the most severely affected area die immediately from ischemia. Not understood, however, is the gradual loss of neurons in the region outside the core of the stroke, where the oxygen supply is reduced but not eliminated. Perhaps, some cells that might otherwise recover from the ischemia may be dying because the injury triggers their suicide programs [*Science* 1998; 281:1302–03].

Some scientists question whether the dying neurons are truly undergoing apoptosis, because the cells do not completely fit the textbook description of the process. Perhaps a better description of what is occurring is caspase-mediated cell death. Whatever the phenomenon is called, the cell death may be a promising target for drugs aimed at limiting stroke damage.

The view that apoptosis is the cause of neuronal death received much support from studies of stroke damage induced in mice. Compared to control animals, caspase inhibition decreased the area of stroke damage by up to 50%. Moreover, the neurons were not only preserved but seemed to remain in working order; treated mice had fewer movement and sensory impairments than controls.

Cell suicide may also play a role in Alzheimer's disease, although the benefit of blocking the process is not yet known [*Science* 1998;281:1303–04].

Researchers have found that the brains of Alzheimer's patients contain dying neurons that display characteristic signs of apoptosis, including DNA breaks. Furthermore, three proteins already linked to Alzheimer's pathology, including the toxic protein beta amyloid, seem to drive drug cells into apoptosis under certain conditions. The lack of an acceptable animal model of the disease, however, has prevented tests to determine whether inhibitors of apoptosis can protect against cell death in Alzheimer's patients, as they have in animal models of stroke.

ANGIOGENESIS

Introduction
Angiogenesis and Tumor Progression
Therapeutic Inhibition of Angiogenesis in Neoplastic Disease
Angiogenesis Inhibitors and the Media
Therapeutic Augmentation of Angiogenesis

Introduction. Angiogenesis is the proliferation of endothelial cells to form a primitive vascular bed, which is subsequently surrounded by smooth muscle to form new blood vessels. The process is fundamental to reproduction, development, and repair. The formation of blood vessels involves both positive and negative regulators of the growth of microvessels. Endogenous angiogenic proteins include basic fibroblast growth factor (bFGF) and vascular endothelial growth factor (VEGF). Among known endogenous negative regulators of endothelial-cell proliferation are angiostatin and bFGF soluble receptor.

In adults, active angiogenesis is largely pathogenic and leads to tumor growth and ocular neovascularization. Therapeutic inhibition of angiogenesis may be an effective strategy for treatment of cancer. Conversely, therapeutic acceleration of angiogenesis may hasten wound healing and salvage ischemic tissue.

Angiogenesis and Tumor Progression. In 1971, Judah Folkman postulated that malignant tumors could not expand to a clinically significant size unless they are able to induce nearby vessels to sprout a new vascular network [*N Engl J Med* 1971;285:1182–86]. In the prevascular phase, a tumor rarely grows larger than a few millimeters in diameter. Without neovascularization, the primary clump of cancerous cells depends solely on diffusion for oxygen and nutrients. When certain cells in the tumor, possibly responding to local hypoxia, switch to an angiogenic phenotype, they trigger expression of messenger RNA for VEGF and other growth factors, translation to the protein products, and vascularization.

Neovascularization greatly improves oxygenation and nutrient perfusion of the tumor as well as removal of waste products, thus permitting it to grow and metastasize. Neovascularization also heralds the onset of cancer symptoms. The development of new blood vessels at the tumor site increases the opportunity for malignant cells to enter the circulation, because newly formed capillaries have fragmented basement membranes and are more easily penetrated by tumor cells than mature vessels [*Oncology* 1997;54:177–184].

Therapeutic Inhibition of Angiogenesis in Neoplastic Disease. Researchers are now giving serious consideration to attacking tumors by cutting off their supply lines. Among the strategies for angiogenesis inhibition are: (1) inhibition of release of angiogenic factors from tumor cells and/or neutralization of angiogenic agents that have been released; (2) inhibition of vascular endothelial cell proliferation and migration; and (3) inhibition of the synthesis and turnover of the vessel basement membrane.

Clinical applications of angiogenesis research started in 1989 when interferon alfa was first used for the treatment of life-threatening hemangiomas in infants. Hemangioma of infancy is an angiomatous disorder characterized by a proliferation of capillary endothelium that usually presents as a single skin lesion. Large lesions may be life threatening if a substantial blood volume is diverted to the tumor. Interferons suppress the production of FGFs in human tumor cells. One of the angiogenic proteins over-expressed by hemangiomas is bFGF, and treatment with interferon alfa-2a results in significant tumor regression in patients with advanced disease [*N Engl J Med* 1992; 326:1456–63]

Several drugs that inhibit endothelial cell proliferation and/or migration are under investigation. Among them is the naturally secreted antibiotic fumagillin. Fumagillin inhibits a specific enzyme, methionine aminopeptidase-2, which is believed to play an important role in the proliferation of endothelial cells. TNP-470 is a less toxic synthetic analog of fumagillin and a more potent inhibitor of angiogenesis. The analog was the first angiogenesis inhibitor to be given to humans and is now in phase II trials. A recent communication reports that treatment of metastatic cervical cancer with TNP-470 in a 49-year old patient resulted unexpectedly in complete remission [*N Engl J Med* 1998;338:991–92]. Injection of Kaposi's sarcoma lesions with platelet factor 4 inhibits angiogenesis and growth factor-stimulated endothelial cell proliferation, resulting in regression of the lesions [*Oncology* 1997;54:177–84].

Proliferating endothelial cells express integrin alpha$_v$beta$_3$, an adhesion molecule that enables angiogenic endothelial cells to bind to surrounding tissues and form new blood vessels. Antibodies directed against these surface receptors are antiangiogenic. Results in a phase I clinical trial show that Vitaxin, a humanized form of the anti-alpha$_v$beta$_3$ monoclonal antibody LM609, may be efficacious in stage IV cancer patients with a variety of tumor types [*Nature Med* 1998;4:395–96].

Given its tumultuous growth, a tumor is probably the last place one would look for angiogenesis inhibitors. Defying intuition, however, researchers have found the most potent and effective anti-angiogenesis agents presently known in tumors themselves [*Science* 1997;275:482–84]. Thrombospondin, an anti-angiogenic protein also found in platelets and the extracellular matrix, emerged from this research. In the presence of thrombospondin, endothelial cells are unable to respond to angiogenic stimulation. Preliminary work suggests that breast cancer cells engineered to over-express thrombospondin lose some of their ability to promote angiogenesis.

Following the discovery of thrombospondin, other investigators isolated an angiogenesis inhibitor produced in mice by Lewis lung carcinoma and called it angiostatin. Angiostatin not only stops experimental tumor growth in mice, it also shrinks the tumor [*Nature Med* 1996;2:689–92]. More recently, this research team reported purifying yet another anti-angiogenic factor from a different metastasis-limiting tumor. This protein, called endostatin, is even more potent than angiostatin. It shrinks a variety of tumors in mice to microscopic size and keeps primary tumors and metastases in check during treatment [*Cell* 1997;88:277–85].

Drugs inhibiting angiogenesis seem to offer a treatment that is complementary to traditional chemotherapy, that does not produce resistance, and that is effective against a wide array of tumors. A seminal report by Folkman and his colleagues published in 1997 strongly supports these possibilities [*Nature* 1997;390:404–07]. The report describes the treatment of three different mouse tumors—subcutaneous carcinomas, fibrosarcomas, or melanomas—with repeat cycles of endostatin. On the first cycle, endostatin reduced tumor volume in each case by about 90%. The tumors then grew to pretreatment volume 5 to 14 days after stopping endostatin, at which time the mice again received endostatin. As the cycles continued, the investigators made two remarkable observations. The tumors did not develop resistance during treatment cycles. And after two to six cycles of endostatin therapy, the number being characteristic of the tumor cell type, the tumors did not recur on endostatin cessation. As a control, the investigators showed that the mouse carcinoma quickly developed resistance to chemotherapy with cyclophosphamide.

A commentary on this work noted: "The failure to develop resistance to endostatin during cyclic therapy that lasted from 80 to 200 days contrasts with acquired resistance to cyclophosphamide that develops within 50 days and argues for profound differences in the cellular targets of theses drugs."

The results of cyclic endostatin therapy suggest that drugs targeting angiogenesis and the tumor vasculature may be a new and effective strategy for treating human cancer. Clinical trials, however, are at least two years away [*Nature Med* 1998;4:13–14].

Another important finding that has emerged from laboratory work is that angiostatin enhances the effects of radiation on human tumors grafted into mice. Angiostatin seems to make blood vessels that supply the tumor more sensitive to radiation. The findings suggest a new way of thinking about how radiation works. Radiation was thought to be effective only against actively dividing cells. Because angiostatin inhibits the growth and division of endothelial cells, it had been thought that it and radiation therapy would not work synergistically. The opposite seems true. The study also challenges the idea held by some skeptics that while angiostatin might be effective in preventing new tumors or perhaps the dissemination of tumors, it will not work against established tumors that already have a blood supply. Folkman, commenting on the new work, said he has always envisaged that angiogenesis inhibitors would supplement, not replace, standard treatment with radiation and/or chemotherapy. He added that his studies also suggest that even established tumors should, in principle, be vulnerable to anti-angiogenesis factors [*The New York Times,* July 16, 1998, p A16].

The imaginative pioneering angiogenesis research by Folkman and those in his laboratory has stimulated great interest in other researchers and perhaps brought us to the threshold of a major advance in the treatment of cancerous tumors. Anti-angiogenesis therapy may prove to be a vital addition to chemotherapy in a wide array of tumors. Treatment with angiogenesis inhibitors also promises low toxicity and no acquired resistance.

Angiogenesis Inhibitors and the Media. Studies in angiogensis inhibition, to cut off a tumor's blood supply, has been ongoing for nearly 30 years. Many scientists have kept a keen eye on the progress of the work but, until recently, the research has been largely unheralded. *The New York Times* carried two articles describing encouraging results with endostatin and noted the pioneering work of Judah Folkman in late 1997. But, these reports had relatively little impact.

On May 3, 1998, however, a typical newsless Sunday, it seemed that the entire country was talking about angiostatin and endostatin and an imminent cure for cancer. The trigger was a feature story on the two agents titled: "A Cautious Awe Greets Drugs That Eradicate Tumors in Mice." It appeared above the fold on the first page of *The New York Times*. Gina Kolata, a highly respected science writer, prepared the article. While the story had caveats, noting that the agents have not been tested in humans and that findings in mice often do not hold up in clinical trials, it also contained a lot of hyperbole. The article included statements such as: 'Dr. Folkman will cure cancer in two years,' and '. . . angiogenesis inhibitors are the most exciting things on the horizon for the treatment of cancer and the top priority of the National Cancer Institute,' and attributed them to leading experts. That night, radio and television news programs opened broadcasts by presenting the report in the *Times* as breaking news. The next day, hundreds of newspapers carried hopeful reports about angiostatin and endostatin. In a few days, however, the media frenzy shifted and articles appeared toning down the original reports. On May 5, 1998, the front page of *The New York Times* carried an article titled: "In Excitement over Cancer Drugs, A Caution over Premature Hopes."

According to *JAMA* [1998;279:1936–37]: "The frenzy of coverage in the nation's major newspapers, national news magazines, television, radio, and on the Internet led thousands to besiege their physicians to help them obtain what some perceived as a cure for cancer." Participants in the American Society of Clinical Oncology meeting in May 1998 were troubled by the false expectations raised by the media. Several attendees stressed that bringing the war against cancer to a satisfactory conclusion will require multiple therapies. Nevertheless, almost all participants agreed that "It's a very exciting time for oncologists."

A small pharmaceutical company called EntreMed, which holds licensing rights to the patents on angiostatin and endostatin, was particularly affected by the media event. On the day after the article in the *Times*, the company's shares increased from $12 to $85 and then dropped back to close at $50. Shares of other companies developing related agents also benefited from the sudden attention.

Since the media event in May, Dr. Folkman has been hailed, received awards and citations, and rubbed elbows with the rich and the famous. A growing number of research groups, however, suggest that celebration is premature [*The Wall Street Journal*, November 12, 1998, pp A1,A18].

In science, confirmation is paramount. The crucial test of experimental data is whether scientists working independently can reproduce findings. Researchers at the National Cancer Institute (NCI) and Genentech report that they cannot replicate Folkman's results. And for more than two years, scientists at Bristol-Myers Squibb could not produce consistent results with angiostatin. One batch showed some anti-angiogenic activity while the next demonstrated little or no activity. Only recently has the company succeeded in making small batches that slow tumor growth in mice consistently. Some scientists in the company express fear that angiostatin is no more than a laboratory curiosity. A consultant to EntreMed, who once worked in Folkman's laboratory, says that he has been able to harvest many endostatin variants that slow the proliferation of blood vessels, but they are only modestly effective. He wonders whether an unknown containment might have been responsible for the dramatic effects seen in Folkman's laboratory.

Dr. Folkman is highly respected and seems to have little interest in the monetary rewards his findings might bring. However, some researchers who have worked with him say, ". . . he is single-minded in promoting his theories . . ." and perhaps ". . . he has promised too much too soon." Folkman has also struggled for many years to keep his very costly laboratory afloat and has been compelled to emphasize positive findings to secure funding from the drug industry.

Dr. Folkman strenuously defends his discoveries and says that the results have been reproduced again and again in his own laboratory. If others have had difficulty reproducing his experiments, he says it is because of the technical difficulties of isolating and working with the complex anti-angiogenic molecules. Everyone hopes the controversy will soon be put to rest. Dr. Folkman has invited the NCI to send a team of scientists to his laboratory to learn firsthand about the methods used to produce the reported results.

Therapeutic Augmentation of Angiogenesis. Patients with atherosclerosis and gradual occlusion of coronary arteries often develop collateral circulation. Neovascularization improves clinical outcomes but is almost always inadequate to compensate fully for the flow lost to occlusion. Studies in animal disease models have encouraged clinical trials to test whether angiogenic growth factors provide benefit to patients with ischemic heart disease. Patients with severe disease who are not candidates for mechanical revascularization (e.g., patients with occlusion of vessels too small to be bypassed and those who are not surgical candidates) might benefit from the application of angiogenesis-based therapy.

The first report of angiogenic therapy of human coronary heart disease appeared in *Circulation* earlier this year [1998;97:645–50]. The randomized trial involved patients with three-vessel coronary artery disease, 20 of whom received rhFGF-1 (also called acidic fibroblast growth factor) while the other 20 received inactivated rhFGF-1. The test material was injected directly into the myocardium during bypass graft surgery. Twelve weeks later, angiography showed coronary artery neovascularization extending out from the area of injection and bridging areas of stenosis. In the 20 patients who received inactivated growth factor there was no evidence of myocardial neovascularization on the 12-week angiogram.

An editorial [*Circulation* 1998;97:628–29] accompanying this seminal report observes: "An advantage of this approach is that it induces local angiogenesis and appears to avoid high levels of circulating angiogenic activity that could possibly stimulate plaque angiogenesis and secondary plaque growth." The author marvels at the persistence of neovascularization—for at least 12 weeks—after only a single set of intramyocardial injections and suggests that the persistent effect may result from upregulation of VEGF and its receptors in hypoxic tissue.

Also this year, *The Wall Street Journal* (January 6, 1998) reported the application of angiogenesis augmentation to a 60-year old man with severe atherosclerosis. The patient underwent routine coronary artery bypass graft surgery to reroute blood flow around three arterial occlusions, but a fourth obstruction defied graft replacement. The investigators then injected a gene expressing VEGF, carried by an adenovirus vector, into the myocardium near the occluded artery. The research team hopes new vessels will grow and establish normal blood flow. The *Journal* also reported that Collateral Therapeutics, a start-up company, plans to test a gene expressing fibroblast growth factor. They plan to deliver the gene without surgery into coronary arteries via catheter, also using an adenovirus as the vehicle. Yet another research group, sponsored by GenVec and Parke-Davis, plans to inject a gene for VEGF directly into the myocardium, believing that direct injection provides better dose control than delivering the gene into coronary vessels.

More recently, *The Wall Street Journal* (March 31, 1998) carried preliminary results of Genentech's efforts to biologically bypass occluded coronary vessels by infusing VEGF into coronary arteries. The investigators selected patients with viable but underperfused myocardial tissue who were not ideal candidates for coronary revascularization. Thirteen of 15 patients reported improved symptoms and reduced chest pain.

The strategies under study to rescue ischemic myocardial tissue also apply to the treatment of peripheral arterial disease. In 1996 the first report of angiogenic therapy for ischemic vascular disease was the intra-arterial gene transfer of a plasmid encoding for VEGF to a patient with severe peripheral vascular disease in a lower limb [*Lancet* 1996;348:370–74]. Four weeks after gene therapy, angiography showed an increase in collateral vessels at the knee, mid-tibial, and ankle levels that persisted for at least 12 weeks.

More recently, a research team reported that it had successfully used angiogenesis augmentation to bypass stenotic and occluded femoral arteries [*Circulation* 1998;97:1114–23]. The investigators injected naked plasma DNA for the gene responsible for making VEGF directly into skeletal muscle near a blocked artery. Ischemic ulcers healed or markedly improved in four of seven treated limbs. Three patients avoided the limb amputation that had been recommended before treatment. An editorial accompanying the report described the work as an important step in the evolving strategy of angiogenic therapy for severe limb ischemia refractory to conventional therapy [*Circulation* 1998;97:1108–09].

The understanding of angiogenesis developed through Folkman's work has allowed others to recognize that promoting angiogenesis may be a non-invasive strategy for bypassing stenoses and occlusions and for re-establishing perfusion to ischemic areas. We eagerly await the results of clinical studies evaluating these new strategies.

Gene Therapy

Delivering Genes to Target Sites Still a Major Hurdle
In Utero Gene Therapy

Delivering Genes to Target Sites Still a Major Hurdle. Not too long ago gene therapy was a darling of the scientists and investors of the biotechnology industry. Press releases describing very preliminary clinical work were issued regularly and hyped by the media. The inevitable failures went largely unnoticed. In 1996 the National Institutes of Health was compelled to urge researchers to tone down their optimism about gene therapy until efficient vectors were available to deliver genes. Today, although more than 230 gene therapy clinical trials (mostly phase I) are ongoing, there is still no ideal vector. One expert went further, observing: "No form of gene therapy can yet be considered a success and the major problem still lies in delivery mechanisms." Another likened the field of gene therapy to a tool box containing instruments researchers have not quite mastered, and the number of tools in the box—viral and nonviral vectors—keeps increasing. "People are still trying to figure out what tools to use for what disease." Yet another expert suspects that genetic treatment for hereditary disease is years away, while gene therapy for AIDS and cancer is even farther down the road [*The Scientist* May 11, 1998, pp 4–5].

The field has strongly favored viral vectors. RNA viruses (retroviruses) that can integrate a therapeutic gene (transgene) into the host genome of the cell have a good capacity for carrying genes and appear to avoid detection by the immune system. The major disadvantage of most retroviral vectors, however, is that they cannot transfect non-dividing cells. Adenoviruses are DNA viruses that can transfect dividing and non-dividing cells. They are, however, immunogenic; cells containing the virus are rapidly removed from the body. Adenoviruses may also promote inflammation. This problem plagued tests of adenoviral vectors aimed at treating cystic fibrosis. Adeno-associated viruses have most of the benefits of adenonoviruses without the baggage. They are disadvantaged, however, by having a small capacity to carry therapeutic genes.

Some investigators rest their hopes on lentiviruses—a subset of retroviruses that infect non-dividing cells [*Scrip Magazine*, October 1998, pp 43–46]. Human immunodeficiency virus (HIV) is the best known lentivirus. In theory, lentiviruses can deliver transgenes to brain, heart, lung, liver, and muscle. Current pharmaceutical development programs are aimed at treating hemophilia, cancer, and AIDS, as well as single gene disorders such as cystic fibrosis. Future therapies for Parkinson's disease, using lentiviral vectors to deliver therapeutic genes to non-dividing neurons in the brain, could ensure that dopamine is produced only where it is needed. These vectors could also be used for the treatment of cardiovascular diseases by targeting non-dividing vascular endothelial cells or muscle cells in the heart, and for cystic fibrosis by delivering genes to non-dividing lung epithelial cells. Delivery of transgenes to lymphocytes and macrophages could dramatically improve the chances of eradicating HIV infection.

One of the primary concerns of lentiviral vector gene therapy, however, is its safety, particularly since most of the data are for HIV-based systems. Nevertheless, lentiviral vectors hold great promise for future gene-based therapies.

Some researchers have abandoned viral delivery systems and embraced non-viral strategies. Among the vectors under study are cationic and cholesterol-containing liposomes, modified lipoproteins resembling chylomicrons, remnants that transport lipids in the blood, combined peptide-lipids, and combined viral components-liposomes [*Lancet* 1998;351:346]. Other nonviral strategies have been reviewed in *The Scientist* [May 11, 1998, pp 1,6].

One report in 1998 updated information on the application of gene therapy to the treatment of muscular dystrophy [*Scrip Magazine,* June 1998, pp 36–37]. Duchenne's muscular dystrophy (DMD) is a genetic disorder that primarily affects boys and causes a progressive wasting of muscle. Patients with DMD usually die in their teens of cardiac and respiratory failure. The genetic defect results in the failure to produce the skeletal protein dystrophin. In the mid-1980s, there were expectations that delivering the gene for dystrophin would quickly bring about a cure. Today, far fewer research groups work on this problem. Multiple technical barriers and the low prevalence of the disease, which limits profitability, drove many start-up companies out the field.

One barrier is that the gene that encodes for dystrophin is one of the largest known, and therefore, very difficult to fit into viral vectors. There are also immunological barriers that severely limit the duration of effect of a single dose. Those with DMD do not produce dystrophin; the protein itself is foreign and elicits an immune response. Furthermore, the coating of adenovirus, the most commonly used vector, induces a cellular and humoral immune response. The problem of the large size of the gene encoding dystrophin may yield to efforts to use smaller sections of the gene—the so-called minigene. To overcome the immune response to adenovirus, some clinical investigators have been giving patients the immunosuppressive drug tacrolimus (*Prograf*).

Another strategy to attack the disease involves a human gene that expresses a protein called urotrophin, which greatly resembles dystrophin. The urotrophin gene is unaffected in DMD. Preclinical studies suggest that up-regulation of urotrophin, could provide urotrophin-rescue for boys with DMD. Introduction of the urotrophin gene to transgenic dystrophin deficient mice stopped the necrotic process in the muscle fibers. Still another research group is using a nearly dismantled adenovirus that has the capacity to contain the entire dystrophin gene and, in theory, should reduce the immune response to the virus.

A report in *The New York Times* [August 4, 1998, B1, B13] informs that the focus of gene therapy has now shifted from inherited, rare diseases, which involve a single mutation, toward more common, more complex, and more profitable illnesses like cancer and heart disease. The president of the National Organization for Rare Disorders says: "It's only genes for things like obesity and baldness that are spurring further investigations." Of the 244 gene therapy human studies registered since 1989, 150 are aimed at cancer. Only 33 are for diseases caused by a defect in a single gene and half of those are for cystic fibrosis.

In Utero Gene Therapy. In October, a National Institutes of Health advisory committee began a discussion over whether to permit the next step in gene therapy—correcting genetic defects in a fetus before birth [*Science* 1998;282:27]. While the start of studies on fetal gene therapy are two to three years away, the strategy carries new potential risks and ethical implications. Among them is the possibility that transplanted genes could find their way into germ cells—sperm or egg—and be passed on to future generations. The worry is that the transferred gene could cause deleterious mutations.

The advisory panel has before it two pre-proposals for *in utero* therapies. The researchers hope to test fetal gene therapy on two potentially fatal diseases: the hemoglobin disorder homozygous alpha-thalassemia, and severe immunodeficiency disease caused by the lack of adenosine deaminase. The protocol for treating thalassemia involves mixing fetal blood with a retroviral vector carrying a functioning copy of the missing or defective gene that makes the protein alpha globin, and then returning the treated blood to the fetus. The hope is that the virus will insert the gene into stem cells. Because the genetic manipulation would be performed outside the womb, there would be little risk of the gene entering the fetus's germ line.

The likelihood of the vector transfecting germ line cells is much greater in the proposal for correcting ADA deficiency. In this case, the protocol calls for injecting a retroviral vector carrying the functioning ADA gene directly into the fetus's peritoneal cavity. Given prior results in sheep, the researchers hope that the vector will carry the gene into rapidly dividing bone marrow stem cells. For now, committee members asked for more experiments to assess both the risks of the proposed protocols including germ line cell transfection and their chance of success.

Monoclonal Antibodies

Human Antibodies by Design. Almost 25 years have passed since the development of the first monoclonal antibody (MAB). Only now is the technique establishing a beachhead in the clinic. A major obstacle, from the start, is that although murine MABs are easily made, they are often recognized as foreign by patients. Technical difficulties have impeded the production of fully human MABs. A recent review describes the status and relative merits of the different approaches to producing human antibody therapeutic agents [*Nature Biotech* 1998;15:535–39].

To improve the therapeutic potential of rodent MABs, chimeric antibodies have been constructed in which constant regions of the murine antibody are replaced by their human counterparts. A typical chimeric MAB is 60% to 70% human. Although freighted with immunological problems, this strategy is sometimes successful. For example, the use of a chimeric MAB for patients with colorectal adenocarcinoma shows greater persistence after a dose and improved immunogenicity. Immunogenic responses, however, remain an obstacle with chimeric antibody therapy. More than 50% of patients develop an antiglobulin response against the rodent domains after repeated dosing.

Another strategy is the use of humanized MABs, which are technically more complex to develop but seem to hold more promise than chimeric antibodies. Using known structural data, researchers make an iterative series of MABs to identify the optimal humanized MAB that retains a high affinity for the antigen but has the minimal number of foreign residues. The effort to effect a balance between retention of antigen binding and increasing risk of immunogenicity suggests that only a small number of surface-exposed residues might need to be replaced to make the surface of a murine MAB appear human. The first humanized MAB used in the clinic was CAMPATH-1H for the treatment of non-Hodgkin's lymphoma and rheumatoid arthritis. Although this preparation had clinically measurable activity, it evoked an immune response after repeated dosing. Studies with other humanized MABs, however, have shown negligible antiglobulin responses.

The display of antibody fragments on long, threadlike bacterial viruses (phage) has been used to develop the first completely human antibodies. The first human MAB directed against tumor necrosis factor and derived from phage display is in clinical trials for the treatment of rheumatoid arthritis and ocular fibrosis. Transgenic mice offer an alternative approach to the development of fully human MABs. The reviewers conclude: "Humanization has proven to be a powerful method for transferring the specificity and affinity of an existing appropriate rodent MAB into human format." They believe that although the development of so-called magic bullets is today wholly dependent on the existence of rodent MABs, this will change. "With the isolation of more and more fully human MABs from phage display and transgenic mice, it seems likely that the frequency with which rodent MABs are humanized will slowly decline."

PHARMACOGENOMICS

Genetic Strategies to Individualize Drug Therapy. Industry leaders say that genomic science will fundamentally change the way in which drugs are discovered and developed. They predict that in the future we will retreat from developing broad-spectrum drugs and advance the development of medicinal agents for genetically-defined subpopulations. "The vision of pharmacogenomics is that the discovery of genetic variances that affect drug action will lead to the development of new diagnostic procedures and therapeutic products that enable drugs to be prescribed selectively to patients for whom they will be effective and safe" [*Nature Biotech* 1998;16:492–93]. The aim of pharmacogenomics is improvement in the care of individual patients.

Fueling interest in this strategy is a growing number of reports showing marked differences in drug response among people of different genetic makeup. For example, the effects of pravastatin (*Pravachol*) on cholesterol levels are much greater in people with a cholesteryl ester transfer protein B1B1 genotype than in patients with the B1B2 or B2B2 genotype [*N Engl J Med* 1998;338:86–93]. The B1 allele is associated with increased progression of coronary atherosclerosis. Patients with the B2B2 genotype do not appear to benefit from treatment. The frequency of the genotypes in the study population was 35% B1B1, 49% B1B2, and 16% B2B2.

In Alzheimer's disease, differences in apolipoprotein E (APOE) genotype appear to explain differences in response to drug treatment. The response to treatment with tacrine (*Cognex*), which inhibits acetylcholinesterase and preserves acetylcholine in the brain, is better in patients with the APOE *E2* or APOE *E3* allele than in those carrying the APOE *E4* allele. APOE *E4* is inversely associated with residual brain choline acetyltransferase, the enzyme required for the synthesis of acetylcholine. Patients with this phenotype may not have sufficient acetylcholine to benefit from a drug that inhibits acetylcholinesterase [*Scrip*, April 10, 1998, p 22].

Another application of pharmacogenomics is the rescue of a problem drug in development or already on the market. Clozapine (*Clozaril*), for example, was one of the first atypical antipsychotic drugs developed for patients with schizophrenia, and is one of the most effective drugs in the class. Its use, however, is severely restricted because about 1% of patients develops the life-threatening blood disorder, agranulocytosis. Consequently, clozapine is used only when first-line therapies fail. If a test for an agranulocytosis drug-response gene existed to identify at-risk patients, clozapine would be first-line therapy for the 99% of patients who would not develop the side effect [*Scrip Magazine,* May 1998, pp 35–37].

The first product of pharmacogenomics to reach the US market is Genentech's *Herceptin,* a humanized monoclonal antibody aimed at the 25% to 30% of all cases of breast cancer in the US in which a mutated oncogene overproduces a cell surface growth factor receptor called HER-2. *Herceptin* and a HER-2 diagnostic kit were marketed in October 1998. If the vision of pharmacogenomics proves true, the big winner will be the targeted patient, who will realize greater effectiveness and safety from prescribed drugs.

Roche Holding in Basel, the major stockholder in Genentech, has announced its intention to market selected drugs with diagnostic tests. Roche is the first company to implement this novel business strategy. The company hopes that using genotyping methods to determine those at risk, following disease progression, and identifying individuals who are likely to respond to treatment, will eliminate a major share of the uncertainty in prescribing [*Nature Biotech* 1998;16:815].

LATE BREAKING REPORTS

New Products

New Warnings for Remicade. Centocor has issued a "Dear Doctor" letter that warns health care professionals of a potential immune reaction on re-treatment of patients with its new anti-TNF therapy *Remicade* (infliximab) [*Scrip,* November 25, 1998, p 15]. The drug is approved for the treatment of Crohn's disease and in late development for rheumatoid arthritis. The letter alerts physicians that, ". . . the risk of potentially serious delayed adverse reactions should be weighed against the potential benefit of re-treatment after a period of more than two years without treatment." The letter also said: "In those patients tested, antibodies to infliximab have been observed and the levels of infliximab were lower than expected. . . ." The reaction was seen in 10 patients with Crohn's disease; all but one first received a liquid formulation (no longer in use) of the drug. The reaction has not been observed in patients with rheumatoid arthritis.

In the Pipeline

Recombinant Bovine Fibroblast Growth Factor for Burns. Fibroblast growth factors stimulate proliferation and differentiation of endothelial cells and fibroblasts, and may be useful to accelerate wound healing. To study that application, investigators recruited 600 patients with second-degree burns. Patients received either a daily dose of topical recombinant bovine fibroblast growth factor (rbFGF) or placebo. Patients treated with rbFGF had faster granulation tissue formation and epidermal regeneration than those in the placebo group. Superficial and deep burns treated with rhFGF healed in a mean of 10 days and 17 days, respectively, compared with 12 days and 21 days, respectively, in patients treated with placebo. No adverse effects were observed. The investigators conclude that rbFGF decreases healing time and improves healing quality. "Clinical benefit would be shorter hospital stays and the patient's skin quickly becoming available for harvesting and grafting" [*Lancet* 1998;352:1661–64].

Photophoresis More Effective than Cyclosporine to Prevent Cardiac Graft Rejection. Cyclosporine-based immunosuppression has dramatically increased survival among organ transplant recipients. However, these regimens have serious side effects, place the patient at increased risk for opportunistic infections and malignancies, and are not uniformly effective. Treatments directed at suppressing donor-specific T-cell clones in recipients have potential to decrease graft rejection without increasing the toxicity of immunosuppressive drugs. One such treatment is photopheresis, an immunoregulatory technique in which lymphocytes are re-infused after exposure to a photoactive compound (methoxsalen) and ultraviolet A light. On photoactivation, methoxsalen binds to DNA bases, cell-surface molecules, and cytoplasmic components in the exposed white cells, causing a lethal defect. On re-infusion, these cells die within two weeks, but during that period they stimulate an autologous suppressor response that targets nonirradiated T-cells of similar clones.

To determine whether this technique decreases rejection episodes, investigators randomly assigned 60 cardiac transplant recipients to cyclosporine, azathioprine, and prednisone alone or with photopheresis [*N Engl J Med* 1998;339:1744–51]. After six months, patients receiving photophoresis had significantly fewer acute rejections per patient. Photopheresis also significantly increased the number of patients with only one or no rejection episodes and decreased the number with two or more rejection episodes. This benefit accrued without an increase in the incidence of infection. The work presents a preliminary look at the potential of photophoresis as an addition to standard immunosuppression in cardiac transplantation.

Therapeutic Strategies

Angiogenesis

Therapeutic Augmentation of Angiogenesis. Presentations at the American Heart Association's national meeting in November 1998 reported progress in the use of gene therapy for the treatment of peripheral and coronary artery disease. A US research team reported on 16 patients with severe refractory angina who had previously undergone bypass surgery or coronary angioplasty. The patients received a direct myocardial injection of the gene for VEGF to stimulate new blood vessel growth. Symptoms improved in all patients and the need for sublingual nitroglycerin decreased substantially. In some patients, benefit persisted for up to 90 days [*Lancet* 1998;352:1603]. A full report of the study was published in the December 22, 1998 issue of *Circulation*. Another growth factor that may be effective in this regard is fibroblast growth factor (FGF-1) [*The New York Times,* December 22, 1998, p A22].

7 Alternative Medicine

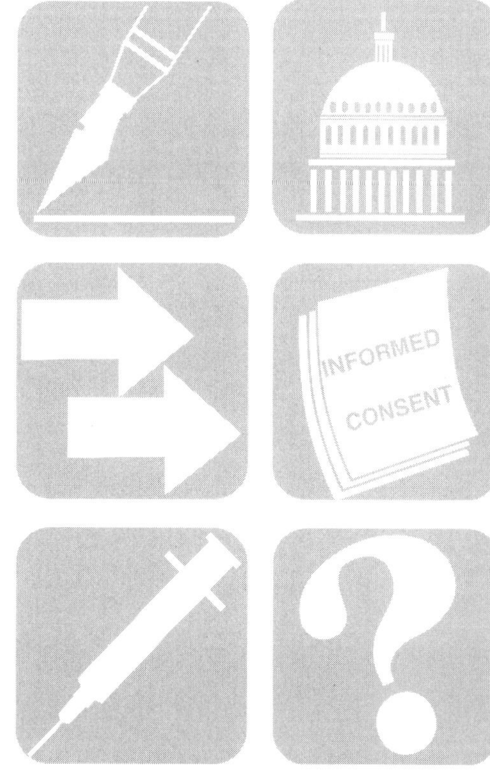

INTRODUCTION

Unconventional or alternative medicine, defined as those practices neither taught widely in US medical schools nor generally available in US hospitals, has been scorned by the medical establishment for decades. Scorn, however, is being steadily replaced by the grudging acceptance of mainstream health professionals and health care institutions. A very large number of medical patients, particularly more educated patients, are using the services and products of alternative medicine in addition to conventional therapies. Moreover, patients willingly pay out-of-pocket for alternative health services and products, because until recently their health insurance plans did not provide reimbursement. In 1993, a survey reported that 34% of adults in the US used at least one unconventional form of health care during the previous year. Today that number exceeds 50% and is growing rapidly. Most of these people also use vitamins, dietary supplements, and herbal remedies regularly.

Conventional health professions schools are no longer denying the existence of alternative medicine. A recent survey of academic or curriculum deans and faculty at each of the 125 medical schools in the US found that 64% of the schools are offering elective courses in complementary or alternative medicine or including these topics in required courses. About one third of the courses were offered by departments of family medicine and 11% by departments of medicine or internal medicine. Common topics include chiropractic, acupuncture, homeopathy, herbal therapies, and mind-body techniques [*JAMA* 1998;280:784–87].

Dissatisfaction with conventional medical therapy because of ineffectiveness, side effects, and high costs has led people to seek alternative forms of health care. A recent survey, however, reveals that people turn to alternative medicine largely because, ". . . they find these health care alternatives to be more congruent with their own values, beliefs, and philosophical orientation toward health and life" [*JAMA* 1998;279:1548–53].

CLINICAL STUDIES

Vitamin E Cuts Risk of Prostate Cancer

Multivitamins, Folate, and Colon Cancer in Women

Vitamins, Homocysteine Levels, and the Risk of
  Cardiovascular Disease

Ginkgo for Dementia

Garlic Has No Effect on Elevated Cholesterol Levels

DHEA for Aging

Selenium May Protect Against Prostate Cancer

Supplementing Fatty Acids in Infant Formula Enhances
  Problem Solving

Cancer Cure Sweeps Italy

Vitamin E Cuts Risk of Prostate Cancer. A large primary prevention trial in 50–69 year-old smokers has shown that a vitamin E supplement in the form of alpha-tocopherol reduces the risk of prostate cancer by about one-third [*J Natl Cancer Inst* 1998;90:440–46]. Cancer of the prostate is the fourth most common malignancy in men. The study panel consisted of 29,000 Finnish men who smoked. The investigators randomly assigned them to 50 mg vitamin E (about three times the recommended daily allowance), 20 mg beta-carotene, both, or placebo and followed them for up to eight years.

At the end of study, there were 246 new cases of prostate cancer that resulted in 62 deaths. Incidence was 32% lower and mortality was 41% lower in men taking vitamin E than for those not taking the vitamin. There was a higher incidence of hemorrhagic stroke among men receiving vitamin E, but the difference was not statistically significant. The reduction in prostate cancer incidence was evident within two years after starting supplementation; this led researchers to suggest that vitamin E may influence the transformation phase of cancer from latent to clinical. Beta-carotene was without significant effect, but trended toward a higher incidence of prostate cancer and a higher mortality. Previous work by these investigators in the same population associated beta-carotene supplementation with a higher incidence of lung cancer.

A co-author of the report observed that more detailed analyses of the results indicate that vitamin E might provide some protection against colorectal cancer and, after five years of supplementation, some protection against lung cancer. The degree of protection, however, was not at the level seen for prostate cancer. He suggests that a pattern of a broad cancer preventive effect from vitamin E supplementation is developing. An important question remains: Will vitamin E also protect against prostate cancer in men who do not smoke?

In an earlier report on the same cohort of male smokers, the investigators found that those taking vitamin E experienced a reduction in deaths from coronary heart disease and ischemic stroke. The amount of vitamin E used in these studies may be reached by consuming foods rich in vitamin E rather than a supplement, but this would require a high intake of dietary fat.

Multivitamins, Folate, and Colon Cancer in Women. Long-term use of multivitamins reduces the risk of colon cancer by 75% according to an analysis of food questionnaires given to 88,756 women participating in the Nurses' Health Study [*Ann Intern Med* 1998;129:517–24]. The benefit, however, is slow to evolve and was realized only after 15 years of use. The researchers suggest that folic acid in the vitamin preparations may explain their protective effects.

Vitamins, Homocysteine Levels, and the Risk of Cardiovascular Disease. The potential role of elevated levels of homocysteine in the pathogenesis of cardiovascular disease was first recognized nearly 30 years ago. Most clinical and population studies find that a moderately elevated level of homocysteine is an independent risk factor for coronary heart disease (CHD), stroke, and peripheral arterial occlusive disease, comparable in importance with an elevated level of cholesterol, smoking, and hypertension. A more recent study, however, of more than 15,000 men and women with atherosclerosis finds that homocysteine levels in plasma are not an independent risk factor for coronary heart disease [*Circulation* 1998;98:204–10]. Other epidemiological studies associate deficiencies of folate, vitamin B_6, and vitamin B_{12} in the diet, and low plasma levels of these vitamins, with elevations of plasma homocysteine. Conversely, folic acid supplementation and diets rich in folate and other B-complex vitamins reduce levels of plasma homocysteine [*N Engl J Med* 1998;338:42–50].

Does a reduction in plasma homocysteine lower the risk of CHD? A recent report, while not the final word, supports that premise [*JAMA* 1998;279:359–64]. Investigators from the Nurses Health Study, evaluating self-reports from more than 80,000 women, found a significant inverse relation between folate and vitamin B6 dietary intakes and CHD (nonfatal MI and fatal CHD-related event) during a 14-year period. Women in the highest quintile of both folate (median 696 μg/day) and vitamin B6 (4.6 mg/day) intake were 45% less likely to suffer CHD than women in the lowest quintile of folate (158 μg/day) and vitamin B6 (1.1 mg/day) intake. Risk of CHD was also nearly 25% lower among women who regularly used multiple vitamins, a major source of folate and vitamin B6.

The investigators conclude that a daily intake of 400 μg folate and 3 mg vitamin B_6 protects against CHD. They add that the current RDA for folate of 180 μg/day and for vitamin B_6 of 1.6 mg/day may not be sufficient to minimize CHD risk. An accompanying editorial observed: "The findings of the current study encourage the view that with intervention through supplementation, fortification, improved dietary intakes of folate and vitamin B_6, . . . the decline in US cardiovascular mortality and morbidity will continue" [*JAMA* 1998:279:392–93].

Cereal-grain products in the US are now fortified with folic acid (140 μg per 100 g of product). The decision to add folate stems from concern that the intake of food-based folic acid by many American women of childbearing potential is below the recommended dietary allowance (RDA). Inadequate folate may lead to a high incidence of neural-tube defects in their offspring. The FDA estimates that the level of supplementation now required increases folic acid intake by about 100 μg/day.

Will the current level of supplementation with folic acid in cereal-grain products reduce homocysteine levels to a clinically important degree in people at risk? To test that hypothesis, investigators assessed the effects of breakfast cereal fortified with three levels of folic acid in men and women with coronary artery disease [*N Engl J Med* 1998;338:1009–15]. They found that plasma folic acid increases and plasma homocysteine decreases proportionately with the folic acid content of the cereal. Cereal providing 127 μg of folic acid daily decreases homocysteine levels by only 4%, whereas cereals providing 499 and 665 μg of folic acid daily decrease plasma homocysteine by 11% and 14%, respectively. The modest change resulting from the cereal providing only 127 μg of folate daily suggests that levels of fortification higher than FDA's recommendation may be warranted if indeed lower levels of homocysteine reduce heart disease.

A case-control study has recently shown an association between stroke and low circulating levels of vitamin B_6 and folate [*Circulation* 1998;97:437–43]. The investigators measured plasma levels of total homocysteine, red cell folate, and vitamins B_6 and B_{12} in patients less than 60 years of age with documented vascular disease as well as in healthy control subjects.

They found lower vitamin B_6 levels in patients with vascular disease than in healthy controls. Study participants with vitamin B_6 levels in the lowest quintile were almost twice as likely to have heart disease or stroke as those with higher levels of vitamin B_6. Folate levels were also lower in patients with vascular disease than in healthy controls. Study participants with folate levels in the lowest 10th percentile were about 1.5 times as likely to have heart disease or stroke as those in highest 10th percentile.

These associations are possibly related to the effects of folate on the metabolism of homocysteine. However, the investigators also found that the relationship between vitamin B_6 and atherosclerosis was independent of homocysteine levels. An editorial, commenting on the study, cautioned that the results should be considered preliminary. The author warned that an association should not be described as an effect and noted that controlled clinical trials are needed to test the long-term effects of correcting deficiencies in vitamin B_6 to prevent cardiovascular disease [*Circulation* 1998;97: 421–24].

A recent commentary notes that epidemiological studies, no matter how well designed or how large, cannot refute the null hypothesis that there is no causal association between elevated homocysteine levels and risk of vascular disease or atherosclerosis. The test of this hypothesis requires well-controlled clinical trials. The importance of the question compels the authors to urge the initiation of secondary prevention trials, which require smaller sample sizes and shorter follow up times than primary prevention trials. "If secondary prevention trials show a direct benefit of lowering homocysteine with vitamin supplements on the risk of cardiovascular disease, then the causal hypothesis would be greatly strengthened. . . . Trials using intermediate vascular end points may also be of some value" [*Circulation* 1998;98: 196–99].

Ginkgo for Dementia. Extracts made from the leaves of the ginkgo tree (*Ginkgo biloba*) are available in the US as dietary supplements and in France and Germany as licensed drugs for treatment of dementias. In Germany, extracts are standardized for antioxidant content—ginkgo flavonoids and terpenoids. Antioxidants scavenge free radicals, which have been implicated in the pathogenesis of Alzheimer's disease. Studies have shown an effect of ginkgo extract on the electroencephalogram. A drawback is that a terpenoid in ginkgo interferes with platelet aggregation and blood clotting and may lead to bleeding.

A one year controlled trial shows that patients with dementia treated daily with ginkgo extracts score higher on a performance-based cognitive test than those treated with placebo. Rating scales scored by the patients' caregivers also rank the ginkgo group higher than placebo; rating scales scored by the patients' physician, however, show no difference between ginkgo and placebo [*JAMA* 1997;278:1327–32]. Because fewer than half the patients completed the study, its impact is diminished.

An article in the *Medical Letter* [1998;40:63–64] concludes: "Extracts of *Ginkgo biloba* might improve mental function in some patients with dementia, but available data suggest that the benefits, if any, are modest." In a German post-marketing surveillance study the drug appeared to be safe, but serious bleeding has been reported.

Garlic Has No Effect on Elevated Cholesterol Levels. Despite claims that garlic is a "naturally" effective remedy for elevated cholesterol levels, a recent study reports no effects of garlic oil on blood lipid profile [*JAMA* 1998; 279:1900–02]. The investigators enrolled 25 people with moderately elevated total- and LDL-cholesterol levels into a double-blind placebo-controlled, crossover study investigating the effects of taking a commercially available preparation of garlic oil. After a four-week placebo run-in phase, participants received either placebo or garlic oil for 12 weeks. Following a four-week placebo washout period, the participants were crossed over for another 12 weeks. The dose of garlic oil corresponded to 4–5 g of fresh garlic clove daily. The commercial preparation of garlic oil had no effect on serum lipoproteins, cholesterol absorption, or cholesterol synthesis.

Earlier meta-analyses had reported reductions of total cholesterol of between 9% and 12%. Confidence in these data, however, is limited. Many of the studies that met the inclusion criteria of the meta-analysis were of poor quality and because there were so few studies reporting negative results, publication bias is another possible confounder. While the new report clearly rules out a large effect of garlic on serum lipids, the small number of subjects participating in the trial does not allow a complete dismissal of the possibility that garlic has a modest effect.

A second, more robust trial evaluated the effects of garlic powder (*Kwai*) on patients with mild to moderate hypercholesterolemia [*Arch Intern Med* 1998;158:1189–94]. Participants had low-density lipoprotein cholesterol levels no greater than 160 mg/dl and triglyceride levels no greater than 350 mg/dl. They were randomized to 300 mg garlic powder three times daily or corresponding placebo. Twenty-eight patients received garlic powder and 22 received placebo. At the end of 12 weeks, neither garlic nor placebo significantly changed the baseline lipid profile and there were no differences between changes in the two groups. The investigators conclude that 900 mg garlic powder per day is ineffective in lowering cholesterol levels but encourage trials to determine if garlic has effects on fibrinolysis and platelet adhesion, both potential targets for preventing coronary heart disease.

DHEA for Aging. The definition of a dietary supplement adopted by the United States Congress is so broad that it embraces virtually every agent found in nature. One of the more bizarre examples is dehydroepiandrosterone (DHEA). Sold without a prescription, DHEA is said to retard the aging process. The premise of the claim is that natural DHEA concentrations peak in the third decade of life and then decline steadily to about 10% of peak values by age 80. Ergo, supplementation replaces the lost DHEA and returns the body to its youthful vigor.

The results of one of the first studies in humans shows that in a panel of 13 postmenopausal women DHEA increases levels of insulin-like growth factor (IGF-1) in serum [*Fertil Steril* 1998;69:107–10]. This suggests that DHEA might increase muscle mass and strength in older women. A concern, however, is that elevated levels of IGF-1 are linked with breast cancer. Of further concern is that DHEA is converted to androgens and estrogen which could adversely effect glucose tolerance and lipid profile. Androgenic side effects such as hirsutism and acne can also occur.

Despite safety issues, a core of researchers strongly believe that restoring levels of DHEA must result in some benefit. A study is ongoing to determine the cardiovascular consequences of the decrease in circulating plasminogen activator inhibitor type I and tissue plasminogen activator antigen seen in people taking DHEA. Other investigators are studying the potential neuroprotective and antidepressant effects of DHEA. Where these efforts will lead is not evident [*Lancet* 1998;352:208].

Selenium May Protect Against Prostate Cancer. In August, *The New York Times* [August 19, 1998, p A19] reported the results of a case-control study of 181 men with advanced prostate cancer and 181 matched controls. The study found that high levels of selenium in toenail clippings—a measure of long-term selenium intake—are associated with a reduced risk of advanced prostate cancer. Selenium is essential for the activity of glutathione peroxidase, which might protect cellular DNA from oxidative damage. Too much selenium, however, is harmful. A scientist at the National Cancer Institute cautioned that the research was still, ". . . one or two steps away from being able to recommend supplementation."

When comparing the highest to the lowest quintile of selenium levels, higher selenium levels were associated with a 50% reduced risk of advanced prostate cancer. After controlling for family history of prostate cancer, and other relevant risk factors, the investigators found a 65% reduction in the likelihood of advanced prostate cancer among those in the highest quintile compared with those in lowest quintile [*J Natl Cancer Inst* 1998;90:1219–24]. The investigators speculate that selenium might act as an antioxidant or it might stimulate apoptosis—programmed cell death.

An earlier study found that patients who took daily doses of selenium had significantly fewer cases of prostate cancer, colon or rectal cancers, and lung cancer than did those not using a supplement. The study was conducted in patients with histories of basal and squamous carcinomas who were living in areas of the US with low soil selenium content. The participants had a daily selenium dietary intake of only 90 mcg. The investigation determined that men randomly assigned to receive 200 μg selenium daily over 4.5 years had a relative risk of 0.35 for prostate cancer compared with those assigned placebo [*JAMA* 1996;276:1957–63]. The results provide strong support for a cause-and-effect relationship.

A recent commentary in *The Lancet* [1998;352:755–56] called attention to the fact that selenium intakes in the UK have been falling over several decades, largely because of a decrease in imported flour from North American, in favor of the selenium-poor flour of European, countries. A recent survey indicates that the average intake in some regions of the UK may be as low as 30 to 40 μg/day. During this period of declining intakes, prostate cancer incidence and mortality have increased substantially in England and Wales. The report concludes: ". . . the evidence available for prostate cancer seems to justify the further assessment of increasing the selenium intake in the population as a priority for public health."

The current RDA for selenium is 70 μg/day. The amount of selenium that reduces the risk of prostate cancer seems to be 150 to 200 μg/day. Patients should be urged not to exceed a total intake of selenium of 200 μg/day [*Prescriber's Letter*, October 1998, p 58].

Supplementing Fatty Acids in Infant Formula Enhances Problem Solving. Long-chain polyunsaturated fatty acids (PUFAs) may have important functional effects on membrane and cellular properties of neural tissue. Investigators have reported that concentrations of long-chain PUFAs are lower in infants who receive unsupplemented formula than in those infants receiving breast milk or formula supplemented with long-chain PUFAs. It remains uncertain whether this relative deficiency of long-chain PUFAs in formula-fed term infants at a critical time of early brain development has cognitive consequences.

To assess this possibility, researchers randomized 44 term infants for their first four months of life to a formula supplemented with long-chain PUFAs or to a formula with the same composition but not containing long-chain PUFAs [*Lancet* 1998;352:688–91]. Infant cognitive behavior was assessed at ten months of age by a problem-solving test of uncovering and retrieving a hidden toy that required three intermediate steps to achieve the final goal.

At the end of the study, there were no differences between groups in formula intake or anthropometric measures. On the other hand, infants receiving formula supplemented with long-chain PUFAs had significantly more solutions to problems than did infants who received unsupplemented formula. These findings suggest that formula-fed term infants benefit from supplementation and that the effects persist beyond the period of supplementation. The results are important because higher scores on such problem-solving tests are related to IQ in later childhood. That the group receiving supplemented formula had significantly higher scores on the final step of the three-step solution suggests that memory or attention control was improved.

Cancer Cure Sweeps Italy. Earlier this year we learned that a magistrate, moved by the plight of a child with astrocytoma in southern Italy, ordered local health authorities to pay for an experimental cancer treatment that costs up to $6,000 a month. This was especially unusual because the ruling overturned Italian regulations on state funding of medication. Dr Luigi di Bella, an 86-year old Italian physiologist and physician, developed the drug cocktail for the experimental treatment. He claims that the mixture stops tumor growth and avoids the disabling effects of chemotherapy. Di Bella further claims that he has successfully treated thousands of cancer patients with the drug cocktail. The preparation has been dubbed MDB—"Multiterapia di Bella".

The exact composition of MDB varies from patient to patient, but always contains somatostatin and usually includes melatonin, adenosine, and multivitamins. For an individual patient, the mixture may also contain very low doses of cyclophosphamide, parathyroid hormone, corticotropin, bromocriptine, and retinoids [*Lancet* 1998;351:303–04]. Dr di Bella says that MDB does not attack cancerous cells but strengthens healthy ones, making the body more able to fight the disease.

The Italian media heralded the "cure" for months on an almost daily basis, created a frenzy of interest, and lionized di Bella. The press claimed that the state's reluctance to recognize MDB was the result of a conspiracy between the government and the drug industry against the little people. Di Bella said that big drug companies are afraid his therapy might work so well that physicians would no longer want to prescribe their products. Adding their voice to the cacophony, several cardinals said that the treatment should be given free to all those who could benefit from it. They did not, however, offer to open their churches' coffers [*Scrip Magazine,* July/August 1998, pp 7–9].

With considerable emotion, Italians took to the streets to prod the government to establish a generous reimbursement policy for MDB. An academic sociologist in Milan explains, "This is a Catholic country, a country that believes in miracles. Half the country was moved when a Madonna [statue] allegedly cried tears of blood, and in this case we are talking about a cure for cancer" [*The Wall Street Journal,* April 21, 1998]. As excitement spread, the Italian government acquiesced to public pressure and stated its intent to initiate clinical trials of di Bella's unproven method. The companies that manufacture somatostatin provided it at no cost to patients participating in the studies.

Di Bella denounced the initial protocol for the trials as too restrictive. He objected to the requirement that doctors obtain informed consent from patients and provide proof that they have failed other anticancer therapies. He also wanted more treatment options for specific patients. Italy's professional federation for physicians accused di Bella of trying to stop the trials because he was afraid that the treatment would fail when tested rigorously. Nevertheless, the government, under great pressure from the media, the right-wing opposition, and the hundreds of thousands in the streets, agreed to most of the changes stipulated by di Bella and started clinical testing. To satisfy the demands of di Bella, ten different protocols were drawn up and therapy varied depending on the protocol and the type of cancer [*Scrip Magazine,* July/

August 1998, pp7-9]. Agents used in the trial were vitamin A, beta-carotene, vitamin E, bromocriptine, melatonin, and, most important, somatostatin.

By July 1998, enough data had been collected to show that the Italian wonder cure did not work [*Lancet* 1998;352:207]. In one-third of the patients the disease remained unchanged, in half the patients the researchers saw local progression, and in about 15% there were new metastases. Only one of 300 hundred patients showed a partial response and four had a minor response. Adverse effects—nausea, vomiting, and diarrhea—were common.

The Health Minister welcomed the results, hoping that they would put an end to the "squabbles." A well-regarded Italian physician and clinical pharmacologist said the results amount to, ". . . finally proving that donkeys cannot fly, hardly a surprising finding" [*Lancet* 1998;352:460]. Although di Bella approved the protocols, he and his advocates now declare the data invalid. They claim the cocktail did not work because it was given without key ingredients. Italian health authorities have convincingly refuted each claim.

REGULATORY ISSUES

Huperzine for Alzheimer's Disease: End Run Around FDA
FDA Challenges Marketing of Herb to Lower Cholesterol
Medicated Skin Preparations—Drugs or Cosmetics?
Sleep-Aid Found to be Contaminated
The Safety of Dietary Supplements

Huperzine for Alzheimer's Disease: End Run Around FDA. Huperzine is a natural product that has activity similar to the cholinesterase inhibitor donepezil (*Aricept*). *Aricept* is approved by-prescription-only for the treatment of Alzheimer's disease. Huperzine is an alkaloid extracted from a Chinese plant. It is commercially available in China as a prescription drug for dementia. Clinical trials suggest that huperzine improves memory and cognition in the elderly.

Although huperzine has never been tested in the US, it is already being sold over the Internet. Furthermore, Nutrapharm plans to market it as a dietary supplement at stores that sell vitamin and nutrition products under the name *Cerebra*. Under current law, natural products generally can be sold as over-the-counter medication, providing they are safe and that the product label does not characterize them as treatments for disease. The law does not require a demonstration of effectiveness. Data on the safety of huperzine in humans are sparse; Nutrapharm carried out a short-term 20-person tolerance study with huperzine to look for possible side effects and found none. The company was not required to do so.

Nutrapharm makes no claims for *Cerebra* in the treatment of Alzheimer's disease. Packaging refers to enhancements in focus, memory, and concentration. Dietary supplements such as huperzine are regulated largely by the Dietary Supplement Health & Education Act (DSHEA) of 1994. The act defines a dietary supplement as a product (other than tobacco) intended to supplement the diet, that contains one or more of certain dietary ingredients, such as a vitamin, a mineral, an herb, or other botanical, an amino acid, a dietary substance for use by man to supplement the diet by increasing the total dietary intake, or a concentrate, metabolite, constituent, extract, or combination of the preceding ingredients. Of potential concern to physicians and patients is huperzine's possible interactions with drugs routinely used in the treatment of Alzheimer's [*Chem Eng News,* June 1, 1998, pp 45–47].

FDA Challenges Marketing of Herb to Lower Cholesterol. The protracted disagreement between the FDA and Pharmanex, the manufacturer of *Cholestin,* is now in the courts. The outcome may shed some light on the distinction between a drug and a dietary supplement.

Cholestin is marketed as a dietary supplement to lower elevated cholesterol levels. It contains a strain of rice imported from China that is fermented with red yeast. The crux of the debate is that *Cholestin* naturally contains 11 naturally occurring HMG-CoA reductase inhibitors, including lovastatin. Lovastatin is a prescription-only drug sold by Merck under the name *Mevacor.* Patients with coronary artery disease as well as people at a lower risk, when treated with *Mevacor,* realize lower total- and LDL-cholesterol levels, higher HDL-cholesterol levels, and improved cardiovascular outcomes. When first marketed, the *Cholestin* label listed lovastatin as a constituent and made specific claims about lowering cholesterol.

Merck petitioned the FDA to rule that *Cholestin* should be treated as a drug, contending that the product is a disguised version of lovastatin. Some say *Cholestin* is pushing the Dietary Supplement Health and Education Act (DSHEA) to the limit. Others argue that the FDA is over-reaching its authority by trying to regulate *Cholestin* as a drug.

In autumn 1997 the FDA ruled tentatively that *Cholestin* is a drug for the following reasons: (1) it contains lovastatin; (2) its launch *followed* FDA approval of lovastatin as a drug; (3) its label claims that it can reduce or prevent hypercholesterolemia; (4) Pharmanex uses manufacturing processes to maximize and standardize levels of lovastatin in the product; and (5) Pharmanex recommends a daily dose that results in an intake of about 5.6 mg of lovastatin, more than half the minimum recommended daily dose of *Mevacor.* [*Scrip,* 1998, No 2301, p 21].

To assuage the FDA, Pharmanex introduced new labeling with no mention of lovastatin and no specific health claims. The company replaced these statements with a more general claim that *Cholestin* promotes healthy cholesterol levels in combination with a healthy diet and regular exercise. The FDA said that was not enough and on May 22, 1998 announced its intention to ban the sale of *Cholestin.* Three weeks later, a federal judge hearing Pharmanex's appeal ordered the agency to permit the company to continue making *Cholestin* while the court case proceeds. He declared preliminarily that *Cholestin* is a dietary supplement and not a drug [*The New York Times,* June 17, 1998]. The case is viewed as a pivotal battle between the FDA, which is struggling to exert its authority under the 1994 dietary supplement act that left it almost powerless to regulate herbal products. The dietary supplement industry has been growing at a furious pace since the law was passed.

Medicated Skin Preparations—Drugs or Cosmetics? Many of the new cosmetics reaching the market are suggested to have drug-like effects, such as repair of sun damage and reversal of aging skin. These cosmetics are sometimes called cosmeceuticals, a term the FDA does not recognize and does not like. "Cosmetics are defined by law as products not intended to affect the body's structure or functions, and drugs are defined as products that do so" [*JAMA* 1998;279:1595–96].

New or reformulated cosmetic products often contain hydroxy acids, natural substances that induce mild inflammation and accelerate the removal of dead skin. The most widely used of these chemicals are the alpha-hydroxyacids (AHAs) such as glycolic acid. A former director of the American Medical Association's Committee on Cosmetics observes: "A little inflammation isn't bad. It improves skin coloring and evens skin tone. A little edema puffs out fine wrinkles" [*Ibid.*]. Nevertheless, concern remains about decreasing the skin's barrier function or increasing its sensitivity to the sun on long-term use of products containing AHAs.

An independent panel of physicians and other scientists has recently evaluated the safety of glycolic acid and other AHAs. The group concluded that AHAs were safe for use by consumers at a concentration of less than 10% and at a pH of 3.5 or greater. The review panel also found that AHAs increased sensitivity to the sun by an average of 13%, but by as much as 50% in some people. Some members of the panel urged the industry to develop some products that contain both AHAs and a sunscreen. All agreed that people who use these preparations be advised to use daily sun protection, including sunscreens and protective clothing.

The FDA is not convinced that the problem can be solved that easily. The agency has referred AHAs to the National Toxicology Program for a study of phototoxicity, a process that will take several years to complete. Other new cosmetic ingredients alleged to provide therapeutic benefits include vitamins C and E, botanicals such as wild yam extract, and the vitamin A derivative retinol.

Sleep-Aid Found to be Contaminated. Researchers at the Mayo Clinic report finding a potentially harmful contaminant in the popular dietary supplement

5-hydroxy-L-tryptophan (5-HTP). 5-HTP is sold as a remedy for insomnia, depression, obesity, and other ills. The investigators first identified the component—6-hydroxy-1, 2, 3, 4, 4a, 9a-hexahydro-beta-carboline-3-carboxylic acid—in a sample of 5-HTP used by a person who developed symptoms of eosinophilia-myalgia syndrome (EMS). They then found the containment at levels ranging from 3% to 15% in six different samples of 5-HTP purchased from health and nutrition stores in Minnesota and New York [*Nature Med* 1998;4:983].

The researchers' concerns are enhanced because popular books promoting herbal remedies recommend large doses of 5-HTP. The FDA has begun testing samples of the dietary supplement. 5-HTP bears a chemical relationship with another erstwhile dietary supplement, L-tryptophan, which was taken off the market in 1990 following the discovery of an association between its use and an outbreak of EMS leading to serious illness and even death in some patients. Contaminated L-tryptophan from a manufacturer in Japan was said to be responsible for the outbreak, but that was never proved. After L-tryptophan was banned, 5-HTP took its place. In the body, both compounds are converted to serotonin.

The Safety of Dietary Supplements. Six articles in a recent issue of the *New England Journal of Medicine* report that some people using products from health food stores have become seriously ill. The reports describe an array of disorders that result from herbs themselves, toxic contaminants, or adulteration with drugs or hormones. A letter describes an adolescent male with treatable Hodgkin's disease whose family spurned chemotherapy in favor of an herbal product until the disease advanced beyond the efficacy of any treatment. The same report describes a nine-year-old girl who underwent complete resection of a brain tumor. Rather than agreeing to treatment with chemotherapy and radiotherapy after the surgery, her parents opted to treat their child with shark cartilage. Four months later, marked tumor progression was documented and the patient subsequently died. The three-year survival rate after adjuvant therapy for this tumor is more than 50% [*N Engl J Med* 1998;339:846].

Another letter reported that 83 of 260 samples of herbal products from Asia contained heavy metals or other chemicals not listed on the label [*N Engl J Med* 1998;339:847]. A report from Arizona noted that although the FDA has banned the sale of body-building supplements that contain gamma-hydroxybutyric acid, which may precipitate coma and apnea, similar alternative products continue to be marketed. A product called *RenewTrient,* described on its label as a dietary supplement that stimulates the body's own natural production of growth hormone, contains gamma-butyrolactone, a precursor of gamma-hydroxybutyric acid. The authors describe a case of central nervous system depression following a two-ounce dose of *RenewTrient* [*N Engl J Med* 1998;339:847–48]. A brief report noted that a "natural laxative" contaminated with digitalis resulted in the hospitalization of two women who used the product [*N Engl J Med* 1998;339:806–11].

The lead article in that issue of the *Journal* concerned the biological activity of an estrogenic herbal combination used in prostate cancer treatment [*N Engl J Med* 1998;339:785–91]. PC-SPES is a commercially available combination of eight herbs. The product is promoted as a natural nonestrogenic treatment for prostate cancer. To the contrary, laboratory tests and studies in mice show that the product has considerable estrogenic activity. Six of six men with prostate cancer demonstrated decreased serum concentrations of testosterone after using PC-SPES. In eight male patients, the herbal product decreased serum concentrations of prostate-specific antigen. All eight patients had breast tenderness and loss of libido. The investigators conclude: "PC-SPES has potent estrogen activity. The use of this unregulated mixture of herbs may confound the results of . . . therapies and may produce clinically significant adverse effects."

Although the collection of reports involves only about a dozen patients, critics of the dietary supplement industry say that this is only the tip of the iceberg. An editorial in that issue criticized makers of supplements and practitioners of alternative medicine for advocating unproved and potentially harmful treatments [*N Engl J Med* 1998;339:839–41]. The editors of the *Journal* wrote that, "Alternative treatments should be subjected to scientific testing no less rigorous than that required for conventional treatments."

The industry responded to the criticisms by claiming that dietary supplement makers have no more errors and mishaps than do food or pharmaceutical producers [*The New York Times,* September 17, 1998, p A25]. A follow-up article in the *Times,* however, warned that, "Growing numbers of Americans are stepping daily into a potential minefield of substances loosely referred to as dietary supplements, many of which have little or nothing to do with the components of foods people normally consume" [September 22, 1998, p D13]. The September issue of the magazine *New Choices: Living Even Better After 50* cautions against taking five herbal remedies: chapparal, comfrey, germander, lobelia, and yohimbine.

This unplanned collection of reports questioning the safety of dietary supplements is the first gauntlet to be thrown down before the booming supplements industry since Congress acted to limit their regulation in 1994, reigned in the FDA, and signaled the industry that almost anything goes. The new law stipulates that to take a product off the market the FDA must prove it unsafe. Before the law, and still applicable to all pharmaceutical products, a manufacturer must demonstrate safety before FDA would approve a product.

OTHER REPORTS

St. John's Wort for Depression
Kava: The Next Herbal Superstar
Saw Palmetto for Enlarged Prostate
Soy Foods for Perimenopausal Estrogen Deficiency
Androstenedione and Athletic Performance
Horse Chestnut Seed Extract for Varicose Veins
Brand-Name Companies Want a Piece of the Dietary
    Supplement Market
The "Made in Italy" Answer to the Problem of Impotence
Update on Vitamin Supplements
JAMA Devotes November to Alternative Medicine

St. John's Wort for Depression. A commentary in *JAMA* [1998;279;1437–38] alerted family medicine physicians of the wide use of an herbal product called St. John's wort. The preparation is available in health food stores and in many pharmacies. The herbal extract contains a host of pharmacologically active substances. The principle ingredient is thought to be hypericin. Hypericin inhibits reuptake of serotonin, norepinephrine, and dopamine. This inhibition profile overlaps both first- and second-generation antidepressants. Typical of herbal products, the concentration of hypericin in the extract varies widely depending on where the plant is grown, what time of year it is harvested, and what part of the plant is used. An independent survey commissioned by the *Los Angeles Times* tested ten brands of St. John's wort and found that seven had less active ingredient than promised on the label. Three contained less than 50%.

A meta-analysis of clinical trials embracing nearly 1800 depressed patients suggests that St. John's wort is more effective than placebo [*BMJ* 1996;313:253–58]. A few studies show that the herbal antidepressant is about equal in effectiveness to low doses of standard antidepressants, at least in the short term. No controlled studies have compared St. John's wort with standard doses of antidepressants or evaluated the use of the herbal extract for more than 12 weeks. The authors of the *JAMA* article suggest that family medicine practitioners tell patients with moderate to severe depression that conventional antidepressants have well-documented effectiveness and well-defined adverse effects, and that the active ingredients, potency, purity, and safety of the formulations of St. John's wort sold in the US are unknown. St. John's wort is also available as a skin patch. Nothing is known of the transdermal absorption of the herbal extract and the product is best avoided.

Kava: The Next Herbal Superstar. Readers of *The Wall Street Journal* [February 26, 1998, pp B1, B2] learned of the intense interest in kava, an herbal remedy derived from an obscure South Pacific plant. Its known active ingredients are kavalactones, which have muscle relaxant activity and a mildly depressing effect on the nervous system. Promotions suggest that kava is nature's way to reduce stress and heal anxiety. Manufacturers use phrases such as "the solution to the yuppie blues," inviting consumers to "move to another state" and "relax naturally."

The author of the obligatory self-help book on kava and a leading advocate of its use describes his first taste as follows: "A sensuous wave of muscular relaxation washed slowly throughout my entire body like India ink spreading on white paper." Manufacturers are trying to emphasize the remedial qualities of kava and tone down its recreational aura. This will not be an easy task, considering that some brands of kava are called *Rapture* and *Happy Camper*.

In 1996, Americans spent $15 million on kava, and twice that much in 1997. Human studies with kava have been conducted largely in Germany, where investigators find kava helpful in alleviating anxiety, easing symptoms of menopause, and ameliorating sleep disturbances and emotional problems. Although German researchers claim no side effects, kava is not entirely benign. Road signs on some Pacific islands warn against drinking kava and driving. Because it is a depressant, kava should not be taken with alcohol or sedating drugs.

Saw Palmetto for Enlarged Prostate. Saw palmetto is a dwarf palm tree, native to the southeast region of the US. A trade journal, *US Pharmacist* [January 1998, pp 97–102], has reviewed the use of an extract of saw palmetto berries (*Permixon*) as an herbal remedy to reduce the symptoms of benign prostatic hyperplasia (BPH). *In vitro,* the extract is said to inhibit 5-alpha reductase, an enzyme that converts testosterone to dihydrotestosterone which is a potent stimulator of prostate growth. This is the same action as finasteride (*Proscar*), a prescription drug used to reduce prostatic volume in symptomatic men. Current evidence does not support the claim that *Permixon* also reduces prostatic volume.

Soy Foods for Perimenopausal Estrogen Deficiency. According to an article in *The New York Times* [September 8, 1998, p B11], many menopausal women are turning to soybean products—tofu, tempeh, soy milk, and soy-based candy bars—as a substitute for estrogen replacement therapy. Soy contains weak estrogenic components called isoflavones, which are said to mimic some of the effects of natural estrogen. According to reports, soy may help some women to control hot flashes and may be worth a try for women with bothersome symptoms who do not wish to take conjugated estrogens. An academic consultant to the soy industry says that the ability of soy to protect against osteoporosis is, at best, speculative. Most researchers also say that soy consumption does not account for the lower rates of breast cancer in Asian women than in American women.

Androstenedione and Athletic Performance. Some people in the United States believe that record books noting Mark McGwire's prodigious feat—hitting 70 home runs in a single season of baseball—should put an asterisk next to his name. The corresponding footnote should relate that McGwire's achievement was facilitated by his use of a performance-enhancing drug.

McGwire regularly uses a dietary supplement, available without a prescription, that contains a precursor of testosterone, androstenedione. The supplement is taken by hundreds of thousands of Americans and by a large number of baseball players. The principal manufacturer of androstenedione claims that a 100 mg dose increases testosterone levels three-fold and that these levels persist for about three hours. Advocates say that the elevated testosterone levels enable athletes to work out harder and more quickly recover.

There is concern about the safety of androstenedione and no one can vouch for its effectiveness, other than with testimonials. Although the use of androstenedione is permitted in professional baseball, the substance is banned by other sports-governing bodies, including the National Football League and the International Olympic Committee [*The New York Times* September 8, 1998, p B11]. It would come as no surprise if after the current season professional baseball also bans the drug.

Athletes also commonly use drugs ordinarily available only by prescription. They include erythropoietin to increase the production of red blood cells and improve oxygen-carrying capacity and endurance, human growth hormone to promote muscle growth and fat loss, and insulin, by body builders, to increase glucose and amino acid uptake into muscle cells. These agents, however, sometimes have serious risks.

Horse Chestnut Seed Extract for Varicose Veins. The *Prescriber's Letter* [1998;5:17] reports that a new herbal product, derived from the horse chestnut and called *Venastat,* is being heavily promoted for leg swelling due to varicose veins. A division of the German pharmaceutical company Boerhinger Ingelheim is marketing the product. It is very likely that more pharmaceutical firms will start marketing herbal products. A controlled trial reported in the *The Lancet* [1996;347:292–94] compared the efficacy of compression stockings or *Venastat* to reduce edema. Both therapies resulted in significant and nearly equal improvement of edema. The authors suggest that the herbal product is an alternative to compression stocking therapy.

Brand-Name Companies Want a Piece of Dietary Supplement Market. Brand-name manufacturers lured by the billions of dollars in annual sales of herbal remedies and dietary supplements are pushing their way onto shelves of supermarkets, drugstores, and national retail chains, elbowing aside the once dominant but obscure companies with limited ability to distribute products. The new players say that they are simply providing natural solutions for good health in an age of self-medication. Critics scoff at that assertion, saying the brand-name firms are doing just what clothes designer do when they slap their label on lines of generic jeans.

Celestial Seasonings Inc, known for its teas, has introduced a line of herbal supplements, including a product called *Mood Mender* that contains St. John's wort. American Home Products, manufacturer of *Centrum* multivitamins, is seeking to capitalize on that brand name by extending it to herbal products. Bayer, maker of *One-A-Day* vitamin and mineral supplements, has entered the market with a line of products that combines vitamins and herbs. Warner-Lambert is also considering dipping a toe into the water [*The New York Times,* July 23, 1998, p C1, C4].

Nature Biotechnology [1998;16:728–31] has also observed and commented on the growing interest of major pharmaceutical companies in nonprescription dietary supplements and medicinal herbs. The article reports that the drug company Novartis has obtained exclusive rights to develop a plant sterol. The company will market the sterol not as a drug but as a "nutraceutical." A spokesperson said that the acquisition was Novartis's first step in pursuing a science-based nutrition strategy. Johnson and Johnson is collaborating with a company in Europe to market a cholesterol-lowering margarine containing a natural product said to restrict the absorption of cholesterol from the gastrointestinal tract.

Analysts say that the drug industry is realizing that instead of the ten years and $250 million to bring a drug to market, a nutraceutical may take only a few years and a few million dollars. While not obligated to conduct clinical trials to make general claims for a dietary supplement, an increasing number of companies are doing such trials to boost their claims and secure a leading position for their product.

The "Made in Italy" Answer to the Problem of Impotence. *Scrip* [June 5, 1998, p 7] reports that the *Viagra* frenzy has stimulated an Italian company to launch a dietary supplement that it promotes for the treatment of male erectile dysfunction. The product contains zinc, three amino acids, and the botanical agents cola seed and policosanole. The botanicals are reputed to have effects on physical performance. The company is running ads with a message saying: "The tablet that gives you the energy you need for . . . say no more. 'Darling please, I'm tired'." The media is indirectly touting the alternative to *Viagra* with stories headlined "The shadow of death over *Viagra*" and reports of the wonders of the "Made in Italy" dietary supplement.

Update on Vitamin Supplements. In July 1998 the staff of the *Medical Letter* [1998;40:75–77] published its periodic review of vitamin supplements. As we have come to expect from this publication, conclusions are cautious and conservative. The review determines that supplements are necessary to assure adequate intake of folic acid in young women and possibly of vitamin D and B_{12} in the elderly. Supplementing the diet of women of childbearing age with folic acid sharply decreases the incidence of neural tube defects in their offspring. As of January 1998, all enriched cereal grains sold in the United States must contain 140 μg of folic acid per 100 g of grain. This amount, however, is probably inadequate to provide maximum protection. Low intake of folate is also associated with high serum concentrations of homocysteine and a higher incidence of cardiovascular disease and stroke. Vitamin D intake is often insufficient in elderly men and women because of low exposure to the sun and other age-related factors. Current recommendations for vitamin D intake are 400 IU for people 51 to 70 years old and 600 IU for people older than 70. Between 10% and 30% of Americans over the age of 60 cannot absorb vitamin B_{12} and require supplements.

The benefits of taking high doses of vitamin E remain to be established. Studies of dietary intake of vitamin E and the risk of cardiovascular disease conflict. An intervention study reported mixed results. Another intervention study found little difference in cardiovascular risk but a lower incidence of prostate cancer among male smokers. Dietary vitamin E is usually in the form of gamma-tocopherol, whereas vitamin E in supplements is mostly alpha-tocopherol. There is no compelling evidence that supplements of vitamin C prevent disease. Short-term controlled trials show vitamin C supplements do not prevent or mitigate upper respiratory infections.

No one should take beta carotene supplements. An intervention study in smokers found an 18% increase in the risk of lung cancer. Another controlled trial in smokers and workers exposed to asbestos was stopped early because participants receiving combined therapy with beta carotene and vitamin A daily had an excess incidence of lung cancer, cardiovascular mortality, and total mortality.

JAMA *Devotes November to Alternative Medicine.* Alternative medicine is the theme of the November 11, 1998 issue of *JAMA* as well as the annual coordinated theme of the November issues of the nine American Medical Association *Archives* Journals. The editors of these journals sought to provide physicians and other health care professionals with clinically relevant, reliable, and new information on alternative therapies. In response to a call for papers on alternative medicine, investigators from many countries submitted more than 200 manuscripts to *JAMA* and many more to the *Archives* Journals. After peer review, about 80 articles and commentaries were published in the ten journals.

The special issue of *JAMA* includes six randomized trials evaluating various therapies. In one report, investigators found that a Chinese herbal medicine improved symptoms of irritable bowel syndrome compared with placebo [*JAMA* 1998;280:1585–89]. The study randomized 116 patients who received individualized herbal formulations, a standard herbal formulation, or placebo. Compared with patients in the placebo group, those receiving herbal therapy had significant improvement in bowel symptom scores as rated by both patients and gastroenterologists. Herbal preparations individually tailored to the patient were no more effective than a standard herbal therapy.

Another trial demonstrated that acupuncture is no more effective than amitriptyline or placebo for relief of pain associated with HIV-related peripheral neuropathy [*Ibid*, 1590–95]. A third showed that *Garcinia cambogia*, a common component of herbal preparations claimed to facilitate weight loss, lacks efficacy as an anti-obesity agent [*Ibid*, pp 1596–1600]. The issue also carries a systematic review that suggests saw palmetto improves urologic symptoms in patients with benign prostatic hyperplasia. The overall strength of these studies is that they demonstrate that alternative medicine therapies can be evaluated by rigorous scientific methods.

Also in the issue is an updated survey on the use of alternative medicine therapies and procedures in the US [*Ibid*, pp 1569–75]. The investigators report that the prevalence of use of at least 1 of 16 specific alternative medicine strategies during the past 12 months increased from 34% in 1990 to 42% in 1997, that the estimated number of visits to alternative medicine practitioners increased from 427 million in 1990 to 629 million in 1997, and that less than 40% of those who used alternative therapies discussed them with their physician. An estimated 15 million adults in 1997 took prescription medications concurrently with herbal remedies and/or high-dose vitamins. Estimated expenditures for alternative medicine professional services in 1997 were $21 billion, with at least $12 billion paid out-of-pocket. Total 1997 out-of-pocket expenditures for alternative therapies were estimated at $27 billion.

LATE BREAKING REPORTS

Clinical Trials

Echinacea May Not Prevent Upper Respiratory Infections. Investigators compared alcoholic root extracts prepared from two different kinds of echinacea plants with placebo in 302 healthy volunteers to determine prophylactic efficacy. The outcome measure was the time until the first upper respiratory tract infection. Mean time to first infection was about two months in all three treatment groups. About one-third of participants developed an infection; there were slightly fewer in the echinacea groups than in the placebo group. Participants in the echinacea groups reported more benefit from the medication than those in the placebo group. The authors caution that the size of their study does not rule out the possibility of modest reduction in the risk of upper respiratory tract infection [*Arch Family Med* 1998;7:541–45].

Regulatory Issues

Supreme Court Rebuffs Industry's Plea for Health Benefit Claims. The Court declined to review a challenge to a FDA requirement that manufacturers of dietary supplements obtain approval before listing health claims on product labels or promotions. The principal plaintiff was the Nutritional Health Alliance, which represents the natural product industry [*The Wall Street Journal,* December 8, 1998, p A12].

Other Reports

Hormone Replacement Therapy with Phyto-Estrogens. Judging by the abundance of phyto-estrogen-enriched foods in health food stores, the public is convinced of the health benefits of these weakly estrogenic, plant-derived steroids. Japanese women who consume large quantities of soy, a rich source of phyto-estrogens, have a low incidence of breast cancer and few menopausal symptoms. These observations have led to the hypothesis that at the menopause phyto-estrogens act as natural selective-estrogen-receptor modulators (SERMs). Advocates claim that they enhance estrogenic responses in the cardiovascular system, bone, and brain, but dampen responses in the breast and uterus. The most widely embraced claim for phyto-estrogens is cardiovascular disease protections. The others have little or no evidentiary support [*Lancet* 1998;352:1762].

St. John's Wort and Photosensitivity. The December 1998 issue of the *Prescriber's Letter* says that St. John's wort may cause photosensitivity and lead to neurotoxicity. The newsletter notes reports of stinging pain in areas exposed to sun. "Researchers suspect this might be due to photoactive compounds in the herb that may damage the myelin sheath surrounding neurons." Symptoms fade when the herb is discontinued. Until more is known, physicians and pharmacists should probably caution patients taking St. John's wort, especially those with fair skin, to be careful about sun exposure.

Medicine for Children. Pharmacy shelves are beginning to fill with new nonprescription remedies for children with coughs and colds. The novelty of the products is that they taste great, mimicking soft candy and bubble gum [*The New York Times,* December 24, 1998, pp A1,C4]. The industry extols the virtues of these "child-friendly" products, but critics take a far more skeptical view. They say that to treat any medicine as if it were candy is confusing and potentially dangerous for children. Some of these products, such as *Kids-eeze* and *Coughco,* are classified as herbal remedies or dietary supplements.

The manufacturer of *Lolliasthma* represents its product as a homeopathic medical treatment for young asthma patients. The preparation contains infinitesimally small doses of natural "active" ingredients. Another herbal product, *Lollicough,* contains plant-derived belladonna, which is deadly in large doses. *Get Better Bear* lozenges for sore throat are essentially sucrose and pectin. *Cough Pops* contain zinc. A recent study in children concluded that zinc was not effective to ameliorate a cold or any one of its symptoms. Fortunately, most of these products are as unlikely to cause harm as they are to provide benefit.

8 Regulatory Actions and Issues

Drug Recalls and Warnings

Drug Interactions Drive Calcium Channel Blocker from Market. On June 8, 1998, after lengthy discussions with the FDA, Roche Laboratories announced that it would withdraw mibefradil (*Posicor*) from the market because of potentially harmful interactions with other drugs. About 200,000 people in the US were taking *Posicor* when the decision was made. *Posicor,* available in the US for only ten months, was promoted heavily as a safe and effective calcium antagonist with a unique chemical structure and novel pharmacology—a first line therapy for hypertension and angina. The marketing effort was successful and *Posicor* had one of the best initial uptakes of a cardiovascular product in the past decade [*Scrip,* June 10, 1998, p 20].

Mibefradil, however, is also a potent inhibitor of drug metabolizing enzymes and can elevate plasma concentrations of co-administered drugs. More than 25 drugs are now known to be potentially dangerous if used with *Posicor.* The list includes antihistamines, antibiotics, tamoxifen (*Nolvadex*), cyclosporine (*Neoral*), cisapride (*Propulsid*) and several cholesterol-lowering HMG CoA reductase inhibitors, including lovastatin (*Mevacor*) and simvastatin (*Zocor*), and possibly atorvastatin (*Lipitor*) and cerivastatin (*Baycol*).

Many people taking *Posicor* would also receive HMG CoA reductase inhibitors and other cardiovascular drugs, such as amiodarone (*Cordarone*), flecainide (*Tambocor*), and propafenone (*Rythmol*)—all interact with mibefradil. High levels of HMG CoA reductase inhibitors greatly increase the risk of rhabdomyolysis—potentially fatal muscle degeneration. A case report describes severe muscle damage and life-threatening complications in an 83-year old woman treated with mibefradil and lovastatin [*Lancet* 1998; 351:1929–39].

There is also is a report of severe reactions in three patients who had poorly controlled hypertension despite taking *Posicor* and had switched to a dihydropyridine calcium channel blocker (i.e., nifedipine, felodipine, and nisoldipine) [*JAMA* 1998;280:157–58]. The findings also suggest the inhibitory effects of *Posicor* on cytochrome P450 3A4 (CYP 3A4) persist long after stopping the drug. The report prompted Roche to warn doctors to wait as much as two weeks before prescribing alternate drugs for patients who had been taking *Posicor*.

Ordinarily, drug interactions are handled by changes in labeling, but not in this case. According to Roche's CEO, ". . . the number of drug interactions would have become so numerous—and therefore the restrictions on *Posicor* so onerous—that it would have been extremely difficult for physicians to keep track of all the drugs a patient is taking." [*The Wall Street Journal,* June 9, 1998, pp B1, B2] Officials at the FDA said that the effect of *Posicor* on drug-metabolizing enzymes presents an unreasonable risk to patients because there is no evidence that the drug offers special benefits over other antihypertensive or anti-anginal drugs.

The interactions observed in patients taking *Posicor* were predictable from the pharmacology of the drug [*Lancet* 1998;351:1829–30]. When given concurrently with drugs that are metabolized by CYP 3A4, systemic concentrations of these drugs increase and in some cases reach toxic levels. Many drug companies today use human liver microsomes to screen for the drug interaction potential of new drugs before they are studied extensively in people. Indeed, there is a report showing that mibefradil inhibits the metabolism of simvastatin and lovastatin in a human microsomal system [*Lancet* 1998;351:1930–31].

Roche Laboratories' failure to detect the potential problems posed by *Posicor* before marketing the drug is a major blunder. The FDA and its advisory panel must also receive low marks for failing to demand more information on mibefradil before granting approval. Worth noting is that three of the eight experts on the panel declined to recommend *Posicor*. One committee member said that the FDA should have waited for the results of a then ongoing trial in patients with heart failure before considering the approval of *Posicor*. A consumer advocacy group stated that mibefradil is clearly a drug that FDA knew was not needed (*The Pink Sheet* 1998;60 (No24):6–7].

Posicor is the second drug to be withdrawn from the market because of drug interactions. In 1996, Marion Merrell Dow replaced its antihistamine terfenadine (*Seldane*) with an active metabolite, fexofenadine (*Allegra*), which does not interfere with the metabolism of other drugs. Critics accuse the FDA of lowering standards because of intense pressure from Congress to expedite the approval of new drugs.

In November, 1998, the FDA, determined to keep these problems from recurring, issued a draft guidance for the pharmaceutical industry's comments. The guidance, now entitled *In Vitro Drug Metabolism/Drug Interaction Studies—Study Design, Data Analysis, and Recommendations for Dosing and Labeling,* is unusually specific and is likely to be more general when finally adopted.

Long-Term Use of Bromfenac (Duract) Results in Serious Toxicity. Heavily promoted for moderate to moderately serve pain, bromfenac (*Duract*), a new nonsteroidal anti-inflammatory agent launched in July 1997, quickly captured a significant share of new prescriptions for analgesics. Many physicians, however, ignored the manufacturer's recommendation that bromfenac be used for not more than ten days. An unexpected incidence of severe liver damage was the result.

Reports of serious adverse events soon after *Duract* reached the market prompted the FDA to direct Wyeth-Ayerst to include a boxed warning in the labeling that highlighted and emphasized that *Duract* was indicated only for short-term use for the management of acute pain. If physicians wished to use *Duract* for a longer time, they were advised to monitor patients for signs of liver toxicity. The bold warning, however, did not stem the flow of adverse event reports. Physicians continued to prescribe *Duract* inappropriately. Wyeth-Ayerst estimates that 15% of the total number of prescriptions for *Duract* were written for longer than ten days. Severe cases of toxicity included four patients who died while taking the drug and eight patients who required a liver transplant.

In June 1998, just two weeks after the announced withdrawal of *Posicor*, the FDA concluded that it could not control the use of *Duract* by means of labeling and asked Wyeth-Ayerst to withdraw the drug from the market. *Duract* is the third drug American Home Products, the corporate parent of Wyeth-Ayerst, was forced to recall in less than a year. In September 1997, *Pondamin* (fenfluramine) and *Redux* (dexfenfluramine) were pulled because some patients using the diet drugs developed heart valve defects.

A postmortem examination of the rise and fall of *Duract* was the subject of an article in *The Wall Street Journal* [September 30, 1998, pp A1,A10]. Providing insight was a medical officer, since retired, who participated in FDA's review of Wyeth-Ayerst's new drug application (NDA) for *Duract*. The company submitted a rather ambitious NDA in late 1994 and hoped to have *Duract* approved for osteoarthritis, a condition affecting 40 million people in the US and requiring long-term treatment. The medical reviewer found strong support for efficacy but was troubled by Wyeth-Ayerst's safety data. Of 830 patients who had taken *Duract* in clinical trials, 23 had unusually high levels of liver enzymes that were suggestive of hepatotoxicity. His first report stated that *Duract* caused more damage to liver cells than any other analgesic of its kind. Following this report, FDA asked Wyeth-Ayerst to eliminate any suggestions from the proposed label that the drug could be used for chronic pain. The agency told the company that the duration of use of *Duract* must be limited. Wyeth-Ayerst did not protest the spirit of the directive but wished to have the label say merely that the drug was for "short-term" use. FDA insisted that short-term be defined and eventually directed that the label state that the use of *Duract* should generally be limited to ten days or less.

The medical reviewer's report also included the recommendation that the FDA put its most stringent warning on the drug's label. Wyeth-Ayerst mounted a vigorous defense to this proposal. Company officers and well-regarded consultants argued that if taken properly, *Duract* posed no special hazard for short-term use. After seven months of memos and reports, the drug company prevailed. Upon marketing in July 1997, the label carried a mild warning about potential liver toxicity buried in paragraph 19.

Within two months of marketing, reports of serious toxicity emerged. In December 1997, the first transplant was reported for a patient who had taken *Duract* for over two months for osteoarthritis. In January, two more people who had used *Duract* for three months required a new liver. By February, FDA asked Wyeth-Ayerst to issue a new label containing a black-boxed warning in the first paragraph and to distribute a "Dear Doctor" letter informing health care professional of the possible consequences of prescribing

Duract for more than ten days. Four deaths following prolonged use of *Duract* occurred between February and April. On June 22, 1998, the company agreed to withdraw the drug from the market.

The Wall Street Journal observed: "But the rise and fall of *Duract* isn't a tale of the dangers of rushing new science to market. . . . Rather, it's a story about the pitfalls of the drug-approval process. Whether done quickly or slowly, judging the safety of new drugs is an inexact process that doesn't stop when FDA approval is issued. . . ."

Isotretinoin May Promote Depression. The FDA has received reports of depression and suicide among patients treated with isotretinoin (*Accutane*), widely used by adolescents and young adults for the treatment of severe acne. As a result, the agency and Hoffmann-La Roche agreed to highlight the concerns in the drug's labeling. New labeling warns, ". . . isotretinoin may cause depression, psychosis, and rarely suicidal ideation, suicide attempts, and suicide." Of particular concern to the FDA are some 20 reports where the patients' mental states improved on discontinuing isotretinoin, and worsened when the drug was re-introduced. FDA's director of dermatologic and dental drugs suggested the possibility that hypervitaminosis A may be associated with mood disorder. Despite its acquiescence, Roche stressed the lack of proof of a connection between *Accutane* and the reports of mood disorders. They also cited estimates that 20% of young adults have suffered a depressive incident and suggested that the hormones that contribute to the formation of acne can also contribute to depression.

Soon after that coerced agreement, FDA rebuked Roche for promotional material that contradicts the new labeling. The material claims that *Accutane* safely and effectively treats the psychosocial trauma and emotional suffering associated with acne, including negative psychosocial effects such as depression and poor self-image. The agency advised that statements and suggestions that *Accutane* therapy will minimize or improve a patient's psychosocial status, including depression, are false or misleading and an unapproved use, and directed Roche to stop distributing the violative promotion material and to develop a plan to correct the false information. Dermatologists have flown to Roche's defense, pointing out that physicians who prescribe *Accutane* need to be aware that depression occurs frequently in adolescents, and even more often among those with severe acne [*JAMA* 1998;279:1057].

FDA Wants New Drug Interaction Warnings for Astemizole (Hismanal). Interactions between the non-sedating antihistamine terfenadine (*Seldane*) and an array of drugs that inhibit its metabolism may result in potentially fatal cardiovascular adverse events. This serious problem led Hoechst Marion Rousell (HMR) to develop fexofenodine (*Allegra*), a non-interacting active metabolite of terfenadine, and, eventually, to withdraw *Seldane* from the market. Janssen's astemizole (*Hismanal*), another non-sedating antihistamine, has similar drug interaction warnings, but remains on the market.

Like terfenadine, astemizole is cardiotoxic. The drug presents no problems for patients with a full and active complement of drug-metabolizing enzymes because blood levels are low. Inhibition of these enzymes by a co-administered drug, however, elevates the level of unmetabolized astemizole and may pose serious problems.

The FDA has now asked Janssen to revise the labeling of *Hismanal* to include new warnings that greatly expand the list of drugs that should not be taken concurrently. The list now includes clarithromycin (*Biaxin*), most selective serotonin reuptake inhibitors, all of the HIV protease inhibitors, zileuton (*Zyflo*), and grapefruit juice. Janssen is also warning against the use of *Hismanal* for patients with liver disease. Following HMR's lead, Janssen is developing a non-interacting active metabolite of astemizole, norastemizole, but it will not be available soon.

Several months after the safety alert for *Hismanal* in the US, the United Kingdom Medicines Control Agency, acting on a request from the UK manufacturer, proposed that the antihistamine no longer be available without a prescription. Both the company and the agency concluded that the safe and effective use of the drug requires medical supervision. By making *Hismanal* a prescription-only product in the UK, Janssen likely will reduce its exposure to liability claims [*Scrip*, July 8, 1998, p 21].

Safety Concerns Limit the Use of Cisapride (Propulsid). Cisapride (*Propulsid*), available in the US since 1993, has been used by millions of people for the treatment of gastrointestinal motility disorders, such as gastroesophageal reflux disease and nocturnal heart burn. In 1995, Janssen added a boxed warning and cautioned against the use of cisapride with certain antibiotics and antifungal agents because of the possibility of adverse drug interactions. More recently a routine survey of adverse event reports, including serious and sometimes fatal ventricular arrhythmias, revealed to the FDA that there is evidence to support additional restrictions on the use of *Propulsid* [*The Wall Street Journal*, June 30, 1998, p B4].

On June 26, 1998, Janssen informed physicians of a new statement in the labeling of *Propulsid* cautioning that the drug be reserved for patients who do not respond adequately to lifestyle modifications, antacids, H2-receptor blockers, or proton pump inhibitors. The letter also recommended that an electrocardiogram (ECG) should be considered prior to prescribing cisapride. The FDA said that the labeling changes were prompted by serious adverse reactions associated mostly with the use of *Propulsid* in patients taking certain other medications or having particular medical conditions. The new labeling contraindicates use of *Propulsid* with more than 20 drugs. Some of the proscribed agents affect the metabolism of cisapride, while others prolong the QT interval on the ECG and may directly increase the cardiotoxicity of cisapride. Serious cardiac events have also been seen in patients with heart disease taking *Propulsid* without any of the contraindicated drugs [*The Pink Sheet* 1998;60 (No27):5].

Soon after, *The Wall Street Journal* [July 21, 1998, p B13] reported that Sepracor Inc. licensed the rights to develop an enantiomer of *Propulsid* to Janssen's corporate parent, Johnson & Johnson. Norcisapride is a potentially safer form of the drug with similar pharmacological activity. An additional advantage for Johnson & Johnson is that patents will protect the new version until 2014 in the US, seven years beyond the end of the patent life of cisapride.

FDA Seeks to Remove Cancer Warning on Estrogen/Progestin Products. FDA has issued a revised guidance that removes the boxed warning concerning the risk of endometrial cancer from the labeling of estrogen/progestin combination products. The FDA suggests that since progestins are added to estrogen to decrease endometrial hyperplasia, the warning of endometrial carcinoma may not be needed. The boxed warning on estrogen products that cautions against use during pregnancy may also be removed because it applies only to diethylstilbestrol and not to other estrogens that are used now.

Prolonged QT Interval Worries Regulators. There are dozens of drugs across therapeutic classes that list QT prolongation in their labeling. The QT interval—measured from the onset of the QRS to the end of the T wave on an electrocardiogram (ECG)—is an approximation of the refractory period of the ventricles. The QT interval is dependent on heart rate. The heart rate adjusted measure is called the QTc interval. The importance of drug-related prolongation of the QT interval is uncertain. Some think that a prolonged QT interval can increase the susceptibility to arrhythmias. Recent withdrawals of drug products and changes in labeling related to QT prolongation have increased the FDA's concern.

The antihistamine terfenadine (*Seldane*) was withdrawn in February 1998, and the calcium channel blocker mibefradil (*Posicor*) was withdrawn in June, both because of QT interval prolongation. Cisapride (*Propulsid*) and astemizole (*Hismanal*) were relabeled for the same reason. Earlier, Abbott's new drug application for the antipsychotic agent sertindole (*Serlect*) was withdrawn because of QT interval prolongation.

Now, the FDA has asked Pfizer to compare the QTc interval prolongation of its antipsychotic ziprasidone (*Zeldox*) with olanzapine (*Zyprexia*), risperidone (*Risperdal*), and other antipsychotic agents, as a condition for approval [*The Pink Sheet* 1998;60 (No31):19]. Pfizer says it will be late 1999 before it is able to refile the NDA. The comparative study must show a QT interval within an acceptable range and the absence of drug interactions that might increase the duration of the QT interval measured with ziprasidone alone.

Thrombotic Thrombocytopenic Purpura Warning on Ticlopidine (Ticlid) Label. More than four months after a report described 60 cases of thrombcytopenic purpura (TTP) associated with the use of ticlopidine (*Ticlid*), Roche has sent a "Dear Doctor" letter to 70,000 physicians in the US. The letter tells them that revised labeling moves the caution about potentially life threatening drug-related TTP from a bold warning to a more urgent boxed warning.

The boxed warning says that TTP ". . . was not seen during clinical trials but US physicians reported about 100 cases between 1992 and 1997. Based on estimated patient exposure of two to four million, and assuming an event reporting rate of 10%, the incidence of ticlopidine-associated TTP may be as high as one in every 2,000 to 4,000 patients exposed." The boxed warning also says that patients receiving *Ticlid* must be monitored hematologically and clinically for evidence of neutropenia and/or TTP during the first three months of treatment.

Some experts are disappointed that the new label does not address *Ticlid*-associated TTP in patients undergoing a cardiac stent procedure. In this setting, ticlopine is administered for two to four weeks. Although this indication is off-label, it accounts for 50% of the overall use of *Ticlid*. Many stent procedures in the US rely on ticlopidine to prevent complications following the procedure [*Scrip*, August 19, 1998, p 15].

Pediatric Warning on Inhaled Corticosteroids. Oral systemic steroids suppress growth in children. On the introduction of inhaled corticosteroids in

1972, products that are now first-line therapy for patients with asthma, some pediatricians expressed concern about adverse developmental effects in children. For many years, however, the prevailing view was that the amount absorbed from inhaled and intranasal products was too small to warrant concern.

A mounting number of reports, however, has brought this issue to the forefront. Manufacturers have reported statistically significant growth retardation with inhaled budesonide formulations, triamcinolone preparations, and products containing beclomethasone. These products can slow growth velocity by 0.8 to 1.5 cm per year, mainly in prepubescent children [*The Pink Sheet* 1998;60(No31):5].

In July, after studying the evidence of pediatric growth suppression due to inhaled or intranasal corticosteroids, an advisory panel recommended that the FDA develop class labeling that applies to all products. The panel suggested that the new labeling include a general precaution stating that corticosteroids have been shown to cause a reduction in growth velocity when used by children and adolescents. The proposed labeling for the pediatric use subsection would add that suppression of growth has been seen in the absence of hypothalamus-pituitary-adrenal (HPA) axis suppression, as assessed by adrenocorticotrophin hormone (ACTH) stimulation or basal plasma cortisol levels. The evidence suggests that growth velocity is a more sensitive indicator of systemic steroid exposure in children than some commonly used tests of HPA axis function.

Labeling should also state that it remains unclear whether steroid-related growth suppression contributes to shorter stature in adulthood. Because of the limited information, the committee suggested that drug companies with new corticosteroid products should conduct growth impact studies before seeking FDA approval and that the agency should request phase IV studies for products already on the market.

Surveys suggest that inhaled and intranasal preparations of corticosteroids are underused. The head of a patient advocacy group said, ". . . parents would shy away from corticosteroids if more negatives were highlighted." An FDA representative said that the agency, ". . . is not suggesting that oral or intranasal corticosteroids are unsafe for use in children." He added: "These products have tremendous efficacy, but they also carry some risks" [*Scrip*, August 7, 1998, p 17]. Members of the expert panel agreed that suppression of growth velocity in children with asthma should not discourage the first-line use of inhaled corticosteroids.

Authorities Restrict Use of Cough/Cold Preparations. Local authorities are moving to restrict sales of popular cough/cold preparations—*Dristan, Sudafed, Actifed, Tylenol Cold, Nyquil,* and *Contac*—that contain ephedrine and pseudoephedrine, used in the making of methamphetamine, the recreational drug of choice in some circles [*The Wall Street Journal,* August 25, 1998, pp B1, B4]. In San Diego it is illegal to buy more than three packages of most nonprescription cold and allergy preparations. Similar steps are being taken in more than a dozen other cities. According to the US Drug Enforcement Administration (DEA), the nation's thousands of small methamphetamine laboratories depend on over-the-counter medication for their source of ephedrine and pseudoephedrine. However, the agency says that most methamphetamine is made in "super labs" in Southern California and Mexico. These manufacturers have access to bulk shipments of pharmaceutical grade ephedrine and pseudoephedrine.

The law stipulates that chemical manufacturers must report to the DEA bulk sales of ephedrine and pseudoephedrine that they believe might be used to synthesize methamphetamine. The same law says drug companies must sell products containing these agents in unit dose blister packs to hamper attempts to gather large quantities. The pharmaceutical industry argues that the efforts are misdirected and fears the development of a patchwork of rules and regulations across the country.

FDA Cautions about Use of Albumin in Seriously Ill Patients. A meta-analysis prepared by the UK Cochrane Center, part of an international endeavor to promote evidence-based medical practice, challenges the routine use of albumin in critically ill patients [*BMJ* 1998;317:235–40]. The investigators conclude: "There is no evidence that albumin administration reduces mortality in critically ill patients with hypovolaemia, burns, or hypoalbuminaemia and a strong suggestion that it may increase mortality." A series of letters to BMJ, however, many from those working in intensive care, were critical of the review. The director of the UK center observed: "The opinions and attitudes reflected in most responses to the albumin and colloid review does not inspire confidence that those working in intensive care have yet acknowledged sufficiently the need for reliable evidence about the effects of their care on outcomes that matter to patients." In October, the *Prescriber's Letter* [October 1998, p 59] reported that the FDA, prompted by the new findings, is now cautioning about the use of albumin or plasma protein fraction in seriously ill patients. Alternatives are dextran, hetastarch, or crystalloid solutions.

FDA Halts Distribution of Drug Used to Sterilize Women. In June 1998, the front page of the *The Wall Street Journal* carried an article about the use of intravaginal quinacrine pellets to sterilize tens of thousands of women in 20 countries, sometimes without their knowledge or consent. Quinacrine prevents pregnancy by scarring the fallopian tubes. It also causes cellular mutations that may lead to cancer. In 1993, the World Health Organization stated that without more information on safety, quinacrine should not be used to sterilize any woman in any country.

In October, the FDA sent a warning letter asking the two individuals who are distributing the drug to destroy all existing supplies of quinacrine pellets and to do so under agency supervision. The distributors were give 15 days to comply. The FDA has jurisdiction over quinacrine pellets in the US as well as their export overseas. Current agency rules say that certain drugs that are not approved in the US, such as quinacrine, may be exported, but only when they are legal for use in a foreign country and do not present a hazard to public health. One of the distributors said arrangements have already been made to manufacture and distribute quinacrine overseas, out of the reach of the FDA [*The Wall Street Journal,* October 19, 1998, B11].

Alcohol Warnings for OTC Analgesics. The FDA has issued a final rule stating that over-the-counter (OTC) pain relievers and fever-lowering agents—preparations that contain aspirin or other salicylates, acetaminophen, ibuprofen, naproxen, or ketoprofen—must carry a label warning against their use by heavy drinkers. The acting head of the FDA said that consumers with a history of chronic alcohol use need to know the risk of taking OTC analgesics/antipyretics. The new warning is aimed particularly at people who regularly consume three or more alcoholic drinks per day and take products containing acetaminophen, because the combination can lead to severe liver damage. In 1994, Johnson & Johnson became the first manufacturer of acetaminophen to voluntarily add a general warning to the labeling of all *Tylenol* products. Manufacturers of products containing aspirin or other NSAIDs complain that there is little evidence to justify a warning on their products. FDA counters that the risk of stomach bleeding may increase when heavy drinkers use them.

REGULATORY ISSUES

Promotion of Pharmaceutical Products. A regulatory affairs expert recently reported on the history of the Food and Drug Administration's regulation of drug labeling, advertising, and promotion [*Clin Pharmacol Ther* 1998; 63:607–16]. He notes that while the law does not require manufacturers to obtain the permission of the FDA to place promotional material, the agency has kept a close eye on all aspects of pharmaceutical promotion and been quick to correct a perceived misdeed. On occasion, the FDA has required the manufacturer to place a corrective ad when a promotional piece was particularly misleading

A recent example of FDA's *modus operandi* concerns the promotion of a first-generation nonsteroidal anti-inflammatory drug. In an attempt to differentiate nabumetone (*Relafen*) from other NSAIDs, SmithKline Beecham (SKB) claimed a more favorable side-effect profile: minimal gastrointestinal adverse events, lack of effect on platelet aggregation, and lack of significant effect on renal function. In some ads, SKB suggested that based on cell culture studies, nabumetone selectively inhibits cyclooxygenase-2 (COX-2) and therefore is less toxic than older NSAIDs.

FDA's current policy holds that there is insufficient evidence to suggest anti-inflammatory agents that selectively inhibit COX-2 would allay the signs and symptoms of inflammation without causing the type of adverse events associated with the use of currently marketed NSAIDs. The agency requires a drug manufacturer to provide clinical data to support such claims. The FDA challenged each of SKB's safety claims for nabumetone and directed the firm to send a corrective letter to all health care providers, institutions, and organizations who received the violative material and further, to publish a paid advertisement in all journals that carried misleading ads for *Relafen*.

Until recently, drug advertising was limited to placements in medical and other professional journals and material given or sent to individual physicians to persuade them to prescribe the product. Several years ago, however, the FDA came under political pressure and relaxed its guidelines to allow direct-to-consumer (DTC) advertising. The revised rule permitted promotion of a prescription product directly to the public provided that the ad contain extensive labeling material to present a balanced view of risks and benefits. This requirement effectively closed the broadcast media to pharmaceutical promotions. In the absence of labeling information, a radio or television ad for a drug could only state the name of the product or its indication, but not both.

More recently, again under pressure from the drug industry and members of Congress, the FDA agreed to relax requirements for DTC broadcast ads of prescription drugs. Now, radio and television advertisements can identify the drug and explicitly discuss its therapeutic use, without including copious labeling material. To achieve balance, the ad must mention the most significant limitations of a drug product and also include sources for more information.

Physicians have strong opinions both for and against DTC promotions. Many physicians and managed health care plans believe that DTC advertising is unethical and should be limited or, better yet, stopped. Critics fear that DTC promotion leads to inappropriate prescribing because physicians do not wish to deny a patient's request. Especially vulnerable to this type of force is the prescribing of antibiotics to children with viral infections. Drug companies, on the other hand, say that advertising and other marketing techniques provide information that helps patients overcome their problems. Supporting the industry are the results of a recent survey conducted by *Prevention* magazine. Of the adults surveyed, 37% reported having seen an ad for the drug they were taking. About three-quarters of those who saw an ad said that the promotion made them more likely to take their medicines and that it reminded them to have their prescription filled [*The Pink Sheet* 1998;60(No33):6–7].

A *Time* magazine survey in September found that one third of consumers believe they can choose medication without a physician's advice and 28% said they are prepared to change physicians to get a desired medication [*The Pink Sheet* 1998;60(No37):6]. The FDA Drug Marketing, Advertising and Communications Division Branch Chief said that there is a problem if these ads are encouraging a person to believe that he or she can make these kinds of decisions. The survey also revealed that 81% of consumers took some form of action in response to DTC promotion, ranging from speaking with a health care professional to calling the 800 number cited in the ad or discussing the ad with a friend. Twenty-nine percent of consumers who discussed an advertised drug with a physician received a prescription for the product.

The pharmaceutical industry is convinced that DTC promotion will prompt patients to ask their doctor to prescribe specific products and that many physicians will comply. The industry estimates that as many as 12 million people asked for and received a prescription medicine as a direct result of a DTC ad. *The Pink Sheet* [1998;60(No38):26] reported recently that pharmaceutical companies spent $530 million on DTC promotions between January and May 1998. That is a $90 million increase over the same period in 1997.

For the industry as a whole, television is the favored medium. Most heavily promoted in the first two months of 1998 were valaciclovir (*Valtrex*) for herpes and pravastatin (*Pravachol*) for hypercholesterolemia [*Scrip*, June 10, 1998]. A great deal of money is also being spent to promote psychotherapeutic drugs [*The New York Times*, February 17, 1998, pp A1, C3].

In September, a vice-president of Cigna Healthcare told participants at an Institute for International Research conference that some managed care organizations (MCOs) are considering, while others have begun to implement, restrictions on direct-to-consumer advertised drugs to control increasing costs driven by patient demand [*The Pink Sheet* 1998;60(No38):25]. He said some MCOs are excluding DTC-marketed drugs from their formulary in favor of similar drugs not marketed in this manner. He also pointed out that Group Health Cooperative of Puget Sound has never added any DTC-marketed allergy drugs, such as *Claritin*, and thereby has much lower antihistamine costs. MCO's are increasingly convinced that DTC advertising increases their drug costs.

Over the past five to ten years the pharmaceutical industry, with the help of friends in Congress, has dismantled much of FDA's program to control drug promotions. The industry's next target was FDA's rule that prohibited the promotion of drugs for uses other than those approved by the FDA. While physicians were free to prescribe drugs off label, drug companies were not allowed to promote drugs for off-label uses. That rule was the victim of the FDA Modernization Act of 1997. A provision of the legislation allows companies to distribute unabridged, peer-reviewed journal articles to physicians on off-label uses of approved drugs and medical devices, provided they had filed, or agreed to file, supplemental new drug applications (sNDAs) for the nonapproved uses [*Scrip*, June 12, 1998, p 18].

Since 1994, the Washington Legal Foundation (WLF), a pro-industry group, has embroiled itself in a first-amendment lawsuit against the FDA because of the agency's restrictive policies on non-approved uses. Although the FDA Modernization Act addressed many of the issues raised by the WLF, the foundation, believing that the FDA would interpret the act's provisions on promotion of off-label uses as narrowly as possible, continued to seek relief from the courts. In August 1998, a federal judge ruled that while the FDA is more restrictive than it need be, the agency has a substantial interest in adding off-label uses of approved drugs to product labeling [*The Pink Sheet* 1998;60(No31):8]. The judge found that requiring pharmaceutical companies to get new uses on-label does, on balance, promote public health. He pointed out that whether it does or it doesn't, Congress has spoken and said that it benefits the public health to require manufacturers to get all promoted benefits and uses approved by the FDA. He also cited a Supreme Court decision that the requirement is not subject to exceptions based on the difficulty of obtaining approval, the cost, or the conceded benefits of the approved use. The Court concluded that because restrictions on the distribution of information on off-label uses do provide an incentive for manufacturers to have approved drugs evaluated by the FDA for safety and effectiveness of an off-label use, a degree of restriction directly advances a substantial interest of the government.

Despite these caveats, the WLF came away with a victory. The judge agreed that FDA's approach to off-label information included in journal reprints, textbooks, and continuing medical education (CME) programs is too restrictive and therefore is an unconstitutional impediment to free speech. While seeming only to reiterate provisions of the FDA Modernization Act, the ruling directs the FDA to interpret the provisions broadly. The decision enjoins FDA from stopping distribution of reprints from peer-reviewed professional journals or textbooks sold by independent publishers. FDA has strongly opposed the distribution of material from textbooks. The court also enjoined FDA from preventing sponsors from suggesting content or speakers to independent CME providers [*The Pink Sheet* 1998;60(No31):9].

Following the Court's decision, a lawyer for the Pharmaceutical Research and Manufacturers of American (PhRMA) told the Food and Drug

Law Institute that FDA's proposed rule regarding dissemination of off-label information on approved products is in need of major revision [*The Pink Sheet* 1998;60(No38):28]

FDA to Require Pediatric Data on Drug Products. Pediatricians often say that sick children are therapeutic orphans because of the appalling lack of information on the effects of drugs in this population. Until recently, pharmaceutical development of new drugs rarely took use by children into consideration. The large majority of products on the US market carry the disclaimer— safety and efficacy not established in children. The American Academy of Pediatrics estimates that only 20% of all medications marketed in the US carry labeling directing use in infants, children, and adolescents. Voluntary efforts by several drug companies have improved the situation but too slowly to satisfy the Clinton Administration and the FDA.

With the White House providing the impetus, the FDA issued a proposed rule that would require drug companies to provide data on the effects of a new drug or biological in children if physicians are likely to prescribe the product for this population. To support the need for a new rule, FDA cited ten products marketed since 1994 and widely used in children that carry a disclaimer as to use in children. They include albuterol solution for nebulization, fluoxetine, cromolyn sodium, and methylphenidate. There are legitimate technical, ethical, and economic issues that make it difficult to study new drugs in children. For example, guidelines published by the American Academy of Pediatrics Committee on Drugs call for active drugs as controls in trials involving children. Placebo controls may only be used in limited situations [*Lancet* 1998;352:630].

In May 1998, the FDA issued a Pediatric Priority List containing the names of 493 drugs that are commonly used, or could be potentially used, in children and infants, but which are not specifically approved for that use. The document also redefines standards of evidence needed before a license will be granted to cover pediatric age-groups. Furthermore, drug companies conducting a pediatric study at FDA's request or with FDA's approval gain an additional six months of market exclusivity. It is not clear whether the agency has the authority to compel a company to carry out a study. Given the incentive, this point may not matter much. An extra six months of market exclusivity would provide a great deal of additional revenue for a top-selling drug and delay competition from generic products [*Scrip,* June 3, 1998, p 20].

The following month, *Scrip* [July 8, 1998, p 15] reported that the FDA issued additional guidance to the industry on how companies can qualify for an extra six months of marketing exclusivity. To secure this benefit, a drug manufacturer must receive a FDA Written Request to conduct one or more studies of a product in a pediatric population. A company will be able to self-initiate this process by submitting the agency's Proposed Pediatric Study Request, asking the agency to send a Written Request. At this time, a company need not comply with the Written Request initiated by the FDA.

An example of how the new rule will work is the approval of a syrup formulation of midazolam (*Versed*) for use in children [*The Pink Sheet* 1998;60(No43):25]. Up until now, only an injectable form has been available. The injectable has been used widely off-label as an oral solution in clinical practice. The approval extends the exclusive marketing period for *Versed* by six months to June 2000. *Versed* injection for pediatric use received approval in March 1998, but FDA issued a Written Request for more data. The pediatric study for *Versed* syrup was conducted under that Written Request. It involved 400 patients ranging in age from six months to 16 years who received the syrup containing midazolam or a placebo before undergoing a diagnostic, therapeutic, or endoscopic procedure or before induction of anesthesia. More than 90% of patients receiving midazolam at doses of 0.25 mg/kg or 0.5 mg/kg were sedated and free of anxiety.

After reviewing comments on its proposed draft guidance for studies in children and despite strenuous objections from the drug industry, the FDA issued final rules [*The New York Times,* November 28, 1998, ppA1,A10]. The rules are published in the Federal Register and take effect on April 1, 1999. Now, pharmaceutical companies must study the safety and effectiveness of drugs and vaccines in children, ". . . if the products are likely to be used in a substantial number of pediatric patients or if they provide a meaningful therapeutic benefit over existing treatment for children."

Mindful of the new rules' impact on the pharmaceutical industry, the FDA may allow a company to defer testing in children until clinical trials suggest that a new drug is safe and effective for adults. In some cases, pediatric testing will occur after a new drug has been approved for use in adults. FDA may ask for pediatric studies whenever a drug company seeks approval for a new drug, a new use for a drug, a new dosage form, or a new way for patients to take the drug. If a company violates the new rule, FDA will seek injunctive relief.

Drug Industry Proposes Guidelines on Pharmacoeconomic Analysis. In June 1998, the Pharmaceutical Research and Manufacturers of America (PhRMA) sent a proposal to the FDA on the use of healthcare economic information for drug promotion. The proposal is based on provisions in the 1997 FDA Modernization Act, which are less stringent than those observed by the agency in the past. Before the legislation, the FDA felt that resource utilization claims must be supported directly by data from well-controlled trials.

The FDA has not yet issued guidance on how it plans to interpret the new rules. PhRMA suggests that the agency use a more flexible standard of substantiation of claims than it now uses to judge promotional claims for efficacy and safety. Current interpretation of the law requires advertising for prescription drugs to be based on adequate and well-controlled clinical trials. The industry-supported group wants the FDA to use the rules applied to the promotion of non-prescription, over the counter, medication. These regulations require advertising to be based on the considerably less restrictive standard of "competent and reliable" scientific evidence.

According to the congressional committees that wrote the FDA Modernization Act, the methods for establishing economic costs and consequences used to construct healthcare economic information would be evaluated using standards widely accepted by economic experts, not by experts in evaluating the merits of clinical trials [*Scrip*, July 3, 1998, p 11].

Not too long ago, the FDA would have rejected PhRMA's proposal out of hand. The FDA reform bill, however, has softened the agency's previous ban on the use of financial data from epidemiological analyses and mathematical modeling to claim a medicinal product results in fewer visits to a physician's office, fewer days off from work, or less hospitalization [*Scrip*, September 16, 1998, p 15]. Be assured that today the FDA will take the industry's proposal into consideration.

Generic Drug Industry Wants Rule Changes. Since the early 1970s, health care plans have made an effort to reduce the cost of prescription medication. This, in turn, stimulated interest to produce generic versions of drugs no longer protected by patent. Until 1994, however, there was no formal approval process routinely used by the FDA to evaluate the safety and efficacy of generic products. On passage of the Waxman/Hatch legislation, however, the pharmaceutical industry agreed to accept the marketing of generic products provided they were bioequivalent to an innovator's product. In return, the legislation extended the period of marketing exclusivity for the innovator's product. A bioequivalence study compares the rate and extent of absorption, called bioavailability, of the generic product with the innovator's product. A commentary on the current status of generic drug product equivalence was recently published [*Am J Managed Care* 1998;4;1183–89].

Representatives of the generic drug industry claim, with justification, that the spirit of Waxman/Hatch has been fundamentally altered since 1994. They say that innovator firms that had agreed not to oppose generic competition once their patents ran out now spend untold amounts of money to manipulate the legal and regulatory system to their end [*Scrip,* June 17, 1998, p 16]. Some companies in the generic drug industry believe that the only way the abuses can be halted is by a re-opening of Waxman/Hatch by Congress. This, however, is a two-edged sword. Indeed, Representative Waxman (D-Calif) has cautioned generic manufacturers that a re-opening of the act could harm the generic industry.

An example of the aggressive strategies used by innovator firms to delay market penetration of lower-priced generic products is provided by DuPont Merck's defense of its anticoagulant *Coumadin* (warfarin). In March 1998, Barr Laboratories filed suit against DuPont Merck for allegedly impeding market acceptance of Barr's generic version of warfarin. Barr claims that DuPont Merck published false and misleading statements about the equivalence, effectiveness, and safety of generic warfarin. The FDA has also found DuPont Merck's allegations to be false and misleading. The agency has issued two letters to physician organizations and state boards of pharmacy reiterating that Barr's product is bioequivalent in every respect to *Coumadin*. The key issue is whether the generic product and DuPont Merck's product are interchangeable. Barr and the FDA believe they are, with no need of additional coagulation tests or closer monitoring when a patient on *Coumadin* is switched to the generic product [*Scrip,* March 13, 1998, p 9].

A more recent report says that Barr's generic warfarin is gaining acceptance by managed care organizations (MCOs) [*Scrip* August 21, 1998, p 17]. The largest MCO in the US, Kaiser-Permanente, with nine million members, has placed the generic product on its drug formulary after completing an independent clinical study comparing it with DuPont Merck's *Coumadin*. Kaiser is now switching anticoagulant patients from *Coumadin* to the generic. Shortly after Kaiser's announcement, Group Health Cooperative of Puget Sound also said that it would convert its patients requiring anticoagulation to generic warfarin. It too has completed an independent in-house study. In still another action favoring Barr's product, the Minnesota Drug Formulary Committee has delisted generic warfarin from a negative formulary. This means that for Minnesota Medicaid patients, Barr's warfarin must be substituted for *Coumadin.*

Another pitched battle continues between Wyeth-Ayerst, the manufacturer of *Premarin,* and generic drug companies who seek to launch a version of conjugated estrogens. Until recently, the monograph on conjugated estrogens in the United States Pharmacopoeia (USP) described *Premarin*. However, when two generic companies developed products that met USP standards and were bioequivalent to *Premarin,* based on rate and extent of absorption of the five estrogenic components listed in the USP, Wyeth-Ayerst informed the FDA of two additional estrogenic components, not identified by the USP. While *Premarin* contained these additional components, the proposed generic products did not. Consequently in May 1997, the FDA rejected the abbreviated new drug applications for the generic products. Rather oddly, the agency ruled that *Premarin* must be better characterized, presumably by Wyeth-Ayerst, before its active ingredients can be definitively identified and that, until that time, no synthetic generic can be approved.

One of the generic companies thwarted in 1997, Duramed, has filed a new drug application for conjugated estrogens as described in the USP [*Scrip,* August 19, 1998, p 11]. On the heels of the application, Wyeth-Ayerst filed a FDA Citizens Petition seeking to prevent Duramed from classifying its synthetic conjugated estrogens product as "conjugated estrogens." Duramed has now responded to the petition. The response points out that the agency has determined that Duramed's NDA for a synthetic product containing five estrogen components for the treatment of vasomotor symptoms in postmenopausal women is sufficiently complete to proceed with a substantive review. Therefore, the FDA should deny any effort by Wyeth-Ayerst to impose additional requirements for NDA approval.

In its petition, Wyeth-Ayerst says that the approval of NDAs for a five-estrogen mixture product labeled as "Conjugated Estrogens USP" would confuse the public, as it is likely to lead to their use as substitutes for *Premarin* not only for vasomotor symptoms but also in long-term estrogen replacement therapy. Wyeth-Ayerst asked the FDA to recognize that the proposed product contains some, but not all, of the active components of *Premarin* and ask for the revocation of the current USP monograph for conjugated estrogens. Wyeth-Ayerst alleges that the monograph is inaccurate and inconsistent with the agency's May 1997 decision on the composition of conjugated estrogens.

In the future, generic drug makers may face a higher hurdle in gaining FDA approval. In 1997 the agency issued a draft guidelines for comment in which a new concept of prescribability and switchability is proposed. As summarized in a commentary in *The Lancet* [1998;352:85–86], two drug products could have the same mean bioavailability and not be equally prescribable because one could be more variable than the other.

FDA Not Protecting the Public, Say Critics. The unusually high number of drug product withdrawals from the market and the host of additional warnings for recently marketed products provide ammunition for the critics of the FDA and the drug industry. An article in *The Wall Street Journal* [June 14, 1998, p B4] relates the dissatisfaction with FDA's system for monitoring the safety of drugs after marketing. MedWatch is a completely voluntary system that encourages physicians, pharmacists, and nurses to report untoward effects of drugs, particularly newly marketed products. Consumer advocates say that for every dollar the FDA spends on evaluating new drugs for marketing, little more than six cents is spent on monitoring drugs that are already on the market. FDA counters that the timely withdrawal of the analgesic *Duract* (bromfenac) is evidence that MedWatch is working. The critics are not as-suaged. They argue that FDA's system is too reactive, too dependent on drug-company data, and inadequate to monitor the roughly 250,000 reports each year. Some physicians report that they wait to prescribe new drugs for up to one year after marketing to learn what happens when large numbers of people are exposed to the new agent.

An editorial in *The New York Times* [July 2, 1998], that appeared after the recall of *Posicor* and *Duract,* suggested that the FDA ". . . may be having trouble balancing political demands to speed up the drug approval process while maintaining its tradition of rigorous safety review." The opinion piece concludes: "The FDA moved to take *Duract* and *Posicor* off the market because they are not lifesaving drugs and because there are other options that do not pose the same safety risks. That standard might best be applied before the drugs are approved."

FDA Establishes Post-Marketing Office. The Food and Drug Administration has completed the organization of the new Office of Post-Marketing Drug Risk Assessment and named an acting director [*The Pink Sheet* 1998;60(No34):3–4]. Consumer groups have emphasized the need for a separate office to address post-marketing drug safety. They want the office to have the funds and the capacity to use the major tools of public health prevention, including case-control and cohort studies, patient surveys, and data from existing information systems, and the already established MedWatch system. Consumer advocates also ask that the FDA strictly enforce the public reporting requirements of the FDA Modernization Act of 1997 to assure that sponsors are meeting their phase IV commitments. The American Society for Clinical Pharmacology recommends that FDA scientists who are independent of the review and approval process conduct post-market surveillance. There is also a distinct sentiment that the US should separate its drug safety and review function on the model of the UK.

Citizen's Group Petitions FDA on Inaccurate Patient Information. A high-profile consumer advocacy organization, Public Citizen's Health Research Group, has filed a petition with the FDA calling for the immediate recall of all patient information leaflets containing incomplete safety information. The group says that a large proportion of these leaflets—produced by commercial information vendors and distributed by pharmacists to consumers as a free "service" at the time prescriptions are dispensed—are incomplete and misleading. A report in *Scrip* [June 24, 1998, p 14] says that 2.5 billion prescriptions were dispensed in the US last year and about three-quarters of patients received some kind of patient leaflet with them.

Administration Nominates New FDA Commissioner. *The Wall Street Journal* [June 24, 1998, p A14] reported that the Clinton administration's nominee to head the FDA is Dr. Jan Ellen Henney, a cancer specialist, who served as the vice president for Heath Sciences at the University of New Mexico. She is not new to the agency. In 1992, her predecessor, Dr. David Kessler, asked her to be one of his chief deputies. For the next two years, Dr. Henney managed the daily activities of the FDA, and then returned to academia. She hired many of the top officials who now work at the FDA. According to all reports, Dr. Henney's style is very different from Dr. Kessler's who was seen as an anti-industry crusader. Kessler battled repeatedly with Republicans in Congress who wanted the agency to help the pharmaceutical industry to bring products to the market. Nevertheless, the administration geared up for a potential clash in the Senate.

To prepare for the confirmation hearings, the Senate Labor and Human Resources Committee asked Dr. Henney to respond to a list of 140 questions. Most of the questions addressed issues related to the implementation of the FDA Modernization Act. In some quarters this was viewed as political and inappropriately intrusive. The legislative director of the Consumer Federation of America complained that the questions posed to Henney reflect strong industry input and represent an, ". . . unprecedented effort to tie the hands of the commissioner in advance of proper study of the issues" [*The Pink Sheet* 1998;60(No34):6].

Two queries concerned FDA's review of the abortifacient mifepristone. Henney's predecessor, to the dismay of House and Senate conservatives, worked with the Clinton Administration to secure an agreement with European manufacturer Roussel-Uclaf to surrender patent rights to the drug in the US. The agency then worked with the Population Council to develop the drug. Approval of mifepristone is stalled because of difficulties in finding a manufacturer. An amendment to the House version of the FDA appropriation bill would forbid the agency from spending any more money on the review [*The Pink Sheet* 1998;60(No32):3–6].

Dr. Henney's response to questions at the hearing seemed to reassure most Republican members of the committee, particularly in areas related to meeting the letter and spirit of the FDA Modernization Act, adhering to deadlines for reviewing investigational new drug applications and promotional material, and the dissemination of information of off-label uses of drug products. The questions posed to Dr. Henney clearly revealed the implicit expectation of a majority of the committee members that she differentiate herself from her predecessor, Dr. Kessler [*The Pink Sheet* 1998;60(No36):3–4].

One senator, Mike Enzi (R-Wy), said he would not confirm the nomination because of displeasure over Dr. Henney's responses to questions about medical abortion. He repeatedly asked the nominee why the FDA did not consider the harm to the fetus caused by administering mifepristone. Henney attempted, with little success, to dance away from the question. She cited the statute directing the FDA to review a drug's safety and efficacy for its intended use. For mifepristone the intended use is to terminate an early pregnancy. This response seemed to confuse several other members of the committee as well [*Scrip*, September 9, 1998, p 17].

In early September, concern was raised as to the time needed to consider the confirmation of Dr. Henney's nomination before Congress's scheduled adjournment on October 9. Chairman Jeffords (R-Vt) told Dr. Henney that unless, ". . . things come together very quickly and everybody says they love you and there will be no debate on the floor, it will be very difficult to move forward" [*The Pink Sheet* 1998;60(No36):7–8]. Furthermore, Republican leadership has no urgency to give the Clinton administration an opportunity to make headlines with the first woman commissioner of the FDA. After much wrangling, the Senate Labor & Human Resources Committee scheduled a confirmation vote for the nominee.

On September 23, 1998, the Labor & Human Resources Committee voted in favor of the nomination with a single dissension from Senator Enzi [*The Pink Sheet* 1998;60(No36):7–8]. The trade journal observed that Dr. Henney approaches the final hurdle with little visible opposition but also with no aggressive support. There was fear that the lack of an effective champion in the Senate could scuttle the appointment. Indeed, on the floor of the Senate, the Majority Whip, Don Nickles (R-Okla), sought to block the nomination because of concerns about Henney's position on tobacco regulation and mifepristone. With the help of Republican senators, however, and an 11th hour endorsement from the Biotechnology Industry Organization, the Clinton administration convinced Nickles that his concerns were groundless and cleared the way for the Senate to approve the nomination before adjournment [*The New York Times,* October 21, 1998, p A20].

LATE BREAKING REPORTS

Regulatory Actions

FDA Issues Final Off-Label Promotion Rule. The final rule on dissemination of information on non-approved uses of approved drugs was published in the Federal Register in November 1998. FDA requires that the information include a description of the study design and conduct, data presentation and analysis, summary of results, and conclusions pertaining to the new use. The requirement stringently limits the dissemination of information contained in textbooks. The agency will not permit dissemination of abstracts of a publication, data from phase I studies in healthy people, or observations in too small a number of patients. The drug industry association, PhRMA, objects to the new rule on the grounds that it virtually bans the use of reference texts and defines new uses too broadly. The Washington Legal Foundation, which won an injunction against the FDA's proposed guidance on off-label promotion, still considers the regulation illegal. The judge who decided the case has not yet told the FDA whether his ruling also covers the "new use" provision of the FDA Modernization Act [*Scrip,* November 25, 1998, p 11].

Regulatory Issues

Exemptions to Pediatric Corticosteroid Warning. Schering-Plough reports that mometasone (*Nasonex*), its recently approved steroid nasal spray, has no effect on linear growth, unlike most other nasal steroids. The company reviewed data from a 12-month placebo-controlled pediatric study and on the strength of the findings, proposes that any intranasal or inhaled corticosteroid product that meets a 12-month safety criteria should be exempt from class labeling. A waiver from the requirement for *Nasonex* would be a major marketing advantage for the company [*Scrip*, November 18, 1998, p 17].

Citizen's Group Charges that FDA Relents on Safety. A report by Public Citizen's Health Research Group (HRG) maintains that FDA medical officers have been pressured to withhold opinions or data that could have influenced advisory committees against recommending approval of a drug product. According to HRG, 19 medical officers identified 27 drugs approved in the past three years that they felt should not have been approved. Twelve others identified 25 drugs that they felt were approved too quickly. HRG targets Congress as a source of inappropriate pressure on the agency.

9 Biomedical Ethics

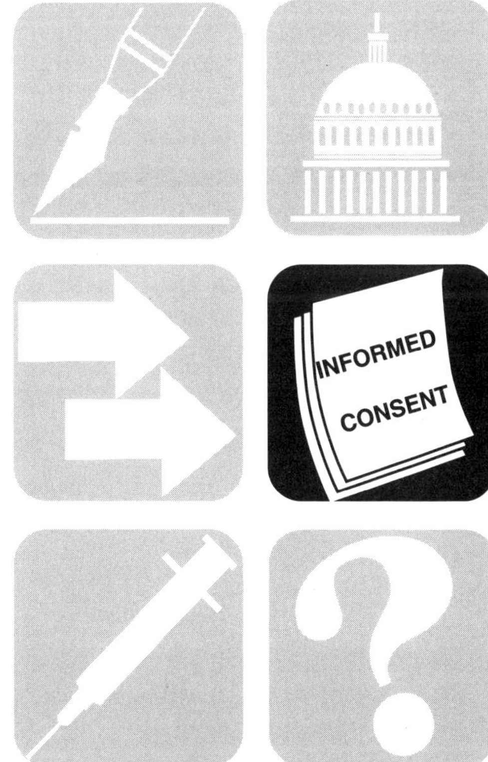

BIOMEDICAL ETHICS

New Marketing Practices Threaten Privacy
Pharmaceutical Companies and Academic Researchers
Protecting Human Research Subjects
AIDS Vaccine Trials in the Third World
Placebo-Controlled Clinical Trials
Treatment of Patients with Terminal Disease
Drug Companies Find Novel Ways to Thwart Generic
    Competition
Rationing Scarce Drugs

New Marketing Practices Threaten Privacy. The Holy Grail of marketing today is targeted promotion aimed at individuals most likely to respond. To do this effectively, the marketer wants to learn as much as possible about an individual: her or his age, occupation, health status, medications, and so on. The drive to acquire information is in direct conflict with the strongly held wish of most Americans for privacy especially concerning their health. Many now feel that the erosion of privacy has gone too far and are calling for federal legislation to ensure confidentiality.

Triggering the latest round of controversy is a February 15, 1998 report in *The Washington Post* revealing that two chain drug retailers have used third parties to send drug company-sponsored reminders to refill prescriptions, as well as information about new products, directly to patients. The report led the two pharmacy chains to terminate their programs. The initial concern was that the stores turned over confidential patient records to an outside marketing firm without the patients' consent. Presumably, if the pharmacy retailer, rather than the third party, sends the information to the patient, there is no breach of patient confidentiality. That may be true, but a question of professional ethics remains. Providing drug company-sponsored information to patients about new drugs that may be of benefit to their condition is often called a switch letter. Drug companies reward stores for encouraging patients to switch from one drug to another.

One of the letters sent out by pharmacy retailers promoted Glaxo Wellcome's new smoking cessation product *Zyban* (bupropion). It was targeted at patients from the chain's database who had had prescriptions for competing smoking cessation products. The letter, printed on the store's letterhead, said that the pharmacy hoped the patients had already quit smoking, but if they had not, they might consider *Zyban*.

Using pharmacies as a conduit for targeted promotion is only one strategy used by drug companies. Often, drug manufacturers obtain the names of people who suffer a specific health problem from the patients themselves. For example, last year, Reader's Digest Association mailed out a survey to its 15 million US subscribers, asking them to disclose medical information about themselves and their families, including prescription medicine in use in the home. The magazine sorted responses and created mailing lists of people with specific diseases and medical conditions. The magazine plans to send to the people on each list a disease-specific booklet that will carry relevant information as well as four pages of ads from a single drug company sponsor. The sponsor will have some control over what the entire booklet contains, but the degree of control has not been determined [*The Wall Street Journal,* April 17, 1998].

Pharmaceutical Companies and Academic Researchers. There is a growing concern that too many academic biomedical researchers are beholden to industry. Evidence of this surfaced recently in reports concerning the safety of calcium channel blockers. A review of editorials, commentaries, and letters showed that 96% of authors who wrote in defense of calcium antagonists had financial ties to manufacturers of these drugs, compared with 37% of authors who wrote critical pieces [*N Engl J Med* 1998;338:101–06]. The investigators concluded: "The medical profession needs to develop a more effective policy on conflict of interest. We support complete disclosure of relations with pharmaceutical manufacturers for clinicians and researchers who write articles examining pharmaceutical products." In a similar study, researchers found that the conclusions of review papers on the effects of passive smoking are strongly associated with the affiliations of their authors [*JAMA* 1998; 279:1566–70]. Overall, 37% of reviews concluded that passive smoking is not harmful; authors with tobacco industry affiliations wrote 74% of these papers.

The policies developed by scientific journals on financial disclosure by authors have divided editors who disagree on whether such policies really improve scientific integrity and manage conflicts of interest [*JAMA* 1998; 280:225-26]. Those who oppose obligatory disclosure argue that, ". . . the mere existence of a financial interest does not imply a conflict and the potential for financial gain is only one of many factors that can generate such conflicts. . . ." Among other factors are academic competition and "intellectual passion." Nevertheless, the International Committee of Medical Journal Editors has identified financial relationships with industry as the most important conflict of interest [*Lancet* 1993;341:472]. Editors who embrace full disclosure say that the way a scientific journal deals with financial conflicts of interest can affect the credibility of published papers.

Another study surveys the frequency, importance, and potential implications of research-related gifts from companies to academic life scientists [*JAMA* 1998;279:995–99]. The survey reveals that 43% of the respondents received a research-related gift in the last three years, independent of a grant or contract; two-thirds of them considered those gifts important to their research. The most frequently received gifts were biomaterials, discretionary funds, research equipment, and trips to meetings. About a third of the respondents said that the donor wanted pre-publication review of any reports stemming from the use of the gift and about 20% reported that the donor expected ownership of all patents that might result from supported research. The investigators also learned that recipients frequently think that donors place restrictions and expect returns that may be problematic for recipients and their institutions. Universities need to develop guidelines concerning gifts as they have for grants and contracts [*JAMA* 1998;279:1031–32].

A commentary on this work observed: "The *JAMA* report is a clear warning that researchers who take money or resources from the private sector in exchange for restrictions on publications or ownership rights may well be on a collision course with their universities and the scientific community" [*Nature Biotech* 1998;16:495]. Corporate gifts to academic researchers may also be used as a means of bypassing existing institutional safeguards relating to management of research grants and contracts.

The FDA will put into effect in 1999 a rule requiring disclosure of financial interests by those who conduct clinical trials. Under the new rule, drug and device companies must inform the agency when researchers have proprietary interests, such as a patent, in the products under review. FDA also wants to know whether clinical investigators have more than $50,000 equity in the company and whether the company has given the researcher more than $25,000 in consulting fees, grants, or equipment. When the rule is in effect, the FDA may refuse to accept marketing applications from sponsors that have not made the required disclosures or certified that no such financial arrangements exist [*Scrip*, February 7, 1998, p 15]. The pharmaceutical industry describes the FDA's ruling as unnecessary, overly intrusive, burdensome, and a hindrance to clinical research.

The Pharmaceutical Research and Manufacturers of America (PhRMA), the lobbying group for major pharmaceutical companies, petitioned for reconsideration of FDA's rule, urging that investigators and institutions involved in large randomized studies be exempted from the financial disclosure. This privilege is already granted for large open studies and other clinical investigations with large numbers of investigators, where no single investigator has major responsibility for the data. PhRMA argues that the same reasoning should apply to large, multicenter controlled trials. It asks that the FDA insert the sentence: "A large multicenter study in which a single investigator contributes less than 20% of the data is not a covered clinical study" [*The Pink Sheet,* 1998;60(No32):13].

Critics who find the industry-academia relationship unwholesome are disappointed with the new rule because it does not go far enough. Consumer advocacy groups urged the FDA to forbid clinical investigators from owning an equity interest exceeding a threshold amount, or from receiving large payments from the sponsor. They are also unhappy that the public will not learn of the disclosures unless the FDA determines there is a conflict of interest.

Also of interest was the announcement from the Securities and Exchange Commission in April 1998 that it had begun to crack down on classic insider trading by biomedical researchers. Most cases have involved clinical investigators who were either privy to or involved first-hand in drug development trials. This information permitted them to profit from imminent and significant changes in the price of a stock [*Nature Biotech* 1998;16:495].

Protecting Human Research Subjects. According to law, research proposals that receive federal dollars and include studies in human subjects must be examined and approved by an institutional review board (IRB) before implementation. The same applies to clinical studies supporting applications to the FDA for approval of drugs and devices. There are more than 3000 locally managed IRBs empowered to protect volunteers in studies at hospitals and clinics throughout the United States. Each IRB, composed of at least five unpaid members including one nonscientist, is responsible for vetting the ethical aspects of research projects within its purview. Specifically, IRBs should review protocol design, examine the risk to benefit ratio for the patients, and ensure that informed consent of trial subjects has been obtained. Some think, however, that the system to protect human subjects in the United States is showing signs of wear and tear [*Nature Biotech* 1998;16:714].

An article in *The Wall Street Journal* [May 30, 1998, p A8] reported that patients who participated in clinical trials of new drugs were sometimes exposed to unsafe and unethical practices because IRBs are overwhelmed with work. Indeed, the burden for members of IRBs has increased by 42% in the past five years [*Science* 1998;280:1830–31]. Some of the reasons for this are increased commercialization of research and the proliferation of multicenter trials.

According to the Inspector General of the Department of Health and Human Services (DHHS), IRBs review too much, too quickly, with too little expertise, and often fail to protect the interests of research subjects. She says that clinical investigators on behalf of drug companies often recruit human subjects with misleading advertisements that stress inducements (i.e., cash payments or free treatment) but downplay or even ignore the risks. Because of the large number of government- and drug industry-supported clinical trials that are now ongoing, subject recruitment is a competitive business and some are using aggressive and sly marketing techniques. She also said that, ". . . review boards were riddled with potential conflicts of interest because they were under pressure to accommodate the needs of academic health centers that depend heavily on the money they receive for clinical research from drug companies and other businesses" [*Ibid.*].

Other criticisms levied by the Inspector General's report include the failure of review boards to visit research sites and query patients about their understanding of the research in which they are participating, the lack of a system to monitor departures from the research protocol originally approved by an institutional review group, and the practice of some drug companies and researchers to seek approval of another, sometimes commercial, review board if dissatisfied with the decision of the institution's review board. She also believes that IRBs should include more nonscientific participants and more members from outside the institution. The report proposes an IRB education program in which members would be trained in technical and ethical issues.

Her report concludes that the system for protecting human research subjects seems to be breaking down and calls for a fundamental re-examination and re-engineering of the process. Defenders of the current system say that it is not in jeopardy and that there is no evidence that patients have been harmed or are at risk. The pharmaceutical and biotechnology industries, in particular, say that the system is not in need of major revision. They fear that implementation of the report's recommendations could lead to closer scrutiny of research protocols, thus making it more difficult to obtain IRB approval.

Punctuating the Inspector General's report was a feature story carried by *The New York Times* (May 19, 1998, pp B11, B14], entitled "Psychiatric Researchers Under Fire." It tells of a patient with manic depression who in 1994 agreed to be a research subject at the National Institute of Mental Health. He hoped he could learn more about his disorder and get superior treatment. Instead, he was taken off his medicines, subjected to stressful tests, and given a variety of agents to study his response. The patient also says that consent forms and explanations of experiments were distributed casually, with little attempt to determine that he understood them.

Clinical trials of drugs for mental disorders frequently require that patients stop current medication. And in some studies, patients may receive chemicals to provoke relapse. Psychiatric researchers argue that their studies are important to the understanding and future treatment of mental disorders and that patients can be deprived of medication for short periods with little harm.

Attempting to address this problem, which critics believe is pervasive, the National Bioethics Advisory Commission is considering proposals that would require researchers to determine first whether potential research subjects have the capacity to give informed consent. Another proposal would require research institutions to include a patient advocate as well as someone familiar with psychiatric research on their IRBs and ensure that patients truly understand the research protocol. One member of the advisory commission offered harsher criticism: "Some of these consent forms contain outright deception."

The New York Times story cited one study in which men and women with schizophrenia were not only taken off their medication, but they were also injected with ketamine to provoke psychiatric symptoms—hallucination, disorientation, paranoia—so the provoked responses could be studied. In another study patients were given methylphenidate (*Ritalin*), which quickly precipitated a severe psychotic episode in more than half of them. Some of the research concerning the commission is carried out in children with behavioral or mental disorders. In light of the attention focused on human research, investigators and institutions expect DHHS to make important changes in the regulations guiding the activity of IRBs.

Despite these criticisms, a recent survey suggests that clinical investigators can anticipate a large reservoir of trust concerning medical research from most patients and potential study participants. The survey involved nearly 2000 patients in the waiting rooms of oncology and cardiology outpatient clinics at 16 institutions across the country. The patients were interviewed about their attitudes toward medical research. Ninety percent had a favorable attitude about medical research in general. Patients reporting that they had participated in medical research expressed the most positive attitudes. African-Americans, however, who suffered the most egregious episode of human research abuse in our history, were more likely than others to believe that medical research usually or always involves undue risk [*IRB* 1998; 20(No4):1–7].

AIDS Vaccine Trials in the Third World. Public health officials all over the globe agree that the only hope for stemming the tide of the AIDS epidemic in the third world is to develop an effective vaccine. In the past, ethical guidelines have required that vaccines be tested in developed nations with comprehensive health care delivery systems before they are used in emerging nations without a safety net. With HIV infection, the international medical community has waived the requirement for the first time. There is a broad consensus that urgency must temper ethical standards [*The New York Times,* October 1, 1998, ppA1,A6].

Uganda, with 20% of its population infected with HIV, is a designated center for current placebo-controlled HIV-vaccine trials. In the country where only six dollars per person annually is spent on health care, the principal question weighing heavily in the minds of Ugandan health officials is what will happen to people who become infected and sick after volunteering for the trial. The risk of infection is high for both the placebo and active intervention groups because the vaccine is not expected to prevent the development of infection, but may only slow progression. Will infected Africans receive state-of-the-art medical care, as they would in the US and France, other vaccine-testing sites? If they do, who will pay? If not, will they be treated like any other Africans—"given aspirin, good wishes, and no hope?" Furthermore, if Ugandans are given the best medical therapy after infection, the investigators will not be able to assess an ameliorating impact of the vaccine on the course of the disease.

Informed consent is another thorny issue. Informing a representative of a village of the details of participation in a clinical trial is unacceptable in the US, but Ugandan officials say they cannot reach individuals and have no other choice. Criticism from some individuals in developed nations that African health officials are not sufficiently sensitive to basic human rights have been met with anger and accusations of patronization.

Another concern facing Uganda and most other developing countries is the possibility that vaccine testing in Africa may result in an effective product that will be too expensive to buy. Health officials insist that if that occurs, "foundations, international relief agencies, pharmaceutical companies, and governments will have to band together to come up with enough money to buy vaccines for poor countries."

Placebo-Controlled Clinical Trials. A commentary on the Nuremberg Code of 1947 that was formulated by Americans sitting in judgment of physicians and scientists accused of murder and torture while conducting medical experiments in Nazi concentration camps, raises provocative and timely issues [*Lancet* 1998;351:974-77]. The author contends that while obtaining truly informed consent is crucial to ethical human research, it is not sufficient to justify research on human beings. Intervention trials with HIV-infected pregnant women in Africa, Thailand, and the Dominican Republic, successfully concluded in 1998 provide an example. These trials, sponsored by the National Institutes of Health and the Centers for Disease Control and Prevention, sought to evaluate a simple and relatively inexpensive drug regimen to prevent maternal-to-infant transmission of HIV. The protocol used in the United States and other developed countries to prevent vertical transmission, which reduces the incidence of HIV infection in newborns by two-thirds, is too expensive and complex to be useful in developing countries.

These third world trials have been harshly criticized for including a placebo. Although an effective treatment is available, the offspring of women assigned to placebo would surely face a sizable risk of acquiring the infection. Many researchers in the US and medical leaders in developing countries reject this criticism, arguing that researchers truly did not know at the trials' initiations whether abbreviated protocols would prove effective; this uncertainty demanded rigorous evaluation and justified the use of placebo.

A "Viewpoint," appearing in *The Lancet* [1998:351:286–87], provided by the Gambia Government/Medical Research Council Joint Ethical Committee, offers the following thoughts: "The need to improve health in developing countries requires informed public-health decisions that will sometimes mean re-examining interventions proved effective under different conditions in resource-rich countries. Stopping trials in Africa that are trying to help improve the health of poor people so that those in affluent countries can have piece of mind seems a tortured form of ethical logic."

Placebo-controlled trials are under attack not only in the third world but also in developed nations. There are few medical conditions that resist amelioration by some form of therapy. Therefore, withdrawing medication and assigning a patient to placebo prevents that person from getting the "best medical treatment available" for the condition. Even IRBs are turning back proposals for placebo-controlled trials enrolling patients with arthritis, mental disorders, and other conditions.

In April 1998, a representative of Public Citizen's Health Research Group told the House Government Reform and Oversight Committee that active-control clinical studies should be required by law when a known therapy exists for a disease [*The Pink Sheet,* April 27, 1998, pp 8–9]. The citizen's group says that drug companies would rather demonstrate that their product is better than nothing, than take the chance that it may be no better, or possibly worse, than existing treatment. The group argues that not only do placebo trials violate accepted ethical guidelines, they often fail to provide information that is most useful clinically—Which is the best treatment?

The citizen's group apportions some of the blame for the emphasis on placebo-controlled trials to the FDA. The agency protests, saying that according to regulations, clinical trial designs may employ five different kinds of controls: placebos, no treatment, active agents, historical controls, or dose comparisons. Despite protestations, the "gold standard" design for the past 30 years has been the placebo-controlled double-blind trial [*The Scientist* 1998;12(No18):1,7,14].

Representatives of the FDA have spoken out often on the importance of placebo-controlled studies to strengthen statistical evaluation of the findings. To support that position, the FDA has provided examples where drug A is significantly more effective than placebo, drug B is "equivalent" to drug A, but drug B is not significantly more effective than placebo. In response to the group's allegations, the FDA says that it does not typically require placebo-controlled trials in therapeutic areas such as infectious disease and oncology, but placebo-control is used more commonly in others.

Treatment of Patients with Terminal Disease. The decision to pursue aggressive chemotherapy for patients who are almost certainly terminal bristles with ethical considerations because of the added pain and suffering. Many view aggressive treatment in the last days of life as a physician's personal battle with death and disregard for the patient's well being. We now know that this is not often the case. A new report says that most terminally ill patients appear to believe that their odds for survival are greater than they really are [*JAMA* 1998;279:1709–14].

The research involved 917 adult patients hospitalized with advanced lung or colon cancer, metastasized to the liver. Experts concur that at this stage of cancer, the disease is generally incurable and associated with a short life expectancy. Each patient and physician was asked to rate the patient's chance of surviving at least six months. Patients were then asked to choose between life-extending cancer therapy or therapy directed at relief of pain and discomfort—comfort care.

The majority of patients said they believed that they had at least a 90% chance of surviving for another six months, though less than half actually lived that long. Patients who thought they were going to live for at least six months were more than twice as likely to favor aggressive therapy over comfort care, compared with patients who thought there was at least a 10% chance that they would not live as long as six months. Patients overestimated their chances of surviving six months, while physicians estimated prognosis correctly about 70% of the time. Patients who preferred life-extending therapy were more likely to undergo aggressive treatment but their six-month survival was no better.

The researchers suggest that a likely reason for the patients' unwarranted optimism is that physicians do not give patients enough information about their conditions. An author of an editorial that accompanied the study report in *JAMA*, who is an expert on the subject of doctors and dying patients, said that some physicians justify withholding information from patients because the patients do not ask. He believes that physicians are obliged to tell the patient and the patient's family the truth, whether or not they ask [*The New York Times*, June 9, 1998, p B10].

Drug Companies Find Novel Ways to Thwart Generic Competition. It is often said, although the source is lost in antiquity, that the term business ethics is an oxymoron. Supporting that cynical conviction are the actions of Hoechst AG, the maker of a widely prescribed, sustained-release form of the calcium antagonist diltiazem called *Cardizem CD. Cardizem CD*, widely used for the treatment of hypertension and angina, ranks among the top 20 best-selling drugs in the United States.

The product is no longer protected by patent and one would expect Hoechst to be fighting to protect its market share from cheaper generic competition. The company, however, has avoided that problem, at least up until now, by striking a deal with Andrx Corp, a generic drug manufacturer. Andrx receives from Hoechst $40 million dollars a year (a small percentage of the *Cardizem CD* sales) to keep their version of extended-release diltiazem, the first generic to be approved, off the market. A group of US consumers finds this arrangement collusive and has filed a class action lawsuit in Superior Court to test their convictions [*The Wall Street Journal*, August 21, 1998, pp B1, B4].

The suit alleges antitrust violations and claims that the arrangement lets Hoechst in fact overcharge patients for diltiazem. Further, Hoechst has placed other potential competitors in regulatory limbo because continuing litigation between Hoechst and Andrx is holding up FDA action to approve other generic versions of *Cardizem CD*. A US drug law gives the first company to reach the market with a generic version of a drug six months of exclusivity before any other generic firm can enter the same market. Two companies have applications before the FDA but the agency will not approve them while the patent is in dispute. As long as Andrx does not start selling its generic product, no other company can. Many observers see this consequence as anticompetitive.

Andrx was poised to release the generic version at the end of 1995. A suit by Hoechst, however, claiming patent infringement, triggered a regulatory provision that blocked the launch for 30 months. The requisite delay ended in July 1998, giving Andrx the right to market the product even though the patent suit is pending. But Andrx decided not to go to market in exchange for Hoescht's payment of $10 million a quarter.

The plaintiffs call the arrangement an "outright bribe" and an "unconscionable and *per se* illegal restraint of trade that assures that [Hoechst] will continue to set and maintain artificially high prices" for *Cardizem CD*. A spokesman for Hoechst said that the deal does not harm consumers because a variety of less expensive calcium antagonists are available. The company posits that the arrangement is an acceptable, legal agreement. If the class action suit fails, other pharmaceutical companies will follow in Hoechst' path.

Also in the courts is a class action lawsuit against BASF/Knoll over levothyroxin (*Synthroid*), used as replacement therapy for people with hypothyroidism. Plaintiffs are the nearly 420,000 patients who used *Synthroid* between 1990 and 1997. They allege that Knoll suppressed publication of a study that found two, less expensive generic levothyroxin products equivalent to *Synthroid* and, in so doing, controlled the US market for thyroid hormone-replacement products. Knoll decided to settle the class action in August 1997. A US Federal Court judge, however, has rejected the settlement after hearing protests from consumer groups, third-party payers, and state attorneys general. The proposed settlement would leave the estimated 5 million potential claimants with only $14 each after the lawyers take $28 million in legal fees [*Scrip,* September 9, 1998, p 13].

Rationing Scarce Drugs. Before the approval of trastuzumab (*Herceptin*), a novel monoclonal antibody for the treatment of a certain kind of breast cancer, Genentech made a small amount of the drug available for compassionate use by means of a lottery. There simply was not enough drug to respond to all requests from women with breast cancer, many in the last stages. The have-nots were bitterly disappointed. The episode prompted a columnist at *The Wall Street Journal* [September 28, 1998, p B6] to question the fairness and ethics of the way the pharmaceutical industry rations scarce, experimental treatment. But she offered no solution.

The rules of Genentech's lottery required patients to have breast cancer that had metastasized, to test positive for the HER-2 oncogene, and to have relapsed after two regimens of chemotherapy. Furthermore, patients also had to be judged strong enough to make monthly trips to a research center. While the lottery was guided by the imperative to "save" the sickest patients, this group may not experience the greatest benefit from *Herceptin*.

LATE BREAKING REPORTS

Questionable Anti-Generic Strategy Could Affect Merger Plan. The FTC has initiated an investigation of charges that Hoechst AG engaged in anti-competitive practices by paying Andrx $40 million a year to keep its generic version of Hoechst's slow-release calcium antagonist diltiazem (*Cardizem CD*) off the market. The findings could influence the agency's review of the drug company's proposed merger with Rhone-Poulenc SA [*The Wall Street Journal*, December 10, 1998, pp A3, A6]. The planned merger is subject to approval by the FTC because both companies, though based in Europe, have sizable US operations.

Protecting Human Research Subjects: An Update. The Human Research Ethics Group reviewed the status of existing human subjects protection and made recommendations to improve and reform the regulations that were last revised in 1981. Their report appears as a policy perspective in *JAMA* [1998;280:1951–58]. The group reached consensus for reform of three key areas—protecting subject populations with special needs and vulnerabilities, oversight by institution review boards, and regulatory policy.

10 Therapeutic Controversies and Dilemmas

CARDIOVASCULAR DISEASE

Hypertension: Dramatically Undertreated
The Treatment of Hypertension: Is There a Role for Calcium
   Channel Blockers?
Underprescribing of β-Blockers After a Heart Attack
TPA for the Treatment of Stroke

Hypertension: Dramatically Undertreated. The message of the National High Blood Pressure Education Program in 1972 was prophetic: Treating high blood pressure would save lives. For the next twenty years a substantial lowering in mortality rates from stroke and coronary heart disease was observed. More recently, however, the news is less encouraging. The risk of stroke is slowly climbing, the decline in heart disease is leveling off, and kidney disease and heart failure are on the rise. At least part of these worrisome trends may be the consequence of not taking hypertension seriously. It is a silent disease without symptoms. Of the 50 million Americans suffering from hypertension, only 34 million are diagnosed, and just 27 million seek treatment. Still worse, only half of those who seek treatment achieve blood pressure levels under 140/90 mm Hg [*The New York Times,* July 14, 1998, pp B9, B12].

We often lay the blame for undertreatment of elevated blood pressure on patients' poor compliance. Some patients, however, are not receiving the most effective drug therapy. Considering that 65 different drugs and 29 combination products are available for the treatment of hypertension, astute prescribing is a challenge. Some physicians do not monitor closely enough to ensure that initial therapy achieves a satisfactory drop in blood pressure. Many patients need more than one drug to reach the goal. The addition of a diuretic is often sufficient but these agents are underprescribed in the US. Some patients may benefit from more aggressive treatment to lower blood pressure to 120/80 mm Hg. Patients must learn about the dire consequences of hypertension and pay attention to prescribed therapy, physicians must pay more attention to individual patients, and public health officials need to increase the volume of their message.

The Treatment of Hypertension: Is There a Role for Calcium Channel Blockers? In May 1998, the American Pharmaceutical Association issued a special report—A Review of the Sixth Report of the Joint National Committee (JNC) on Prevention, Detection, Evaluation, and Treatment of High Blood Pressure. The approach to treatment of hypertension is more flexible in JNC VI [*Arch Intern Med* 1997;157:2413–2446] than in JNC V. Issued in 1993, the fifth report recommended only diuretics and β-blockers as first-line antihypertensive therapy unless contraindicated. They were the only classes of drugs shown in long-term trials to reduce cardiovascular morbidity and mortality.

While retaining the recommendation for use of diuretics as initial therapy for patients without co-morbid diseases that indicate the need for a different class of antihypertensive agents, JNC VI also recognizes the wide range of circumstances in which other classes of drugs may be useful. Four compelling indications dictate the use of a specific class of antihypertensive medication, unless otherwise contraindicated.

For patients with type 1 diabetes and a decline in renal function, the JNC favors ACE inhibitors because they have been shown to slow progressive renal failure. β-blockers are the choice after a heart attack because they reduce the risk of re-infarction or sudden death. For patients with systolic dysfunction after a heart attack, ACE inhibitors prevent subsequent heart failure and reduce morbidity. For patients with heart failure, ACE inhibitors, either alone or combined with digoxin and diuretics, also reduce morbidity and mortality.

JNC VI favors diuretics for isolated systolic hypertension (ISH), common in the elderly, because they significantly reduce the incidence of stroke and major cardiovascular events. A recent controlled trial in elderly patients with ISH reported a 42% reduction in fatal and nonfatal stroke with nitrendipine, a calcium antagonist that is not available in the US. Although the benefits of nitrendipine were not as robust as those of diuretics, the report led the JNC to recommend that other long-acting calcium antagonists may be used as an alternative to diuretics for treatment of ISH.

The inclusion of calcium antagonists in the new recommendations, albeit circumscribed, is hotly debated among experts, and caused several JNC panelists to resign in protest. Dissenters argue that the evidence of benefit with calcium antagonists for patients with ISH is too weak to support the recommendation. They also say there is an absence of reliable evidence about the effects of calcium antagonists on mortality and morbidity in patients with hypertension, and no evidence of beneficial effects of calcium antagonists in patients with coronary heart disease [*J Hypertension* 1997;15:1201–04]. The critics point to The American College of Cardiology-American Heart Association Task Force on Practice Guidelines [*J Am Coll Cardiol* 1996;

28:1328–1428]. The guidelines state: "Calcium channel blocking agents have not been shown to reduce mortality after acute MI, and in certain patients with cardiovascular disease there are data to suggest that they are harmful. . . ."

Those who wish to have calcium channel blockers prescribed only for very specific indications have focused on the potential harm of these agents in patients with coronary heart disease. The most recent report emerged from the Nurses' Health Study [*Circulation* 1998;97:1540–48]. In analyses of data from nearly 15,000 women who regularly used antihypertensive medication, adjusted only for age, the investigators found a significant increase in the relative risk of myocardial infarction in women who used calcium channel blockers compared with those who did not. Confounding the study, however, is a higher prevalence of ischemic heart disease at baseline in women who received a calcium antagonist than in those who were prescribed a different type of antihypertensive agent. On covariate-adjusted analysis, the investigators found that calcium channel blockers increase the risk of heart attack in women who smoke but do not increase risk in nonsmokers.

Some observational studies suggest that calcium antagonists may also increase the risk of cancer. A prospective analysis of more than 3,000 American women who were at least 65 years old, shows that those taking calcium antagonists have twice the risk of developing breast cancer than other women [*Cancer* 1997;80:1438–47]. When women used both estrogen and a calcium antagonist, the relative risk (RR) of breast cancer increased to 4.5. The largest RR (8.5) was in women using both estrogen and an immediate-release form of a short-acting calcium antagonist. The investigators believe that calcium channel blockers stimulate apoptosis in some tissues but inhibit it in hormonal tissues such as the breast, thus disabling a natural defense mechanism against cancer. In a comment on the report, the National Heart, Lung and Blood Institute emphasizes that the findings are preliminary, derive from an observational study with only 75 cases of breast cancer, and relate primarily to short-acting agents and not to the longer-acting drugs and formulations now used by most patients. The Institute, however, stresses that the results of the new study are consistent with previous findings that link short-acting calcium antagonists with an excess risk of cancer, as well as an increased risk of heart attack.

A more recent case-control study based on hospital data arrives at a different conclusion [*JAMA* 1998;279:1000–04]. The study involved about 9500 patients with cancer and 6500 controls admitted for nonmalignant conditions. The investigators found that the use of calcium channel blockers was not related to the risk of cancer overall (RR, 1.1) nor was use associated significantly with increased risk of individual cancers, except cancer of the kidney (RR, 1.8). The use of β-blockers and ACE inhibitors was also associated with kidney cancer (RR, 1.8) but not with any other cancer. The authors suggest that the use of calcium antagonists is unrelated to an increased risk of cancer, except kidney cancer, which has, for unknown reasons, been associated with hypertension and with drugs used to treat hypertension. The conclusions of this report are limited by the relatively small number of cancer cases in patients using calcium antagonists for five or more years. Overall there were 97 cases of cancer, and only 27 cases of breast cancer.

An editorial in *Cardiovascular Drugs and Therapy* [1998;12:145–47] attempts to summarize the available evidence of the safety and efficacy of calcium antagonists. The report concludes that (1) nifedipine and other short-acting agents cannot be considered safe for the treatment of hypertension and ischemic heart disease; (2) among the medium-duration and long-acting dihydropyridines, nitrendipine prevents stroke and cardiac events in patients with isolated hypertension, and these agents prevent anginal attacks in stable disease; and (3) verapamil and diltiazem can be used in the treatment of supraventricular tachycardia, atrial fibrillation, angina pectoris, and to reduce blood pressure and prevent cardiac events in postinfarct patients without congestive heart failure. More information is needed about calcium antagonists in patients with heart failure and in those who succumb to sudden cardiac death.

Underprescribing of β-Blockers after a Heart Attack. Long-term administration of β-blockers after acute myocardial infarction (AMI) improves survival. Two new studies, however, provide more evidence that far fewer patients receive these agents than would seem appropriate. Physicians seem to be reluctant to prescribe β-blockers, particularly for older patients and those with chronic pulmonary disease, left ventricular dysfunction, or non-Q-wave AMI.

In one study, researchers abstracted the medical records of more than 200,000 patients with AMI. Using a statistical model that accounted for multiple factors that might affect survival, they compared mortality among patients treated with β-blockers with mortality among untreated patients during the two years after a heart attack. They found that only 34% of patients received β-blockers. The percentage was lower among the very old, blacks, and patients with low left ventricular ejection fraction (LVEF), heart failure, chronic obstructive pulmonary disease (COPD), renal impairment, and type 1 diabetes. Mortality, however, was lower in every subgroup of patients treated with a β-blocker than in untreated patients.

In patients with AMI but no other complication, treatment with β-blockers resulted in a 40% reduction in mortality. The same reduction was seen in patients with non-Q-wave infarction, and those with COPD. A lower percentage reduction was seen in blacks, patients 80 years of age or older, and those with LVEF below 20%, serum creatinine greater than 1.4 mg/dl, or diabetes. The authors note, however, that because of the higher mortality rates in these subgroups, the absolute mortality was similar to or greater than that among patients with no additional risk factors. They conclude: "This analysis strongly indicates that β-blockade is an underused therapy for patients who have had a myocardial infarction. In addition to otherwise healthy patients, those with nontransmural infarction, heart failure, pulmonary disease and older age are likely to benefit when given β-blockers after a myocardial infarction" [*N Engl J Med* 1998;339:489–97].

An accompanying editorial criticizes the report because it does not provide adequate information about the severity of the conditions that have been considered by specialists to be contraindications to β-blocker therapy. "For example, because chronic obstructive pulmonary disease can range in severity from mild to life-threatening, grouping all patients with this condition may bias the results in favor of β-blocker therapy. Patients with more severe disease, who have a higher risk of death, are less likely to be given β-blockers." [*N Engl J Med* 1998;339:551–52]. Widely accepted treatment guidelines specify severe COPD as a contraindication to β-blocker therapy, not merely the presence of the condition. Consequently, the authors conclude that ". . . the interesting findings . . . cannot serve as the basis for expanding the recommendations for β-blocker therapy after myocardial infarction."

The other report concerns a retrospective cohort study using data from medical charts and administrative files [*JAMA* 1998;280:623–29]. The study group consisted of 115,000 eligible patients aged 65 years or older who survived an acute MI, at least until hospital discharge. Among the 45,000 patients without contraindications to β-blockade, 50% had a β-blocker prescribed at discharge. Prescribing a β-blocker to otherwise healthy heart-attack patients, however, varied widely across the country. In Connecticut, 77% of candidates received a β-blocker compared with about 30% in Mississippi. Of the some 37,000 patients who were not receiving β-blocker therapy on admission, 44% had therapy initiated on or before discharge. Curiously, patients who received a discharge prescription for a calcium channel blocker had only a 25% probability of receiving a prescription for a β-blocker.

After adjusting for potential confounding variables, β-blockers were associated with a 14% lower risk of mortality at one year after discharge. The authors conclude: "Many ideal patients for β-blocker therapy are not prescribed these drugs at discharge following AMI . . . Elderly patients who are prescribed β-blockers at discharge have a better survival rate . . ."

The results of a study by the National Committee for Quality Assurance (NCQA) show that during 1997 in the US, the administration of β-blockers after a heart attack ranged from 60% of managed care enrollees in the South Central region to 90% in New England [*The Pink Sheet* 1998;60(No39):6]. NCQA estimates that if industry-wide performance improved to the 90th percentile, more than 2,000 cardiac deaths would be avoided among managed care enrollees each year.

TPA for the Treatment of Stroke. Although the FDA has approved the thrombolytic agent alteplase (TPA, *Activase*) for use within three hours after an ischemic stroke, the number of patients treated in the US with *Activase* is small and few European neurologist believe that alteplase provides a net benefit. The drug is not licensed for stroke in any European nation [*Scrip Magazine,* March 1998, pp 29–32].

The results from the NINDS trial, a study that randomized carefully-selected patients to active drug or placebo, were the basis of approval of alteplase for the treatment of stroke in the US [*N Engl J Med* 1995;333:1581–87]. On presentation, patients underwent a computed tomographic (CT) scan to rule out cranial hemorrhage. Alteplase can be fatal if used in patients with hemorrhagic stroke. These patients were excluded as well as patients with blood pressure exceeding 185/100 mm Hg. The use of aspirin and heparin was prohibited for the first 24 hours to further reduce the risk of bleeding.

The investigators found no difference between alteplase and placebo in the percentage of patients with neurologic improvement at 24 hours or in survival at 90 days. However, despite a highly significant excess of intracerebral hemorrhages compared with placebo, intravenous alteplase improved clinical outcome at three months. Approximately 30% more patients were alive and free of disability in the active treatment group than in the placebo group (51% vs. 38%). The NINDS study is the only positive trial of a thrombolytic agent in the treatment of stroke. Other trials with alteplase and all trials with streptokinase have failed to show a net benefit.

An editorial accompanying the report warned that the risk of cerebral hemorrhage should discourage the use of alteplase unless patients meet clearly defined criteria. Absolute requirements are a short time from the onset of the ischemic event to treatment and the absence of any sign of brain injury on CT [*N Engl J Med* 1995;333:1632–33]. Shortly after the approval of the new indication for alteplase in 1996, an expert panel issued guidelines for its use in the treatment of stroke, emphasizing the importance of patient selection [*Circulation* 1996;94:1167–74].

The use of alteplase in an evolving stroke, even in carefully selected patients, requires deliberation. The evidence indicates that although alteplase provides a 12% absolute increase in the number of patients surviving without disability, there is also a 6% increase in the number of patients with symptomatic brain hemorrhage, about half of whom will die. The question that must be answered by the patient's family is: Do you wish to risk a 12% chance of a favorable neurologic outcome at three months against a 6% chance of hemorrhagic stroke and a 3% chance of early death? [*JAMA* 1996; 276:995–96]

Some neurologists in the US do not believe that alteplase is an appropriate treatment for all patients with acute ischemic strokes. The October 30, 1997 issue of the *New England Journal of Medicine* published a clinical debate on this issue. The dissenters argued that many patients with ischemic stroke do not have occlusive blood clots in large arteries, lysis of which is the presumed mechanism for the effectiveness of alteplase [*N Engl J Med* 1997;337:1309–10]. In response, other experts said that the use of alteplase for patients with stroke provides an opportunity to help patients who up until now have been helpless. They cautioned, however, that improvements will not occur without radical changes in the way hospitals and medical centers manage stroke [*N Engl J Med* 1997;337:1310–13].

On a more positive note, a group of neurologists recently reported on the feasibility, safety, and efficacy of using alteplase in the treatment of ischemic stroke in their practice at two hospitals in the one-year period immediately after its approval [*Stroke* 1998;29:18–22]. Following a strict protocol, they treated only 30 patients presenting with ischemic stroke. These patients represent 6% of all patients hospitalized with ischemic stroke at the university hospital and only 1% at the community hospital. The average time from stroke onset to administration of treatment was 157 minutes. The rates of total, symptomatic, and fatal intracerebral hemorrhage were 10%, 7%, and 3%, respectively, almost the same as in the NINDS study. Eleven patients recovered to fully independent function.

The results were very encouraging. Of course, they only apply to the very small number of patients with ischemic stroke who meet the imposing selection criteria. The authors conclude: "When treatment guidelines are carefully followed in an urban hospital setting, intravenous t-PA for acute ischemic stroke is feasible, and shows safety and efficacy comparable to the results of the NINDS study." There is doubt, however, that the results of this study, conducted by clinical investigators experienced in the use of alteplase for the treatment of ischemic stroke, apply to other urban hospitals.

While early treatment with alteplase may benefit some patients with ischemic stroke, it is unlikely to have a major impact on morbidity in the stroke population. Many other strategies are under investigation. Of considerable interest is a combination of low-dose alteplase with one of the new glycoprotein IIb/IIIa antiplatelet agents—*ReoPro, Integrilin, and Aggrastat.* This approach may improve safety and may be more effective than alteplase alone.

The applicability of administering a thrombolytic agent in patients with emergent stroke would increase dramatically if alteplase were to provide benefit as late as five or six hours after onset. That hope was dashed, however, in July when *The Wall Street Journal* [July 21, 1998, p A8] reported an announcement by Genentech that *Activase* did not show efficacy in an interim analysis of a trial of patients with ischemic stroke when administered between three and five hours after the onset of symptoms. The analysis determined that there was only a small chance of demonstrating a net clinical benefit by enrolling an additional 500 patients as initially planned. Genentech has now abandoned efforts to seek a label extension for use of alteplase beyond three hours.

In the most recently reported trial, ECASS II, investigators randomized 800 patients to alteplase at the same dose used in NINDS or placebo [*Lancet* 1998;352:1245–51]. Patients were enrolled if they were able to receive treatment within six hours of onset of symptoms. The cut-off point in NINDS was three hours. The results do not demonstrate a statistically significant benefit for alteplase, but a trend toward efficacy may support its use. The researchers conclude that, "Despite the increased risk of intracranial hemorrhage, thrombolysis with alteplase at a dose of 0.9 mg/kg in selected patients may lead to a clinically relevant improvement in outcome."

A commentary on the report presents a less sanguine view [*Lancet* 1998;352:1245–51]. The author muses on the future of alteplase and suggests that "A reasonable starting position is that thrombolysis does work . . . but that this point has not yet been proven beyond reasonable doubt." Given the adverse effects of alteplase in this setting and that patients likely to benefit cannot yet be identified, he believes that there should be no rush to license alteplase for acute ischemic stroke in the UK or the European Community until more compelling evidence is available.

INFECTIOUS DISEASE

Prophylactic Acyclovir and the Risk of Developing Drug-Resistant Herpesvirus. Genital herpes caused by herpes simplex virus is the most prevalent sexually transmitted disease in the world. It is an incurable infection. Acyclovir (*Zovirax*) has good activity against herpes simplex virus type 2 (HSV-2) and is used to treat episodic outbreaks of genital herpes. Acyclovir also offers benefits when used for prevention.

Despite effective therapy, genital herpes is untreated in many developing countries. In the US, only 10% of cases are treated. There is fear that widespread use of antiviral agents to treat genital herpes may result in the emergence of drug-resistant herpes strains. The question then is: "To treat or not to treat?" [*Nature Med* 1998;4:664–65]. Up until now, the answer has been no. An effort to increase the use of acyclovir by marketing a product that could be sold without a prescription was blocked by the FDA because of the fear of antiviral resistance.

More recently, investigators have developed a mathematical model that predicts the emergence of drug-resistant virus as treatment rates for patients with genital herpes are increased [*Nature Med* 1998;4:673–78]. The model suggests that it should be possible to increase treatment rates in the HSV-2 infection population while keeping the emergence of drug-resistant strains in check. According to the model, at least five drug-sensitive infections are prevented on average for each resistant case that emerges. Unless the net cost of treating a drug-resistant infection is at least five times greater than that for treating a drug-sensitive infection, it is cost-effective to treat. The researchers argue that many painful outbreaks of genital herpes could be avoided by increasing treatment rates.

Treatment of Infection for Secondary Prevention of Cardiovascular Events. Ample evidence exists of an ongoing inflammatory process in patients with atherosclerosis. This association has led to the suggestion that coronary artery disease may be an inflammatory disease. The stimulus for inflammation, however, is not clear. Data gathered in recent years suggest that infection may initiate the inflammatory process. At the same time, there is a growing understanding that the traditional risk factors, such as smoking, an unfavorable lipid profile, hypertension, and diabetes, do not explain the occurrence of coronary atherosclerosis in a large proportion of patients. Some researchers believe that in certain genetically susceptible people infection with common organisms such as *Chlamydia pneumoniae* or cytomegalovirus may lead to localized infection and a chronic inflammatory reaction [*J Am Coll Cardiol* 1998;31:1217–25]. One cardiologist says: "The evidence that bacteria are found in plaque needs to be taken seriously." If this relation were causal, treatment for coronary artery disease would change dramatically [*Science* 1998;281:35–36].

A debate persists concerning the finding of chlamydia antigen or DNA in coronary atheroma. Its presence may reflect a relatively late-onset "passenger" role of the organism as it migrates within macrophages to the site of disease, rather than an early role in the endothelial injury thought to initiate atherosclerosis. A recent report furnishes serological evidence showing that *C. pneumoniae* frequently precedes both the earliest and more advanced lesions of coronary atherosclerosis that harbor the pathogen. These findings suggest a chronic infection and a developmental role for chlamydia in coronary heart disease [*Circulation* 1998;98:628–33].

If patients with infectious atherosclerosis could be identified, treatment aimed at eradicating the organism may be appropriate. Two small trials to evaluate macrolide antibiotics for prevention of cardiovascular events in people with coronary artery disease (CAD) have yielded promising results [*Circulation* 1997;96:404–07; *Lancet* 1997;350:404–07]. Larger and better-controlled trials are ongoing or planned. A major question in developing protocols for these trials is how long subjects should be treated. The biology of chronic chlamydia infection suggests that short treatment periods, one month or less, will be inadequate for lasting benefit. There is an infectious nonreplicating form of the organism that is not susceptible to the action of antibiotics and that persists in the body for weeks or longer. On the other hand, long-term antibiotic therapy could contribute to resistance. One expert recommends that the treatment period be one year [*Circulation* 1998; 97:1169–70].

Another recent report offers an alternative explanation for the favorable effects of macrolides on cardiovascular outcomes [*Lancet* 1998;351:1858–

59]. The authors suggest that macrolide antibiotics may suppress macrophage activity by blocking a potassium channel, and stabilizing atherosclerotic plaques in coronary arteries.

At the March meeting of the American College of Cardiology investigators described results from a trial of azithromycin in 300 patients with heart disease. The antibiotic did not reduce heart attacks or ischemic episodes after six months, but it did reduce inflammatory cytokines in plasma. The investigators say that six months may be too soon to see a benefit. The largest ongoing study in this arena is the Wizard trial supported by Pfizer to evaluate azithromycin in 3500 patients who have documented atherosclerosis and have tested positive for *Chlamydia* antibodies. The patients will be followed for at least three years [*Science* 1998;281:36–37].

Drug-Resistant Microbes. For the past decade, scientists at the Centers for Disease Control and Prevention and infectious disease specialists from all over the world have been warning about the growth of antibiotic resistance, a problem accelerated by patients who demand antibiotics at the first sign of an upper respiratory infection and by physicians who give in to such demands. The list of virulent drug-resistant microbes now includes organisms that cause pneumonia, childhood ear infection, meningitis, tuberculosis, and gonorrhea. Of greatest concern is the recent report of vancomycin intermediate-resistant staphylococcus aureus (VISA). Vancomycin has long been considered the ultimate weapon against staphylococcus infection, which is relatively easy to acquire because the organism is common, living on the skin and in the nostrils. Drug companies are now spending a great deal of money to search for antibiotics with different mechanisms of action than currently available drugs [*The New York Times Magazine,* August 2, 1998, pp 42–47].

A vivid illustration of the almost reckless overuse of antibiotics is the treatment of children with ear infections. Twenty percent of all antimicrobial use in the US is for the treatment of otitis media, for which the average pediatric patient consumes three months' worth of antibiotics during the first two years of life. A recent commentary observed: "Such extensive use of these agents is a major reason for the increasing antibiotic resistance among the bacteria implicated in this infection—*Haemophilus influenzae, Streptococcus pneumoniae,* and *Moraxella catarrrhalis.*" The authors add: "The diminished susceptibility of the pneumococcus to penicillin is especially worrying, since few alternatives exist" [*Lancet* 1998;352:672].

There are two camps that hold very different views of the issue of antimicrobial resistance. One says that research towards a better understanding of the problem is necessary before specific recommendations on prescribing habits can be given. The other says that enough is known about antibiotic use and abuse, its consequences, and how to control it to allow action now on a broad front [*Nature Med* 1998;4:985]. Included in the first camp is the pharmaceutical industry. An abrupt change in the current overprescribing of antibiotics would seriously damage the bottom line of several large pharmaceutical firms.

Principles of Therapy of HIV Infection and Guidelines for Use of Antiretroviral Agents. With the development of tools to monitor HIV replication, the risk for disease progression can be assessed and the effectiveness of anti-HIV therapies can be determined directly. Potent antiviral therapies, often called "highly active antiretroviral therapies" (HAART), can bring about prolonged suppression of detectable levels of HIV replication and thwart the tendency of the virus to develop drug-resistant variants.

In light of the complexity of anti-HIV therapies, the Office of AIDS Research of the National Institutes of Health (NIH) sponsored the NIH Panel to Define Principles of Therapy of HIV Infection. This panel delineated 11 principles that address issues of basic importance for the treatment of HIV infection [*Ann Intern Med* 1998:128:1057-78]. A brief summary of these principles follows.

1. Unchecked HIV replication leads to immune system damage and progression to AIDS. Current therapies are unlikely to result in true long-term survival free of clinically important immune dysfunction.

2. Plasma HIV RNA levels indicate the degree of HIV replication as well as the rate of CD4 T cell destruction. CD4 T cell counts indicate the extent of immune damage already suffered. Frequent measurements are needed to determine when to initiate or modify antiretroviral therapies.

3. Rates of disease progression differ among patients, and treatment decisions should be individualized based on available information.

4. Therapy that suppresses viral replication below the levels of detection limits the potential for selection of drug-resistant HIV variants, the most important factor limiting the ability of therapies to inhibit viral replication and delay disease progression.

5. Prolonged suppression of HIV replication is best achieved with combinations of anti-HIV drugs that the patient has never received and that are not cross-resistant with agents the patient has received.

6. Physicians should prescribe and patients should take each of the drugs in combination therapy according to optimum schedules and doses.

7. Because there are only about a dozen antiretroviral agents available, having only one of two mechanisms, cross-resistance can develop between drugs. Any change in anti-HIV therapy limits future therapeutic options.

8. Women should receive optimal antiretroviral therapy regardless of pregnancy status.

9. The same therapeutic principles apply to children, adolescents, and adults infected with HIV.

10. Persons identified during acute primary HIV infection should be treated with combination therapy to suppress viral replication to levels below the limit of detection.

11. Patients with HIV infection, even those with no detectable viral load, should be considered infectious.

The foregoing principles provide the basis for specific treatment recommendations made by the Panel on Clinical Practices for the Treatment of HIV Infection, a group of experts sponsored by the Department of Health and Human Services and the Henry J Kaiser Family Foundation. [*Ann Intern Med* 1998;128:1079–99].

Their report recommends that medical care should be supervised by an expert and makes recommendations for monitoring, with particular emphasis on measurement of viral load. It also provides guidelines for therapy, including when to start, what drugs to use, when to change therapy, and options when changing therapy. Antiretroviral drug regimens are complex, have major side effects, and challenge compliance. The development of drug-resistant strains of HIV may result from nonadherence to the drug regimen or suboptimal levels of anti-HIV agents.

The report recommends that treatment should be offered to all patients with acute HIV syndrome and all with symptoms ascribable to HIV infection. However, for patients with asymptomatic infection, the panel says that treatment is discretionary, based on the patient's willingness to receive treatment, probability of compliance, and prognosis as predicted by viral load and CD4 T cell count. The report adds that treatment should be offered to individuals with fewer than 500 CD4 T cells per mm^3 or plasma HIV RNA levels exceeding 20,000 copies per ml based on the reverse transcriptase polymerase chain reaction assay. Some practitioners disagree with this recommendation and choose to initiate highly active therapy for anyone who is HIV-positive, regardless of viral load or CD4 count.

Consistent with the principles of antiretroviral therapy for the treatment of HIV infection, the panel urges that once the decision has been made to start therapy, the goal is maximum viral suppression for as long as possible. Clinical trials suggest that the goal is best achieved with a protease inhibitor combined with two nucleoside reverse transcriptase inhibitors (NRTIs). An alternative is the combination of saquinavir and ritonavir plus one or two NRTIs. Failure of therapy—plasma HIV RNA levels greater than 500 copies per ml at four to six months—is often ascribed to one of several factors, but is not well understood. Patients who fail therapy should receive at least two new agents that are unlikely to show cross-resistance with drugs given previously.

Understanding and Treating HIV Infection: A Survey. Good news and bad news were in store for scientists arriving in Chicago in early February for the 5th Conference of Retroviruses and Opportunistic Infections. The take-home message of the meeting was the more that we know about the workings of HIV, the more complicated the picture gets. For example, at the conference, the understanding of an inverse relation between viral load and the competence of the immune system as measured by CD4 cell counts was revealed as too naïve. Until new findings were presented at the conference, a rebound in viral load to measurable levels during aggressive treatment was taken as a signal of treatment failure. Researchers reported, however, that immune cell counts can remain high even when the virus re-emerges [*Science* 1998; 279:1133–34].

One research group described a study of 45 patients taking a combination of anti-HIV drugs, including a protease inhibitor. Viral loads dropped sharply on initiation of treatment, but after six months, bounced back to nearly original levels. Nevertheless, after 18 months, their CD4 counts were still about 125 cells higher than they were before treatment. Gains of that magnitude may ward off opportunistic infections. No one knows, however, how long the extended benefit lasts. One theory as to why strong CD4 cell counts persist in the face of emerging virus is the development of mutant viruses, resistant to drugs but less able to destroy the immune system.

Other investigators said the answer lay elsewhere. They estimated CD4 production rates in people with HIV infection, some receiving aggressive therapy and others receiving only reverse transcriptase inhibitors (RTIs), and in uninfected people. Production rates varied from 0.7 billion CD4s per day to 12 billion. Those on the most potent drug regimens produced new CD4 cells at the highest rates, while uninfected people made them at the lowest rates. Treatment may stimulate CD4 production directly and the extent of damage to the immune system may determine how someone responds to treatment. These researchers do not believe that anti-HIV drugs work simply by preventing the virus from killing CD4 cells.

This good news was offset by reports of an odd, recently recognized side effect of therapy that could complicate treatment. Twelve different research groups reported that long-term therapy with protease inhibitors causes a redistribution of fat—lipodystrophy—which could presage more serious side effects. One group found that 64% of 116 patients treated with protease inhibitors for an average of ten months had fat wasting of the limbs and face, and fat accumulation in the abdomen. Others reported fat accumulation in the breasts of women and over the cervical vertebra ("buffalo hump") in men and women, as well as elevated plasma levels of triglyceride and cholesterol.

Experts at the meeting were uncertain about the cause of the condition. Later in the year, however, investigators offered a hypothesis for HIV protease inhibitor-associated peripheral lipodystrophy, based on the discovery that the catalytic region of HIV protease, to which protease inhibitors bind, has about 60% homology to regions within two proteins that regulate lipid metabolism [*Lancet* 1998;351:1881–83]. Inhibition of one of the proteins results in reduced differentiation and increased apoptosis of peripheral adipocytes, with impaired fat storage and lipid release. Inhibition of the other leads to central obesity, breast fat deposition, and insulin resistance.

The success of aggressive therapy with anti-HIV drugs—undetectable plasma levels of HIV RNA in up to 90% of chronically infected patients—prompted some scientists to muse over the possibility of a cure if treatment were given for a few years. This provocative speculation was based on the assumption that cellular reservoirs of HIV have a short half-life and that they are accessible to currently available drugs [*JAMA* 1998;279:1343–44].

These thoughts were banished by two reports published at the end of 1997. One research group found that although the amount of HIV fell to undetectable levels in blood following highly active anti-retroviral therapy (HAART), constant amounts of the virus remained latent in resting blood cells—CD4 T cells and macrophages. Even when given as early as ten days after the onset of primary infection, HAART is not sufficient to prevent latent HIV infection of resting CD4 cells [*Proc Natl Acad Sci USA* 1998;95:8869–

73]. The findings underscore the rapidity with which latent reservoirs are established.

Resting cells have the viral genome woven into their own but do not actively produce new copies of the virus. Another study found that the latent virus can be reactivated, and that a low level of viral replication may continue during a regimen of highly active therapy. The biologic function of resting cells is to persist for years and provide immunologic memory. They represent a potential long-term reservoir of HIV. Researchers estimate that eradication of infected resting cells would require five years of treatment at a minimum and 20 years in the worst case scenario. There is a question as to whether current anti-HIV treatment can be given for five years or more without provoking viral resistance or unacceptable toxicity.

Several strategies are being explored to address the problem posed by the resting virus [*Nature Biotech* 1998;16:15]. One group hopes to activate the resting memory cells and accelerate their rate of decay by using monoclonal antibodies targeting CD3 markers on the surface of memory cells. Another strategy is to use a mixture of cytokines such as interleukin-2 (IL-2) plus IL-6 and tumor necrosis factor to activate the latently infected cells, while preventing further viral replication with HAART [*Science* 1998;280:1866–67]. At a scientific meeting at the end of February, researchers suggested that administering OKT3, an antibody that, at low doses, specifically signals T cells to replicate, might flush latently infected T cells. Others suggested that latently infected macrophages might be forced out of hiding by giving immune system messengers such as granulocyte-macrophage colony-stimulating factor (GM-CSF) [*Science* 1998;279:1854–55].

In March, an article in the Medical News and Perspectives section of *JAMA* [1998;279:641–42] reported on the early impact of HIV infection and effects of treatment. Studies suggest that starting treatment with a potent combination of drugs as soon as possible after infection, within the first six months, may be critical to preserve an important element of the immune system—virus-specific helper T cells. These key cells are eliminated early in the course of infection. Without early intervention, some of the damage may be irreversible. Studies in long-term "nonprogressors"—HIV-infected people who have lived up to two decades without disease progression—show that the body's ability to control viral load is correlated with a strong response by HIV-specific CD8 cytotoxic T lymphocytes (CTLs). This level of activity by CTLs depends on a strong response by helper T cells, which secrete cytokines that activate CTLs. Anti-HIV helper T cell response is absent in people with progressive HIV infection because the virus preferentially infects them and many are eliminated during the early stages of the infection. Salvaging the helper T cells and CTL components of the immune system may allow people with HIV infection to stave off illness on their own without continued reliance on drug therapy. Currently under study is another strategy to prompt re-emergence of helper cells through the intermittent injections of a vaccine (*Remune*) that is based only on proteins inside the core of HIV [*The Wall Street Journal,* July 6, 1998, p A18].

In July, JAMA devoted an entire issue to HIV infection and treatment. One article in that issue concerns reservoirs of HIV in patients receiving HAART [*JAMA* 1998;380:67–71]. The authors conceptualize two types of reservoirs—cellular and anatomical. "Cellular sanctuaries may include latent CD4 T cells containing integrated HIV provirus; macrophages, which may express HIV for prolonged periods; and follicular dendritic cells, which may hold infectious HIV on their surfaces for indeterminate lengths of time." A key anatomical reservoir of HIV appears to be the central nervous system. "An understanding of the nature of HIV within these reservoirs is critical to devising strategies to hasten viral eradication."

Another article discusses the recovery of the immune system when infected people are treated with HAART [*JAMA* 1998;380:72–77]. Suppression of viral replication is associated with favorable changes. During the first three months of therapy for people with relatively advanced disease, there is an increase in circulating memory CD4 and CD8 T lymphocytes and B lymphocytes. A deficit in CD4 cells reduces antigen responsiveness and the production of helper T cell cytokines. CD8 cells are important effectors of cell mediated cytotoxicity. After three months there continues to be an increase in CD4 and CD8 cells, but at a slower rate that persists for at least the first year of therapy. "Although incomplete, considerable immune recovery occurs, sufficient to provide adequate protection against most AIDS-associated opportunistic infections." Recovery of the immune system is directly related to the degree of suppression of HIV resulting from therapy. Assuming that an individual is able to continue taking anti-HIV combination therapy, one researcher estimates that it would take four to eight years for full reconstitution of the immune system to occur [*The New York Times,* July 3, 1998, p A13].

The July 1, 1998 issue of *JAMA* also carried a consensus statement titled "Antiretroviral Therapy for HIV Infection in 1998." The report contains updated recommendations of the International AIDS Society-USA Panel

[*JAMA* 1998;280:78–86]. After many meetings and considerable deliberation, the panel continues to support early institution of potent antiretroviral therapy for patients with HIV infection. A variety of combination regimens—a protease inhibitor and two nucleoside RTIs, a nonnucleoside RTI and two nucleoside RTIs, two protease inhibitors, a protease inhibitor and a nonnucleoside RTI, and three nucleoside RTIs—are efficacious, thereby expanding the treatment options for initial therapy. The panel also recommends alternative regimens in the event of treatment failure, but notes that the HIV RNA levels that define failure are uncertain. The panel also continues to recommend initiation of treatment for any patient with HIV infection and HIV RNA levels greater than 5000 to 10,000 copies per milliliter as soon as possible.

Also in that issue of *JAMA* is a therapeutic debate as to when to start antiretroviral therapy. [*JAMA* 1998;280:93–95]. Almost everyone agrees that there is considerable benefit in aggressively treating acute or primary infection before seroconversion. Lowering viral load dramatically within days of exposure may arrest the establishment of HIV infection by preserving the cellular immune response to the virus. Concern lies in the administration of drugs to individuals who have been infected for several months to years. The published recommendations by national groups dealing with clinical care call for administration of potent combination therapy to asymptomatic patients with viral RNA levels greater than 5000 and a CD4 cell counts less than 500. Some physicians now prescribe intensive therapy even for individuals with a much lower viral load.

A recent article in *The Lancet* [1998;352:982–983] presents the view that "early treatment with antiviral drugs starts the clock ticking too soon," limiting future options and necessitating therapy for the lifetime of the patient, with its attendant known and unknown toxicities. The author believes that anti-HIV therapy either compromises the immune system or puts it out of service. "Without exposure to a sufficient amount of viral antigens, the ability to recognize replicating HIV is lost." Thus, the patient taken off suppressive therapy cannot respond effectively to a re-emergence of productive virus infection by the cellular reservoirs of HIV not directly affected by antiviral therapies.

The author suggests that until we have a good surrogate market presaging irreversible damage to the immune system or a means of inducing an anti-HIV immune response, a delay in initiating therapy should be considered. He urges that intensive combination therapy be reserved for those patients who have symptoms or whose CD4 cell counts have dropped substantially. Specifically, the author finds it plausible to start treatment when CD4 cell-counts fall below 400 and viral loads are above 30,000. These levels of infection and immune status have been associated with what appears to be an early demise of the immune system but one that can be reversed. He holds that administering drugs under these conditions is the best strategy because the virus can be controlled and the immune system can recover.

The global community concerned with understanding, treating, and preventing HIV infection met in Geneva from June 28 through July 3 for the 12th International Conference on AIDS. Unlike the 11th conference in Vancouver, the meeting in Geneva provided no quantum leaps in the areas of therapeutics and pathogenesis. Reports of dramatic improvement in prognosis for patients infected with HIV were tempered by the many challenges that remain. A more pensive and even pessimistic outlook replaced the buoyant mood of Vancouver. This turnabout prompted an article on the op-ed pages of *The New York Times* [June 27, 1998, p A27] written by a leading researcher, David Ho. The piece was titled "Too much pessimism on AIDS therapies." Ho challenged the doomsday scenario, described by a number of scientists and commentators, wherein patients on combination therapy deteriorate one after another in rapid succession, because of the emergence of viral strains that are resistant to drugs. He argues that the exaggerated portrayals hurt HIV research, and scolds those who say that the obstacles posed by deep HIV reservoirs are insurmountable.

The first report from Geneva concerned drug-resistant strains of HIV [*The Wall Street Journal*, July 1, 1998, pp A3, A8]. Researchers reported the emergence of new strains of HIV that are resistant to some drug combinations. In several cases, patients contracted the mutant form rather than developed it. While the problem is not rampant, it is a wake-up call. The prevention of both the development of HIV drug resistance and the transmission of drug-resistant variants of the virus is a central issue of public health importance [*JAMA* 1998;279:1977–83], and there are several strategies available to minimize the development of resistant strains [*Ann Intern Med* 1998; 128:951–54]. Another report forecasts that drug-resistant HIV will increasingly challenge physicians and public health agencies [*JAMA* 1998;279: 2000–03]. "The challenge to pharmaceutical companies is to develop drug combinations with once-a-day or twice-a-day dosing to improve adherence." Many believe that compliance with the prescribed regimen of anti-HIV medication—avoiding missed doses and drug holidays—is the most efficient way to prevent the emergence of drug-resistant virus.

Some researchers at the conference said that it might now be essential for physicians treating newly infected people to use a rather expensive test to identify whether a person carries drug-resistant HIV strains. A consensus statement is available on antiretroviral drug resistance testing for adults with HIV infection [*JAMA* 1998;279:1984–91]. The expert panel that prepared the statement concluded that testing for drug resistance before initiation of therapy in treatment-naïve patients cannot be recommended for routine use at this time. Decisions concerning initial therapy should be made on the basis of plasma HIV RNA level, CD4 cell count, and clinical status. Although evidence suggests that viral resistance and treatment failure are closely linked, the panel does not recommend resistance testing as the primary assay to decide when to change therapy. Rather, an increase in plasma HIV RNA level should be the main trigger when considering a treatment change. The pitfalls of resistance testing following treatment failure are described in another report [*Science* 1998;280:1871–73].

Shortly after the conference, a report in *The New England Journal of Medicine* [1998;339:307–11] described a case of sexual transmission of HIV with mutations in the protease and reverse-transcriptase genes. The mutations conferred resistance to zidovudine, lamivudine, saquinavir, ritonavir, indinavir, and nelfinavir. The message is clear: "The availability of highly active antiretroviral therapy cannot be relied on as primary prevention" [*N Engl J Med* 1998;339:341–43].

Researchers at the AIDS conference also discussed the importance of reconstituting the immune system. While all agreed that immune cell reconstitution in addition to antiretroviral therapy is needed to effectively attack HIV infection, there was debate over how best to achieve this. One virologist argued that it will require a better understanding of basic biology. Evidence now suggests that in addition to a decline in the number of CD4 cells due to infection with the virus, there is also an impairment of uninfected CD4 cells and a loss of CD8 (killer T cells). The uninfected but impaired CD4 cells proliferate if the HIV-transactivator transcription protein (TAT) and alpha-interferon are removed [*Scrip*, August 5, 1998, p 27]. This could be an effective strategy for immune reconstitution. Another researcher explained that CD8 cells have two functions in HIV infection. They can kill infected cells or suppress replication without killing the cell by producing soluble proteins such as CD8 antiviral factor (CAF). CD4 cells produce interleukin-2 (IL-2), which in turn boosts levels of CD8 which then produce CAF. Agents that can stimulate CAF could be very useful. Administration of IL-2 may also be a promising approach.

A post-mortem report at the close of the international meeting in Geneva said that, ". . . the nearly 14,000 participants heard that researchers are now scrambling to find new treatment strategies, as the first-line drugs begin to fail in some patients, that drug side effects are mounting, and that new drug-resistant strains of HIV are emerging. Remission, not cure, is the new buzzword" [*Science* 1998;280:281–82]. Most frustrating for the participants was the lack of progress being made in the development of a preventive vaccine.

ONCOLOGY

High-Dose Chemotherapy and Autologous Bone Marrow
    Transplantation for Breast Cancer
Rationing Taxol in the UK

**High-Dose Chemotherapy and Autologous Bone Marrow Transplantation
for Breast Cancer.** Estimates for 1997 were that breast cancer occurs in more
than 180,00 women in the US and that about 25% die of the disease. Mortality
has declined modestly in the 1990s, because of early detection and improved
therapies. On the other hand, only about half of patients with lymph node-
positive breast cancer remain free of disease at five years. The prognosis for
women with metastatic breast cancer is grimmer. Clearly, more effective
treatment is needed.

Myeloablative high-dose chemotherapy (HDC) followed by autologous
cell rescue (ACR) by means of bone marrow transplantation or peripheral-
blood stem-cell transplantation has been proposed as a promising strategy
for breast cancer. HDC/ACR is based on the hypothesis that high-dose
chemotherapy will overcome drug resistance, eradicate metastatic disease,
and increase the proportion of women with breast cancer who survive for at
least five years after treatment. In general this is a largely untested proposition.
Nevertheless, the strategy has captured the interest of oncologists and the
procedure is in wide use, particularly for women with metastatic disease.
Despite the frequency with which this procedure is used, the effectiveness of
HDC/ACR in the treatment of breast cancer is not well defined. An exhaus-
tive review of the biomedical literature [*J Natl Cancer Inst* 1998;90:200–09]
from January 1983 through May 1997 found only one phase III trial comparing HDC/ACR with conventional therapy. The study found that high-dose
chemotherapy with hematopoietic rescue significantly improves the response
rate and duration of survival [*J Clin Oncol* 1995;13:2483–89].

In an uncontrolled study, investigators observed the effects of standard-
dose chemotherapy followed by HDC/ACR in 85 patients with lymph node-
positive breast cancer. Five-year event-free survival was 71% and overall survival was 78% compared with rates of 28% to 34% and 37% to 48%, respectively
in historical controls [*Proc Am Soc Clin Oncol* 1995;14:317]. However, the
same investigators in a randomized trial failed to confirm the superiority of
HDC/ACR over standard chemotherapy [*Proc Am Soc Clin Oncol* 1996;
15:121].

A more recent randomized trial compared conventional chemotherapy with HDC/ACR in 90 patients with metastatic breast cancer and reported promising results. The investigators found an overall response rate of 95% for HDC/ACR compared with 53% for standard therapy, and complete remission in 51% of patients receiving HDC/ACR compared with 5% assigned to standard treatment [*J Clin Oncol* 1998;13:2483-89]. A commentary questions the rigor of this work, noting that the median follow-up was only 72 weeks, the study was small, and the conventional chemotherapy used in the trial might be judged by some investigators to be suboptimum [*Lancet* 1998;351:386–87].

The commentary concludes that on the basis of clinical studies reported so far, HDC/ACR is not superior to conventional chemotherapy for advanced breast cancer. Another commentary in the *Journal of the National Cancer Institute* [1998;90:200–09] arrives at the same conclusion, but the authors believe that HDC/ACR is likely to make a contribution to the treatment of breast cancer and calls for large, randomized trials to settle the issue. The wide availability of HDC/ACR in treatment centers, however, is making it difficult for researchers to accrue patients to participate in randomized trials.

A recent report in *The Lancet* [1998;352:515–21] brings more discouraging news. Investigators studied the effects of aggressive therapy in 97 women who had breast cancer with extensive axillary lymph node metastases. After randomization, all patients received three courses of chemotherapy. After surgery, stable patients, or those who responded to chemotherapy, were randomly assigned to one of two treatment groups. One group received a fourth course of conventional therapy followed by radiation and two years of tamoxifen (40 patients). The other group received high-dose therapy—identical treatment but an additional high-dose regimen and peripheral blood progenitor cells support after the fourth course (41 patients).

No patients died from the toxic effects of the chemotherapy. With median follow-up of 49 months, four-year survival and disease-free survival for all 97 patients were 75% and 54%, respectively. There was no significant difference in survival between the group on conventional therapy and the group on high-dose therapy. The authors conclude: "High-dose therapy is associated with substantial cost and acute toxic effects, but also has potentially irreversible long-term effects. Until the benefit of this therapy is substantiated by large-scale phase III trials, high-dose chemotherapy should not be used in the adjuvant treatment of breast cancer, apart from randomized trials."

Soon to be published are the results of a study designed to determine whether the addition of two cycles of high-dose cyclophosphamide, etoposide, and cisplatin followed by autologous stem-cell transplantation improves outcomes in high-risk breast cancer [*Lancet* 1998;352:501–02]. All patients received eight courses of conventional chemotherapy, radiotherapy, and a five-year course of tamoxifen, if appropriate. There were no significant differences in four-year disease-free survival (55% vs. 48%) or overall survival (68% vs. 60%) between the high-dose and standard dose groups. These recent studies suggest that if there is a benefit associated with high-dose therapy, either it is not a large one or prevails only in an as yet unidentified subgroup of patients. A recently proposed cellular model of tumor recurrence that emphasizes clonal heterogeneity in drug sensitivity even in early-stage tumors suggests that the benefits of high-dose chemotherapy are likely to be modest.

Rationing Taxol in the UK. Experts in ovarian cancer have enlisted the help of politicians and cancer support groups to demand that all women with the disease in the UK receive paclitaxel (*Taxol*) and cisplatin [*Scrip*, May 27, 1998, p 28]. *Taxol* has been indicated for first-line treatment of ovarian cancer in the UK since 1996, but it is used infrequently because of its high cost. Some UK health authorities have refused to fund the drug but it is used in "centres of excellence" and for private patients.

According to *Scrip*, there are about 6000 cases of ovarian cancer diagnosed in the UK annually; 80% of the cases would be considered candidates for the *Taxol* combination. Fewer than half, however, receive it. An oncologist at the Hammersmith Hospital claims that the National Health Service spends 200 million pounds on constipation each year but just 58 million pounds on chemotherapy. The situation has prompted a panel of experts to develop a consensus statement concluding that the evidence now available shows that *Taxol*-cisplatin provides a survival advantage and should be considered "gold standard treatment."

Pain Management

Undertreatment of Pain Remains a Serious Problem. Once again the media heralds news of a report of shameful undertreatment of patients in pain. This time the report concerns elderly people with cancer residing in nursing homes [*JAMA* 1998;279:1877–82]. The survey, which used records collected by the Health Care Financing Administration, was undertaken because as hospital stays grow shorter and the elderly population increases, more and more old people with cancer are living out the end of their lives in nursing homes. The study population consisted of 13,625 patients who were at least 65 years of age and discharged from the hospital to any of 1492 certified facilities.

Nearly 40% reported daily pain. About one-quarter of the patients in daily pain received no medication. The findings are consistent with other studies that have reported that cancer pain is poorly managed in most settings [*JAMA* 1998;279:1914–15]. Age, gender, race, marital status, depression, and cognitive status were all independently associated with the presence of pain. Undertreatment was worse for patients 85 years of age or older than for patients 65 to 74 years of age, in women than in men, in African-Americans and other minorities than in whites.

One cancer expert said that nursing staff and physicians seem to give up on patients who they know are going to die. Another believed that outright prejudice is at work, particularly for minority patients. Almost everyone agrees that nursing home health-care workers are poorly trained to recognize pain [*The New York Times,* June 17, 1998, pp A1, A25]. The same is largely true for most physicians, except those specializing in pain management. Unrecognized pain is untreated pain—patients must volunteer that they are in pain before health professionals take notice. One study reports that educating outpatients with cancer about pain, and teaching them how to describe their pain and communicate with health care practitioners, improves pain control. The authors of the report join a sizable body of alarmed health-care professionals who say that failure to treat pain effectively at all times is unacceptable and should be considered a primary indicator of poor quality of medical care. None of the reasons given as to why treatment of pain is not a top priority in cancer care justifies untreated or undertreated pain.

Some think that the broad application of patient-controlled analgesia (PCA) may be an effective way to improve pain management. Rather than receiving fixed doses of analgesic at fixed intervals, the patient has immediate access to pain relief, almost on demand. Surveys show that patient satisfaction is high with PCA and the quality of pain relief in general is higher than that achieved with conventional therapy. For reasons of safety, PCA must have a lockout interval to prevent the patient from receiving a dangerously high dose of opioid. The lockout interval should be long enough to allow the onset of pain relief before a subsequent dose is given, but not so long that the second dose is received well after the maximum effect of the first dose has been achieved. Morphine, because of its rapid onset of effect, is the most attractive option for PCA. Fentanyl is also well suited to PCA.

SUBSTANCE ABUSE

Methadone Clinics Challenged in New York City. Methadone has been widely prescribed and distributed in community hospitals and clinics for the last 30 years to blunt opioid craving in addicted individuals. Advocates say that the strategy allows some individuals, perhaps up to one-third of addicts, to function in society, and decreases the societal toll that results from addicted people seeking illicit drugs. Critics maintain that methadone clinics do nothing more than exchange one dependency for another, and that abstinence from drugs is a more moral approach to curing addiction.

In New York City, Mayor Rudolph Giuliani has directed that heroin addicts receiving treatment at city hospitals will generally be allowed to get methadone for no more than three months [*The New York Times,* August 15, 1998, p B17]. Giuliani challenges the effectiveness of existing programs pointing out that barely one-third of methadone patients in the city has found regular jobs. The failure of methadone programs to move addicts in treatment off welfare and into jobs is said to be an important reason the mayor declared war on methadone.

Under the new plan, addicts involved in city programs will be weaned from methadone, instead of taking it indefinitely, as they do now. The program will continue to offer counseling and other services. The decision created a furor in the drug-treatment community. While New York City officials control less than 10% of methadone treatment slots, the program is oversubscribed and the Mayor's policy will have an impact. The president of New York City's Health and Hospital Corporation, supporting Giuliani's policy, said that limiting methadone will liberate heroin addicts from their dependence on opioids and, as in the alcoholic treatment model, move them to abstinence.

An article in *The New York Times Magazine* [September 6, 1998, pp 48–50] rebuts the Mayor's position. The author observes: "Since its introduction in the mid-1960s, studies have consistently shown that the synthetic narcotic cuts addicts' craving for heroin, enabling onetime street junkies to restart their lives. In so doing, methadone helps boost employment, inhibit the spread of HIV, and cut crime. That's why the New York City Mayor's recent attacks . . . have left experts scratching their heads. That methadone is effective is not a matter of opinion. It is a matter of fact." Ironically, the development of methadone was spurred by rampant heroin addiction in New York City barely impacted by detoxification programs.

Despite Mayor Giuliani's tirades, the White House has announced a policy to expand the availability of methadone. Under the plan, physicians would be permitted to administer methadone in the privacy of their offices to patients who request and need the drug. Up until now, methadone has been dispensed only at designated community clinics one dose at a time. Only 115,000 people in the US addicted to heroin or other opiates use methadone. Expanded access might benefit hundreds of thousands more. The government hopes that facilitating access and strongly endorsing the effectiveness of methadone will prompt the eight states that do not permit methadone clinics to start a program and encourage the rest of the states to expand their current programs.

WOMEN'S HEALTH

Birth Control by Means of Emergency Contraception
Low-Dose Estrogen Oral Contraceptives and the Risk of Heart
  Attack
Safety of Third Generation Oral Contraceptives
Mifepristone (RU-486) and Misoprostol to Terminate
  Unwanted Pregnancy
Hormone Replacement Therapy and Secondary Prevention of
  Heart Disease

Birth Control by Means of Emergency Contraception. Some right-to-life advocates regard emergency contraception, also called morning-after pills, as a form of chemical abortion. The more widely held view in the US is that pregnancy starts on implantation of a fertilized egg in the uterine lining. A commentary in *The New England Journal of Medicine* says that any method of regulation of fertility that acts before implantation is not an abortion. Emergency contraception works by altering the endometrium to prevent implantation.

The morning-after strategy requires a woman to take twice the dose of a commercially available oral contraceptive combination within the first 72 hours of coitus and then take another double dose 12 hours later. The FDA has identified six brands of birth-control pills sold in the United States as safe and effective for use as emergency contraception. Taken as directed, these regimens safely and effectively prevent pregnancy about 75% of the time. FDA's action on emergency contraception is unusual in that no drug company has petitioned the agency to approve the new indication. American Home Products and Schering, the companies that manufacture the identified brands of oral contraceptives already on the market, want no part of the new indication [*The Wall Street Journal*, June 26, 1998, pp 1,5]. For the drug companies, the risk of litigation and abortion politics have made emergency contraception an unattractive marketing opportunity.

In July 1998, Gynetics, a start-up company, announced its intention to seek approval for a prescription product expressly developed for emergency contraception. The company proposed to market a combination pill that contains ethinyl estradiol and levonorgestrel, both of which are no longer protected by patent [*The New York Times*, July 21, 1998, p A14]. The FDA approved Gynetic's kit, called *Preven Emergency Contraceptive Kit,* in early

September [*The Wall Street Journal,* September 3, 1998, pp B1, B4]. It contains four birth-control pills, a pregnancy test based on a urine sample, and an information booklet. Women take two tablets within 72 hours of unprotected intercourse and two more tablets 12 hours later. The *Prescriber's Letter* [1998;5:53–54] cautions that women may experience nausea and vomiting because of the high dose of estrogen. The newsletter suggests that first giving an anti-emetic will prevent women from losing the dose by vomiting. The kit costs about $20. Gynetics plans to promote the product directly to consumers. Advocates of post-coital contraception hailed the availability of the kit as an important option for women. Barr Laboratories will manufacture the contraceptives.

The corporate chairman of Gynetics said the company was not concerned about anti-abortion protests because the regimen works before women become pregnant. If a woman is already pregnant, treatment will have no effect on the pregnancy. Nevertheless, to distance *Preven* from abortion, Gynetics is emphasizing its potential to reduce the need for surgical abortion. The company says that the kit could help eliminate 800,000 abortions and 1.2 million unintended pregnancies each year [*The Pink Sheet* 1998; 60(No36):9–10]. The National Right to Life Committee, which opposes abortion, said it has no official position on emergency contraception.

In a novel program in Washington state, where pharmacists have a measure of prescriptive authority, 87 pharmacies throughout the state are offering morning-after pills without the need for a prescription. Specially trained pharmacists screen clients to ensure safety, and council them on the use of the pills. Patients can learn about the location of certified pharmacies any time of day by calling 1-888-NOT-2-LATE. Over a three-month period, Washington pharmacists filled 2,000 orders for emergency contraceptives. Advocacy groups are developing plans to educate women about the availability of emergency contraception.

There is considerable interest outside the US in the use of mifepristone (RU-486) for emergency contraception. Some investigators report that mifepristone is the most effective and best tolerated morning-after contraceptive tested to date. A further advantage is that it can be taken as a single dose. The dose of mifepristone, when used for emergency contraception, is much less than the dose needed to terminate pregnancy [*Scrip,* October 16, 1998, p 22].

Low-Dose Estrogen Oral Contraceptives and the Risk of Heart Attack.
Healthy women using oral contraceptives (OCs) containing low-dose estro-

gen (<50 μg ethinyl estradiol) should have little fear of an increased risk of myocardial infarction (MI). This is the conclusion of a recently reported case-control study [*Circulation* 1998;98:1958–63]. The investigators identified 271 women between the ages of 18 and 44 with a previous MI and matched them with 993 controls. They found that the risk of MI was similar in current and past users of OCs as well as in women who had never used an oral contraceptive. Duration of use was unrelated to MI. The progestin component in the product did not affect the risk of a heart attack. Several studies from the late 1970s, when OCs contained more estrogen than is common today, showed an increased risk of MI with OC use.

Safety of Third Generation Oral Contraceptives. First generation oral contraceptives (OCs) contained estrogen in excess of 50 μg. On learning that many women using these products developed deep vein thrombosis (DVT), drug manufacturers soon replaced them. The culprit seemed to be estrogen. Second generation OCs contain less than 50 μg of estrogen and are the most widely used contraceptive products in the United States. Both first and second generation OCs also contained a progestin, frequently levonorgestrel. Third generation OCs were marketed only recently. They contain less than 50 μg of estrogen as well as one of two new progestins—desogestrel or gestodene. Only products containing desogestrel are available in the US (*Ortho-Cept, Desogen,* and *Mircette*).

In October 1995, following submission of three reports on the safety of OCs to *The Lancet,* health officials in the UK warned physicians that women using third generation OCs were at greater risk for DVT than women using second generation OCs. The announcement created a scare in Britain and many women abruptly stopped using the new products; some had an unwanted pregnancy. The UK and several other countries in Europe restricted the prescribing of the new OCs. Health officials in the US did not evince much concern over the new findings, but did ask manufacturers to note the results in product labeling.

Many clinicians criticized the British government's haste, arguing that the reports stemmed from epidemiological studies that could have been confounded by the prescribing of third generation products to women at greater risk of DVT. This suggestion is plausible because some studies suggest that the new products have a more favorable cardiovascular safety profile than the older products and may reduce the risk of a heart attack. Oral contraceptives that contain desogestrel or gestodene are less androgenic, have less effect on carbohydrate and lipid metabolism, and result in stronger suppression of ovarian activity than older progestins, thus enabling the lowering of the dose of estrogen to only 20 μg [*Ann Intern Med* 1998;128:467–77].

Studies in several different countries now support preferential prescribing of third generation OCs in women at risk for thromboembolism as an explanation, at least in part, for the seeming increased risk of DVT [*Prescriber's Letter* 1998;5:35]. Studies demonstrating preferential prescribing provide a helpful clinical perspective. However, they do not rule out the possibility that desogestrel and gestodene are more likely to result in a DVT than levonorgestrel and other older progestins. Indeed, a biological explanation for this possibility has been proposed. Women with a newly discovered inheritable coagulation disorder, Factor V Leiden, are at increased risk of DVT. Heterozygous carriers have a risk of DVT that is seven times as high as that in the general population; for homozygous carriers the risk is 80 times as high. The mutation causes resistance to activated protein C—a natural anticoagulant. The presence of both Factor V Leiden and OCs increases the risk of DVT 35-fold. OCs alone increase the risk only fourfold. Third generation OCs have greater resistance to activated protein C than second generation OCs. In women with the factor V mutation, third generation OCs increase the risk of DVT more than 50-fold [*Br J Haematol* 1997;97:233–38].

A recent report concerns the interaction of two prothrombotic mutations in the genes encoding coagulation factor V and prothrombin [*N Engl J Med* 1998;338:1793–97]. Both mutations are established genetic risk factors for venous thrombosis. The proportion of carriers of factor V Leiden in the white population varies from 2% to 15%, but is rare in non-whites. The prevalence of the mutation in the gene encoding prothrombin varies from 0.7% to 4%. The abnormality in heterozygous carriers increases the risk of DVT 3- to 6-fold compared with the general population.

The investigators compared the frequency of the mutations and the use of OCs among 40 unrelated patients who had a confirmed diagnosis of cerebral-vein thrombosis with the frequency among 120 healthy control subjects. The prevalence of the prothrombin-gene mutation was higher in patients with cerebral-vein thrombosis than in healthy controls (20% vs. 3%) and was nearly the same as the prevalence in patients with DVT (18%). Similar results were observed for the mutation in the factor V gene. The researchers also found that oral contraceptives are a strong risk factor for cerebral-vein thrombosis (odds ratio, 22). The use of OCs was more frequent among women with cerebral-vein thrombosis than among controls (96% vs. 32%), and among those with DVT (61%). For women using OCs who also had the prothrombin-gene mutation, the odds ratio rose to about 150.

Despite the small number of subjects, the investigators clearly show that mutations in the prothrombin gene and the factor V gene are associated with cerebral-vein thrombosis. The use of OCs is also strongly and independently associated with the disorder. The presence of both the prothrombin mutation and OCs raises the risk of cerebral-vein thrombosis further. Oral contraceptives change the concentrations of hemostatic and fibrinolytic components of the blood and may add to the disturbance in the hemostatic balance introduced by a prothrombotic mutation [*N Engl J Med* 1998;338:1840–41].

While there may be differences in the risk of DVT with different OCs, the absolute risk of DVT among young healthy women is very low, usually less than the risk of DVT during pregnancy. Nevertheless, prudence suggests that a woman who has the Leiden mutation, especially if she is a smoker, should not use oral contraceptives, particularly third generation products. The new evidence indicates that a mutation in the prothrombin gene may also pose a serious risk for women using oral contraceptives.

Mifepristone (RU-486) and Misoprostol to Terminate Unwanted Pregnancy. Many American women do not have access to abortion. The availability of medical abortion could lead to greater access to safer abortion services. Medical abortion is now used by 70% of French women who are seeking abortions and who are no more than seven weeks pregnant. Mifepristone, a progesterone antagonist, combined with a prostaglandin is more than 95% effective in terminating pregnancies 49 days old or less. The prostaglandin causes contractions and fetal expulsion. Most studies of safety and effectiveness have used the combination of mifepristone and gemeprost and some have evaluated mifepristone combined with misoprostol. One study suggests that a combination of methotrexate and a prostaglandin may also be safe and effective.

FDA approved the combination of mifepristone and misoprostol in 1996, but it is still unavailable in the US and is unlikely to be sold in this country until 1999, at the earliest. Abortion opponents vow to boycott any company that makes the drug. As a result, the Population Council, the organization that holds the rights to mifepristone in the US, has had great difficulty finding a manufacturer.

The results of the first study of mifepristone and misoprostol in American women are now available [*N Engl J Med* 1998;338:1241–47]. The investigators gave mifepristone and then misoprostol two days later to about 2000 women with pregnancies up to nine weeks' duration. After observation, the women went home and returned on day 15 for final evaluation. Pregnancy was terminated in 92% of women carrying for 49 days or less, 83% of those carrying for 50–56 days, and 77% of those carrying for 57 to 63 days. Failures as well as adverse effects—abdominal pain, nausea, vomiting, diarrhea, and vaginal bleeding—increased with increasing duration of pregnancy. Almost half the expulsions occurred during the four hours following administration of misoprostol. For women with pregnancies of longer duration than 49 days, vaginal rather than oral misoprostol may be more effective.

There is a sizable minority of the US population that seeks to block the marketing of mifepristone. Their views have prevailed in the House of Representatives. The bill to fund the FDA that squeaked through the House contains a provision prohibiting the agency from using any money for the chemical inducement of abortion. The provision is aimed solely at mifepristone and, if enacted, may prevent final approval of the drug [*Scrip,* July 1, 1998, p15].

Hormone Replacement Therapy and Secondary Prevention of Heart Disease. Many observational studies report lower rates of coronary heart disease (CHD) in women who take postmenopausal estrogen than in women who elect not to receive this therapy. The association appears to be particularly strong for prevention of further complications in women with CHD. For this population, estrogen replacement is associated with 35% to 80% fewer recurrent events. Some clinicians find the association so persuasive they question the ethics of randomizing women to placebo.

Despite the abundance of epidemiological evidence of cardiovascular benefit, observational studies of hormone replacement therapy (HRT)—estrogen alone or with a progestin—are plagued. None can rule out the possibility that reduced risk may be attributable to selection bias. Women who choose to take hormones are usually healthier and have a more favorable CHD profile than those who do not. Regardless of the strength of the association, observational studies cannot resolve this uncertainty.

The results of the first randomized controlled trial of the effectiveness of HRT are now available and they are disappointing [*JAMA* 1998;280:605–13]. Investigators participating in the Heart and Estrogen/progestin Replacement Study (HERS) identified 2,763 women with coronary disease who were postmenopausal, younger than 80 years, and had an intact uterus. The women received either 0.625 mg conjugated estrogens plus 2.5 mg of a progestin (medroxyprogesterone) in a single tablet or matching placebo daily. Follow-up averaged 4.1 years and compliance with active therapy was 75% at the end of three years. The main outcome measure was the occurrence of non-fatal myocardial infarction (MI) or death due to CHD.

Overall, there was no difference between the placebo and active treatment groups: 172 women in the hormone group and 176 women in the placebo group had an MI or died as a result of CHD. The absence of a cardiovascular benefit occurred despite an 11% lower low-density lipoprotein cholesterol level and a 10% higher high-density lipoprotein cholesterol level in the active treatment group. Although there were no net differences between the groups, there were statistically significant time trends, with more CHD events in the hormone group in year one and fewer in years four and five. About 2.5% of the women who received HRT developed a venous thrombo-embolism, compared with an incidence of only 0.9% in women assigned to placebo. Hormone therapy also increased the risk of developing gall bladder disease by about 40% compared with placebo.

The investigators conclude: "Based on the finding of no overall cardio-vascular benefit and a pattern of early increase in risk of CHD events, we do not recommend starting this treatment for the purpose of secondary prevention of CHD." The additional finding of a favorable pattern of CHD events after several years of treatment suggests that women already receiving hormone replacement are safe to continue therapy.

An editorial observes: "These findings are a sobering reminder of the limitations of observational research, the incompleteness of current under-standing of the mechanisms of vascular disease and the dangers of extrapola-tion" [*JAMA* 1998;280:650–51]. The author reminds that there remains an impressive body of observational data on HRT used for primary prevention and cautions that the HERS results should not be extrapolated to women free of CHD. Whether or not HRT is effective for primary prevention will not be resolved until the results of randomized trials, currently underway, are available.

The report is a disappointment to Wyeth-Ayerst, the pharmaceutical company that funded HERS. The firm hoped to add secondary prevention for CHD to the list of indications for their *Premarin* products. Wyeth-Ayerst pointed out, however, that the kind of patients included in the study account for only 6% of the nine million prescriptions written annually for conjugated estrogens. The head of clinical affairs at Wyeth-Ayerst said that typical users of postmenopausal hormones do not have existing heart disease and start therapy at a younger age than those women in the trial [*The Wall Street Journal,* August 19, 1998, pp B1, B4]. Nevertheless, a prevention claim would have bolstered sales.

As it stands now, Wyeth-Ayerst's pursuit of a cardioprotection claim for conjugated estrogens is on hold until 2005 at the earliest. This is when observers expect the results of the historic Women's Health Initiative to be announced. The drug company initially filed for a cardioprotective indication in 1990 based on the results of a meta-analysis including 29 epidemiological studies. The analysis found a 50% reduction in the risk of death from cardiovascular disease for estrogen users compared with nonusers. An FDA panel reviewing the submission voted to recommend the use of conjugated estrogen for lowering the risk of cardiovascular disease for women who had had hysterectomies, but the FDA never acted on the recommendation.

Children's Health

Drugs in Pregnancy
Mandatory HIV Testing of Pregnant Women

Drugs in Pregnancy. Pharmaceutical companies almost never test new drugs in pregnant women to determine effects on the fetus. Consequently, the label of most drugs carries the disclaimer: "Use in pregnancy is not recommended unless the potential benefits justify the potential risks to the fetus." This creates a "Catch 22" situation because physicians caring for pregnant women have little or no information to help them decide whether the benefit of therapy for the mother outweighs the risk to the fetus. A major review concerning the use of drugs in pregnancy appeared in April 1998 [*N Engl J Med* 1998;338:1128–37].

Three drug products—thalidomide, *Bendectin,* and isotretinoin (*Accutane*)—highlight the problems faced by pregnant women and their physicians. Before the development and testing of thalidomide, it was believed that the placenta served as a barrier to protect the fetus from adverse effects of drugs. We learned, however, that fetal exposure to thalidomide during critical periods of development resulted in severe limb defects and other defective organs. Today we believe that every drug has the potential to be a teratogen.

In the late 1950s and through the '60s, *Bendectin,* a combination of an antihistamine (doxylamine) and the vitamin pyridoxine, was the most widely used medication in the US for nausea and vomiting associated with pregnancy. In the 1970s, however, a flood of lawsuits claimed that *Bendectin* was teratogenic and drove the manufacturer to withdraw the product from the market in 1982. The drug was withdrawn despite a large body of evidence that the rate of major malformations among the children of mothers who took *Bendectin* during pregnancy did not differ from the rate in the general population. Upon the withdrawal of *Bendectin,* there was no product available in the US for nausea and vomiting during pregnancy. From 1980 to 1989, rates of hospitalization among pregnant women for severe nausea and vomiting nearly doubled.

Isotretinoin, on the other hand, is indeed a teratogen in both animals and humans. It is widely prescribed and unparalleled for treatment of recalcitrant acne. On approval of isotretinoin, the FDA reasoned that appropriate labeling of teratogenic drugs would be effective to prevent fetal exposure to the drugs. Despite explicit warnings, many children were born with retinoid embryopathy after the drug was introduced. This experience led to the development of a more comprehensive program to prevent teratogenesis—The Retinoid Pregnancy Prevention Program. As part of the program, women are asked to sign a consent form indicating that they agree to use two effective methods of contraception before starting to use the drug, during the use of the drug, and for several months after the use of the drug. The success of this strategy emboldened the FDA to approve thalidomide for use in certain forms of leprosy.

Authors of the review in *The New England Journal of Medicine* conclude: "In addition to the risk associated with fetal exposure to teratogenic drugs, there is a risk associated with misinformation about the teratogenicity of drugs, which can lead to unnecessary abortions or the avoidance of needed therapy. The medical community and drug manufacturers should make a concerted effort to protect women and their unborn babies from both risks."

Mandatory HIV Testing of Pregnant Women. Since the discovery of therapies that sharply reduce the transmission of HIV from a pregnant woman to her offspring, there has been a strident call for mandatory testing of high-risk pregnant women. Mandatory testing of pregnant women would increase the detection of HIV infection and allow the use of antiretroviral drug therapy to reduce vertical transmission of the virus. Almost from the first awareness of HIV disease, however, infected patients, AIDS advocates, and public health officials have rejected the idea of mandatory testing. They argue that some women would avoid prenatal care because they fear HIV testing or resent the mandatory policy. These women would lose the benefits of therapy with antiretroviral therapy for herself and her offspring as well as the benefits of prenatal care. With a voluntary HIV testing policy, some infected women may refuse tests and lose the benefits of anti-HIV treatment but all would receive prenatal care.

Using a decision analysis model, investigators have recently evaluated the relative benefits and risks of mandatory compared with voluntary HIV testing of pregnant women [*Ann Intern Med* 1998;128:760–67]. The results suggest that a voluntary policy is better than a mandatory policy over a wide range of variables used in the analysis. One of the most important variables is the acceptance of HIV testing under a voluntary policy. If, across the country, the acceptance of testing increased to 97%, a goal already reached in some settings, the benefit of a voluntary policy would be greater than that of a mandatory policy. Deterrence rate was another important variable in the model. If mandatory testing deterred 0.5% or more pregnant women from seeking prenatal care, the number of infant deaths resulting from lack of prenatal care would be greater than the number of infants spared HIV infection. The model also suggests that at the current prevalence of HIV infection among women of childbearing age, the voluntary policy is warranted. However, if the overall prevalence increases to 0.58% or more, the question of mandatory testing will require reconsideration.

The authors of the report argue that mandatory HIV testing must be clearly demonstrated to be effective before such a policy is implemented. There is no evidence now that mandatory testing would be beneficial. Moreover, the decision analysis model suggests that mandatory testing might do more harm than good. They urge that future research address strategies to improve voluntary acceptance of HIV testing through counseling and education.

ADVERSE DRUG EFFECTS

Safety of Troglitazone in Patients with Type 2 Diabetes
Are Drug Reactions A Major Cause of Death?
Litigation on Recalled Diet Drugs

Safety of Troglitazone in Patients with Type 2 Diabetes. In January 1997, Warner-Lambert/Parke Davis introduced *Rezulin* (troglitazone) to treat poorly controlled type 2 diabetics who require insulin. It is the first drug in its class (glitazones) to reach the market and many observers hailed its introduction as a significant advance. Most type 2 diabetics produce some insulin but are resistant to its effects. Troglitazone decreases resistance by enhancing the activity of insulin in liver, muscle, and fat cells, thereby lowering blood glucose and insulin levels. Some patients treated with this novel agent can reduce or even eliminate their insulin requirements. Soon after initial approval, troglitazone received a broader indication—the initial treatment of all type 2 diabetics, either alone or with a sulfonylurea. As monotherapy, *Rezulin* works about as well as metformin (*Glucophage*) or a sulfonylurea. Combining *Rezulin* with a sulfonylurea is even more effective.

In late 1997, Warner-Lambert alerted health care professionals about possible hepatotoxicity in patients taking troglitazone. The company urged physicians to check liver function before starting therapy, once a month for six months, every other month for the next six months, and then periodically. Parke-Davis estimated that about 2% of patients will need to stop taking *Rezulin* because of elevated liver enzymes, a sign of liver damage [*Prescriber's Letter* 1997;4:68–69].

In early 1998, the mounting number of reports of hepatotoxicity prompted Glaxo Wellcome, the firm licensed to market troglitazone outside the US and Japan, to withdraw the drug in Great Britain. This sent shock waves through financial institutions keen on the fortunes of pharmaceutical companies. Warner-Lambert, with the full support of the FDA, asserted that *Rezulin* is safe when used correctly. The drug remains on the US market and there is talk that Glaxo Wellcome may re-introduce the drug in the UK [*Scrip*, May 22, 1998, p 21].

The commercial prospects of *Rezulin* were slowed once more in June 1998. The National Institutes of Health announced it would no longer use troglitazone in their Diabetes Prevention Study after the death of one participant who developed liver failure [*The Wall Street Journal*, June 8, 1998, p B9]. The trial was designed to determine if drugs could prevent or delay the onset of type 2 diabetes in patients at risk—a potentially huge market. Investigators were comparing three treatment arms including diet and exercise, metformin, and troglitazone. Medical professionals from Warner-Lambert say that the patient apparently died from complications unrelated to the study and the therapy [*Scrip*, June 10, 1998, p 20]. In the aftermath, Warner-Lambert will have to spend a great deal of money to show that *Rezulin* has an acceptable benefit-to-risk ratio in essentially healthy but at-risk individuals, if it wishes to gain this indication.

Another problem for Warner-Lambert is a petition filed in July by Public Citizen's Health Research Group (HRG) asking FDA to ban *Rezulin* [*Scrip*, July 31, 1998, p 22]. HRG cited information from the FDA that as of June 5, 1998, at least 21 deaths from liver failure and three patients needing liver transplants had been reported among all patients taking troglitazone. The total number of reported troglitazone-related liver toxicities exceeded 500. Warner-Lambert disputes HRG's enumeration. An FDA official said that in the vast majority of documented *Rezulin*-related deaths, patients were not being monitored as recommended in the label. The FDA said that it would review the petition, but it is satisfied with the company's efforts to educate health-care providers about possible adverse effects of *Rezulin*.

Are Drug Reactions A Major Cause of Death? A report in *JAMA* [1998; 279:1200–05] concluded that adverse reaction to appropriate drug therapy— the right patient, the right diagnosis, the right drug, and the right dose—is a leading cause of death in the US. The article shocked pharmaceutical and medical communities. Only a few weeks earlier, a research letter in *The Lancet* [1998;351:643–44] claimed that deaths related to medication error more than doubled from 1983 to 1993, while the number of prescriptions increased by only 40%. The increase over the ten-year period was greater than that for any other cause of death excepts AIDS.

The *JAMA* article concerned a meta-analysis of 39 heterogeneous pro-spective studies, spanning more than 30 years. The investigators tallied only serious adverse drug reactions (ADRs), including those that required hospital-ization, resulted in a permanent disability, or resulted in death. They used the World Health Organization definition of an ADR: "Any noxious, unin-tended and undesired effect of a drug which occurs at doses used in humans for prophylaxis, diagnosis, or therapy." This definition excludes therapeutic failure, overdose, and drug abuse.

The researchers estimated that in 1994 at least 1.7 million hospitalized patients had serious ADRs, and that between 76,000 and 137,000 patients die annually because of ADRs. If 76,000 patients die annually, ADRs rank as the sixth leading cause of death in the US, whereas if the number of deaths caused by ADRs is 137,000 annually, ADRs are the fourth leading cause of death, after heart disease, cancer, and stroke. The findings are astounding and even more so if you consider that the estimates do not include drug misadventures.

The report came under attack from critics who questioned its methods and conclusions. Many observers think the mortality estimates are too high. One expert said that the real number of drug-related deaths might be half that reported [*The New York Times,* April 15, 1998, pp A1, A 19]. Another suggested that there are closer to 50,000 deaths each year in the US caused by adverse reactions to properly prescribed medication [*The Wall Street Journal,* April 15, 1998, p B8]. Even an estimate of 50,000 is very troubling because it is nearly equal to the number of deaths attributed to diabetes each year.

An oddity of these unexpected and disturbing reports is the academic pedigree of the investigators. The authors of the paper in *The Lancet* were from departments of sociology and psychology. The authors of the paper in *JAMA* hailed from departments of zoology, physiology, and public health science. An article in *The New Republic* [June 8, 1998, pp 15–16] raises questions about the objectivity of at least one of the authors. The lead author of the *JAMA* article is an advocate of alternative medicine, a therapeutic nihilist who describes himself as a neuroscientist whose job it is to disprove.

Resolution of the controversy came in a letter written in response to the *JAMA* report [*JAMA* 1998;280:1741]. The communication points out that while the incidence of total ADRs has remained stable over the years, the incidence of fatal ADRs has not. A plot of fatal ADRs over time shows that incidence of drug-related deaths has decreased precipitously during the last 30 years. To arrive at their estimate of the incidence of fatal ADRs, the authors multiplied the total number of drug-related hospitalizations in 1994 by an incidence rate of 0.32%, based on data from all studies published since 1965. Three quarters of these data, however, are 20 to 30 years old. Therefore, the conclusions of the *JAMA* report are erroneous and the estimate of at least 76,000 fatal ADRs each year does not apply to the present. Studies published in the last ten years report a total of only five fatal ADRs among 11,376 hospitalized patients studied, an overall incidence of 0.04%. The re-examination of the data suggests that the incidence of death attributable to ADRs in the US is about 13,000 annually.

Litigation on Recalled Diet Drugs. In September 1997, American Home Products recalled two popular diet drugs—fenfluramine (*Pondamin*) and dexfenfluramine (*Redux*). This followed an announcement by the FDA that about 30% of patients using fenfluramines suffered heart-valve damage, far in excess of the 2% to 6% rate in the general population. The recall led to hundreds of lawsuits that are now in litigation. Before its withdrawal, fenfluramine was used by millions of people, mostly women who were usually prescribed phentermine concurrently (fen-phen).

Six months after the recall, American Home Products released new data claiming that dexfenfluramine is far less dangerous than previously thought. The study was started before the recall and evaluated a new long-acting dosage form of dexfenfluramine. It was stopped right after the recall, when about 1200 patients had been enrolled and taken study medications for a median of 77 days. Within one month of stopping the trial, nearly 1100 patients underwent echocardiography to check for heart valve damage. The investigators found damage in 6.5% of patients taking regular dexfenfluramine, in 7.3% taking long-acting dexfenfluramine, and 4.5% of the patients taking placebo. While there was a trend toward increased and more severe heart valve damage in subjects taking the drug, the estimates of the incidence of drug toxicity are much lower than those suggested by the FDA. Many cardiologists say, however, that the data are not strong enough for definite conclusions to be drawn [*Scrip*, April 3, 1998, p 19].

In September, *The Wall Street Journal* [September 4, 1998, p B6] reported that Interneuron, the company that developed *Redux,* agreed in principle to settle all lawsuits against it for $70 million, plus an estimated $30 million of liability insurance funds. The total is to be paid out over seven years. The deal will cap exposure and leave plaintiffs free to go after American Home Products, which marketed *Redux* as well as *Pondamin,* a company with much deeper pockets than Interneuron. The proposed settlement is contingent on its certification as a class action. All people in the US who used dexfenfluramine and their family members are included in the class. Membership is mandatory. The concept of mandatory participation in a class settlement, which denies dissenters the right to pursue cases individually, is a controversial and untested area of law in the US [*Scrip*, September 8, 1998, p 13].

Soon after the announcement of the proposed settlement, three reports from clinical studies were published in the September 10, 1998, issue of *The New England Journal of Medicine*. They included the seemingly exculpatory trial sponsored by American Home Products and described above. These reports provide the strongest evidence yet linking long-term use of fenfluramines to heart-valve leaks. A cardiologist with the American Heart Association said, "All three studies are concordant and document that [valve disease] in diet-drug users is very real" [*The Wall Street Journal,* September 10, 1998, pp A3, A10]. All three studies, however, also found that the problem affects fewer than the 33% of users estimated by the FDA. The same is true of a study supported by Interneuron. Researchers found that 7.3% of patients who had taken *Redux* had heart valve leaks, as identified by ultrasound tests, compared with 2.6% in a comparison group that had not used a fenfluramine. The study also showed that people with hypertension were more likely to show heart valve problems [*The Wall Street Journal,* November 11, 1998, p B6].

Particularly surprising was the formal publication of the study that seemed to find little evidence of heart-valve defects in people taking dex-fenfluramine for two to three months. The data are presented differently and the results show an excess of early valve disease in treated subjects compared with subjects receiving placebo. The published results show that 17% of subjects assigned to dexfenfluramine compared with 12% of those given placebo had signs of aortic valve leaks [*N Engl J Med* 1998;339:725-32].

In a second study, investigators used echocardiography to examine 233 patients who took dexfenfluramine alone, dexfenfluramine and phentermine, or fenfluramine and phentermine, and compared the findings with those determined in a control group of obese patients who had not taken diet drugs [*N Engl J Med* 1998;339:713–18]. They found that 23% of those who used a diet drug had heart valve abnormalities, compared with 1.3% of the control group. The odds ratio for such cardiac-valve abnormalities was 12.7 with the use of dexfenfluramine alone, 24.5 with the use of dexfenfluramine and phentermine, and 26.3 with the use of fenfluramine and phentermine. It is hard to say whether the addition of phentermine really exacerbated the heart-valve problem because the duration of treatment differed among the three subgroups.

A third study, which analyzed medical records of about 10,000 people who had taken dexfenfluramine, fenfluramine, or phentermine, found 11 cases of newly diagnosed symptomatic heart-valve leaks compared with none for a similar group that did not take diet drugs. Heart-valve leaks were seen only in patients taking a fenfluramine, but the number of patients who took only phentermine was probably too small to rule out a potential effect. The five-year cumulative incidence of cardiac-valve disorder was 7.1 per 10,000 subjects among those who took a fenfluramine for less than four months and 35.0 per 10,000 subjects among those who received either dexfenfluramine or fenfluramine for four or more months. Symptoms among those who developed heart-valve leaks ranged from fatigue to chest pain and heart murmurs [*N Engl J Med* 1998;339:719–24].

An accompanying editorial observed that, ''The additional evidence linking the use of fenfluramine or dexfenfluramine to heart-valve regurgitation reaffirms the wisdom of the FDA's decision to withdraw them from the market.'' The author also points out the need for caution in the long-term use of other agents that act on serotonergic mechanisms [*N Engl J Med* 1998;339:765–67].

It is important to remember that the long-term significance of the heart-valve problem is unknown. Most of the documented cases did not have symptoms; the problem was detected only through echocardiography. Very few cases have required surgery. Nevertheless, some observers believe that the publications could bolster lawsuits against American Home Products. The company said that it expects to conclude a large study of patients who used fenfluramine combined with phentermine, and that the results could shed more light on the issue.

OTHER ISSUES

Optimizing Clinical Trials May Reduce Applicability
Failure to Adhere to Prescribed Drug Regimen

Optimizing Clinical Trials May Reduce Applicability. Randomized clinical trials are costly. Investigators seek to optimize study design and to reduce the number of subjects participating in a study, without a loss of statistical power. Some investigators have used a run-in period (pilot study) before randomization to accomplish that goal. A run-in period before randomization may be used to weed out subjects who are poor compliers, who strongly respond to placebo, or who cannot tolerate the proposed treatment. This strategy may also be useful to select only subjects who have an initial response to treatment and are more likely to benefit from the intervention.

What are the implications of run-in periods for interpreting the results of clinical trials and applying these results to clinical practice? A recent analysis finds that while the results of such trials are valid because randomization follows the run-in period, they apply only to subgroups of patients who are not defined easily by demographic or clinical characteristics [*JAMA* 1998; 279;222–25]. Compared with results that would have been observed without the run-in period, the reported findings overestimate the benefits and underestimate the risks of treatment.

The Physicians' Health Study (PHS) was the first large clinical trial to use a run-in period to eliminate subjects likely to stray from the investigators' directions during the formal trial [*N Engl J Med* 1989;321:129–35]. Poor compliance introduces a major risk of bias in the interpretation of the results of a therapeutic trial [*Controlled Clinical Trials* 1998;19:257–68].

PHS was designed to test the effects of aspirin and beta-carotene in the primary prevention of ischemic heart disease and cancer, respectively. In an 18-week run-in period that screened for poor compliance, one-third of the subjects were precluded from participating in the trial. They were deemed unlikely to take assigned medication and follow the protocol of the trial. Enrolling these subjects would probably have resulted in an underestimate of the effectiveness of the proposed medication.

Reported adherence among the randomized subjects was 90% over the five-year study. Aspirin decreased the risk of myocardial infarction by about 45%. The British Physicians' Study [*BMJ* 1988;296:313–16], however, which did not use a run-in period to exclude poor compliers, achieved only 70% adherence during the study and found no significant difference between groups receiving aspirin and placebo. The efficacy observed in the PHS is a theoretical maximum for the potential effectiveness of the drug in clinical practice, where both compliers and noncompliers are found.

The Tacrine Collaborative Study [*N Engl J Med* 1992;327:1253–59] used a 6-week run-in period to select subjects with Alzheimer's disease who had a favorable response to short-term therapy. Only 34% of those initially recruited were randomized. The Australia-New Zealand Collaborative Group study [*Circulation* 1995;92:212–18], that evaluated carvedilol (*Coreg*) in patients with heart failure, excluded eligible patients who could not tolerate the drug during a two- to three-week run-in period. The reported rate of adverse effects leading to withdrawal from the randomized portion of the study among patients assigned to carvedilol was 14.5%. If the adverse events occurring in patients receiving carvedilol during the run-in period are added to those occurring in the formal trial, the overall incidence is 24.4%, compared with 6.3% in the placebo group.

The Cardiac Arrhythmia Suppression Trial (CAST) is an example of the deliberate use of a run-in period to enhance clinical applicability. Subjects were selected only if they demonstrated significant suppression of ventricular ectopy (e.g., premature ventricular contractions), as determined by a Holter monitor, after administration of an anti-arrhythmic agent. This was the approach used by cardiologists to determine whether or not to prescribe an anti-arrhythmic drug to a patient with irregular heart rhythms. The results of CAST were therefore directly applicable to the prevailing clinical management strategy. This example illustrates that the relationship between the characteristics of the randomized subjects and those of patients encountered in clinical practice determines whether the run-in period enhances applicability or dilutes it. The authors of the report in *JAMA* urge medical journal editors to insist that reports of clinical trials using run-in periods indicate how this aspect of the trial design may affect the application of the results to practice.

Failure to Adhere to Prescribed Drug Regimen. *The New York Times* [June 2, 1998, ppB9, B12] published an article about a medical problem that is pervasive, yet familiar to few readers. The piece was called: "The 'Other Drug Problem:' forgetting to take them." Dozens of studies over the last 20 years show that failure to comply with directions on a prescription—failing to fill a prescription, skipping some doses, doubling up on others and forgetting to refill at the end of the dosing period—is an important, worldwide problem. Large numbers of people—up to 50% depending on the drug, the illness, and the complexity of dosing—take less medication than prescribed and a smaller number take more medication than directed. One expert says that people in general take about 75% of their medications as prescribed. Another says that only 50% of patients take doses correctly.

Discontinuing medication or frequently skipping doses can cause preventable morbidity and impose a considerable clinical and financial burden on the health care system. A study earlier in the decade found that failure to adhere to a prescribed regimen of drug therapy was responsible for 10% to 25% of hospital and nursing admissions in the US. Fortunately, some medications are "forgiving" in that doses may be missed without compromising the well being of the patient. Short-acting medications, however, require good compliance to be effective [*Statistics in Medicine* 1998;17:251–67].

Interest in compliance has been sharpened by new studies showing that treatment of elevated blood cholesterol or asthma is more effective when patients take medications as prescribed. The same is true for hypertension [*Am J Managed Care* 1998;4:957–66]. Failure to comply may be a death sentence for patients with tuberculosis because underdosing promotes the emergence of drug-resistant organisms. For the same reason, some physicians have refused to prescribe anti-HIV therapy for infected homeless people who are unlikely to adhere to the complex directions for administration. Current therapy for HIV infection requires a patients to take up to 24 pills daily, some taken after a meal and others taken on an empty stomach.

The extent of noncompliance by people who are prescribed drugs for dyslipidemias is the subject of a recent cohort study defining all prescriptions filled for lipid-lowering drugs during one year [*JAMA* 1998;279:1458–62]. The cohort consisted of more than 7000 people from New Jersey or Quebec who were older than 65 years and filled one or more prescriptions for a lipid-lowering drug. The investigators determined average persistence to drug therapy, as measured by the mean percentage of days in the study year in which patients had filled prescriptions available.

They found that in both populations, patients failed to fill prescriptions for lipid-lowering drugs for about 40% of the study year. Persistence rates, however, with HMG CoA reductase inhibitors (statins) were significantly higher than those seen with cholestyramine (64% vs. 37% of days with drug available, respectively). These findings may reflect the greater convenience of dosing regimens for the statins, or the different side-effect profiles of the two classes of drugs.

Patients with hypertension, diabetes, or coronary artery disease also had significantly higher rates of persistence than did those free of chronic disease. In New Jersey, the poorest patients had the lowest rate of drug use. A survey of the New Jersey population five years following the study year showed that only 52% of surviving patients who were initially prescribed lipid-lowering medication were still filling prescriptions for this drug class.

The findings depict persistence of drug use ". . . in a set of fiscally generous insurance systems." All patients in the study had comprehensive coverage of drug benefits. It seems that adequate payment mechanisms are not sufficient to guarantee appropriate use of prescribed therapy. Persistence is likely to be even worse when patients must bear the considerable cost of prescription drugs.

Pharmacists seem ideally situated to promote patient compliance with prescribed therapy. A report in *The Pink Sheet* [1998;60(No42):12] shows how this could work. An adherence program involving a chain drug store, Rite Aid, and a pharmaceutical company, Merck, has resulted in a 20% increase in compliance with a prescribed regimen for alendronate (*Fosamax*) to prevent osteoporosis or halt its progression. The program focuses on patients newly prescribed *Fosamax*. Within ten days of their initial prescription, patients receive a counseling call. The next contact is a refill reminder call if a patient is three days overdue for a refill. The second call is repeated throughout therapy. Over the same period of time, women enrolled in the program received and presumably took more medication units than women who did not participate. At the end of 11 months, 61% of those in the program were still taking medication compared with 55% in the control group.

LATE BREAKING REPORT

Substance Abuse

Medical Treatment for Opiate Addiction. The National Consensus Development Panel on Effective Medical Treatment of Opiate Addiction reported their findings in December 1998 [*JAMA* 1998;280:1936–43]. The panel concluded that opiate dependence is a brain-related medical disorder that can be effectively treated. It urges society-at-large to make a commitment to offer effective treatment to all who need it. The panel also opines that all persons dependent on opiates should have access to methadone maintenance therapy. It calls on the US Department of Justice to take the necessary steps to implement this recommendation and on medical schools to improve training for physicians.

INDEX

INDEX

ISBN 0-07-134990-1

9 780071 349901

LIFE UNIVERSITY
1269 BARCLAY CIRCLE
MARIETTA, GA 30060
(770) 426-2688

LIFE UNIVERSITY
1269 BARCLAY CIRCLE
MARIETTA, GA 30060
(770) 426-2688